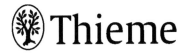

The Bobath Concept in Adult Neurology

Second Edition

Bente E. Bassøe Gjelsvik
Physiotherapist
Specialist in Neurological Physiotherapy MNFF
Member of IBITA
Bergen, Norway

Line Syre
Physiotherapist
Specialist in Neurological Physiotherapy MNFF
Basic Bobath Instructor
Gothenburg, Sweden

207 illustrations

Thieme
Stuttgart • New York • Delhi • Rio de Janeiro

Library of Congress Cataloging-in-Publication Data

Gjelsvik, Bente E. Bassøe, author.
The Bobath concept in adult neurology / Bente E. Bassøe
Gjelsvik, Line Syre. – 2nd edition.
    p.; cm.
Includes bibliographical references and index.
ISBN 978-3-13-145452-2 – ISBN 978-3-13-161772-9
(e-book)
I. Syre, Line, author. II. Title.
[DNLM: 1. Central Nervous System Diseases–physiopathol-
ogy. 2. Central Nervous System Diseases–rehabilitation.
3. Neuronal Plasticity. 4. Neurophysiology–methods. 5.
Physical Therapy Modalities. WL 301]
        RC350.P48
        616.8--dc23
                                            2015032365

© 2016 by Georg Thieme Verlag KG

Thieme Publishers Stuttgart
Rüdigerstrasse 14, 70469 Stuttgart, Germany
+49 [0]711 8931 421, customerservice@thieme.de

Thieme Publishers New York
333 Seventh Avenue, New York, NY 10001 USA
+1 800 782 3488, customerservice@thieme.com

Thieme Publishers Delhi
A-12, Second Floor, Sector-2, Noida-201301
Uttar Pradesh, India
+91 120 45 566 00, customerservice@thieme.in

Thieme Publishers Rio, Thieme Publicações Ltda. Edifício
Rodolpho de Paoli, 25º andar
Av. Nilo Peçanha, 50 - Sala 2508
Rio de Janeiro 20020-906 Brasil
+55 21 3172 2297 / +55 21 3172 1896

Cover design: Thieme Publishing Group
Typesetting by DiTech Process Solutions, India

Printed in Germany by Beltz Grafische Betriebe
                                            5 4 3 2

ISBN 978-3-13-145452-2

Also available as an e-book:
eISBN 978-3-13-161772-9

Important note: Medicine is an ever-changing science undergoing continual development. Research and clinical experience are continually expanding our knowledge, in particular our knowledge of proper treatment and drug therapy. Insofar as this book mentions any dosage or application, readers may rest assured that the authors, editors, and publishers have made every effort to ensure that such references are in accordance with **the state of knowledge at the time of production of the book**.

Nevertheless, this does not involve, imply, or express any guarantee or responsibility on the part of the publishers in respect to any dosage instructions and forms of applications stated in the book. **Every user is requested to examine carefully** the manufacturers' leaflets accompanying each drug and to check, if necessary in consultation with a physician or specialist, whether the dosage schedules mentioned therein or the contraindications stated by the manufacturers differ from the statements made in the present book. Such examination is particularly important with drugs that are either rarely used or have been newly released on the market. Every dosage schedule or every form of application used is entirely at the user's own risk and responsibility. The authors and publishers request every user to report to the publishers any discrepancies or inaccuracies noticed. If errors in this work are found after publication, errata will be posted at www.thieme.com on the product description page.

Some of the product names, patents, and registered designs referred to in this book are in fact registered trademarks or proprietary names even though specific reference to this fact is not always made in the text. Therefore, the appearance of a name without designation as proprietary is not to be construed as a representation by the publisher that it is in the public domain.

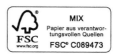

Contents

Foreword to the Second Edition

Knowledge of the central nervous system (CNS), neuromuscular function, and the potential for plastic changes driven by motor experience or lesions to the CNS is increasing, but there is still a lot to learn. We have updated and revised the earlier edition with regard to both the research literature and clinical practice experience. Research evidence as to the effect of various treatment interventions is still sparse, and results from randomized, controlled trials provide information only on the average outcome for the average patient and may therefore not be directly applicable to the patients seen in clinical practice. This book strengthens and broadens the knowledge base with regard to neurophysiology, human movement, and the changes wrought by CNS lesions, thereby enabling therapists to base treatment decisions on strong clinical reasoning and to better evaluate the results for each individual patient.

Bente E. Bassøe Gjelsvik
Line Syre

Foreword to the First Edition

At this time we know more about the central nervous system than ever before, but to bring about the reality of a functional recovery after a lesion is still a very serious clinical challenge to both patients and therapists. In this book Bente Gjelsvik, an acknowledged Bobath Instructor and clinical specialist in neurology, brings all her skills to explain a concept that has evolved over decades to address the complexities of neurodisability. She adopts a problem-solving approach consistent with the definition of the Bobath Concept and its current interpretation of movement control. The basis of the text is to understand the structure and function of the organism, which is expressed through an understanding of posture and movement control. It is a clinically orientated text concluding with two detailed case histories that will be of significant interest to all professionals involved in the management of neurological disability.

Mary Lynch–Ellerington

Preface

About the Authors

Bente Gjelsvik trained as a physiotherapist at the School of Physiotherapy, Royal Victoria Infirmary, Newcastle-upon-Tyne, England, and qualified in 1978. Bente moved back to Norway together with her husband, Olav Gjelsvik, and has worked at the Department of Physiotherapy, Haukeland University Hospital in Bergen, Norway, since July 1978. From 1985 to 1996 she worked in the Neurology Department and since then in the Department of Physical Medicine and Rehabilitation. She completed a master's degree in physiotherapy science in 2010 and a PhD in 2014, both at the University of Bergen. Bente's thesis, "Trunk Control in Stroke: Aspects of Measurement, Relation to Brain Lesion, and Change after Rehabilitation," can be obtained by contacting her directly using the following e-mail address: bente.elisabeth.bassoe.gjelsvik@helse-bergen.no.

The thesis is based on clinical studies reported in the following three articles:

- Gjelsvik B, Breivik K, Verheyden G, Smedal T, Hofstad H, Strand LI. The Trunk Impairment Scale—modified to ordinal scales in the Norwegian version. Disabil Rehabil 2012;34(16):1385–1395
- Gjelsvik B, Strand LI, Næss H, Hofstad H, Skouen JS, Eide GE, Smedal T. Trunk control and lesion locations according to Alberta Stroke Program early CT score in acute stroke: a cross-sectional study. Int J Phys Med Rehabil 2014;S3
- Gjelsvik BE, Hofstad H, Smedal T, Eide GE, Naess H, Skouen JS, Strand LI. Balance and walking after three different models of stroke rehabilitation: early supported discharge in a day unit or at home, and traditional treatment (control). BMJ Open 2014;4(5):e004358

Bente qualified as Basic Bobath Instructor in 1991, and Advanced Bobath Instructor in 2004 through the British Bobath Tutors Association (BBTA), and by Senior Instructor Mary Lynch-Ellerington. She has extensive teaching practice and responsibility and has taught courses in many countries in Europe.

Bente was a member of the executive committee of IBITA from 1994 to 2008, and chairperson for 5 of these years. She received the IBITA Dedicated Service Award when she left the executive committee.

She is a specialist in neurorehabilitation, the Norwegian Physiotherapy Association (NFF), from 1995, and an honorary life member of the Neurology, Orthopaedic and Rheumatology Special Interest Group (NOR). Bente was awarded Physiotherapist of the Year 2015 by NFF in March 2015.

Line Syre trained as a physiotherapist at the University of Wolverhampton, England, and qualified in 1994. She became a specialist in neurorehabilitation in 2007 and an international Bobath Instructor IBITA in 2009, trained through the British Bobath Tutors Association (BBTA), and qualified by Senior Instructor Mary Lynch-Ellerington. Line had extensive practice from hospital work as well as community health services before she decided in 1999 to work solely within the field of neurorehabilitation. She developed her own private practice in 2005 in Sandefjord, Norway. She now has her own private neurorehabilitation clinic in Gothenburg, called VIP Neurorehab, where patients receive intensive rehabilitation. She also assesses and evaluates patients and advises health personnel with regard to individual patients. Line teaches in Norway and Sweden as well as internationally and is a member of the Swedish Association for the Bobath Concept (FBKS). Line can be contacted using the following e-mail address: line.syre@gmail.se.

Carlos Martins Leite wrote Case History 4.2. He qualified as a physiotherapist by Escola Superior de Saúde de Coimbra in 2001, and was awarded a master's degree in neurological rehabilitation—specialty for physiotherapists, by the Universidade Católica Portuguesa in 2011, Portugal. Carlos qualified as a Bobath Instructor in 2014 and is currently working at Centro Hospitalar Tondela-Viseu EPE. He is a professor of neurologic rehabilitation at the Instituto Politécnico de Castelo Branco.

Aims of This Book

This book seeks to improve the therapist's competency in the treatment of individuals with neurological conditions by the following means:
- Building bridges among the following:
  - The structure and function of the central nervous system, the neuro-musculo-skeletal

systems, and the ability for change (plasticity).
- Postural control and movement.
- Treatment of central nervous system conditions.
• Enabling the reader to form hypotheses through clinical reasoning in treatment situations based on a conceptual understanding of the interaction between humans and the environment, between the central nervous system (CNS), the musculoskeletal systems, movement, and function.

Clinical reasoning cannot be learned through reading a book; it is developed through continuous critical evaluation of one's own practice, by pursuing findings, through experimenting, and by improving one's own evidence-based knowledge. We hope that this book may help in this process.

The book is written for physiotherapists and occupational therapists, students, and qualified professionals. It is aimed mainly at the *clinician* working in neurorehabilitation, both acute and long term.

Structure of This Book

The book is meant to be read in the way it is structured. The chapters build on each other, and the reader may miss important information and discussions if it is primarily used as a reference book. I do hope, however, that it will be useful as a reference once read in its entirety.

Chapter 1, Applied Neurophysiology, consists of four parts.
1.1 The organization of the CNS.
1.2 Systems control: systems and structures concerned with movement and sensorimotor integration. This chapter takes a limited view of the structure and function of parts of the CNS, and discusses the interaction between CNS function, muscle function, function, and movement. Consequences of CNS lesions and clinical reflections are discussed throughout.

1.3 Motor learning and plasticity: outlines changes in the CNS as a result of nature and nurture and as consequences of CNS lesions. These changes are the basis for learning and therefore important to understand. Consequences for therapy are discussed, and also theories of recovery after a CNS lesion.
1.4 Lesions and reorganization: consequences of damage to the CNS.

Chapter 2, Human Movement, discusses balance, movement, and deviations from normal human movement, as well as choices therapists may make with regard to interventions.

Chapter 3, Assessment, looks toward the International Classification of Functioning, Disability, and Health as a basis for assessment. This chapter discusses some outcome measures.

Chapter 4, Case Histories, presents two individuals: HS, a patient who has suffered an intracerebral hemorrhage some years prior, and Avelino, a patient with cerebellar ataxia.

The nouns *him* for the patient and *she* for the therapist have been chosen except where photos show differently, although in real life, the situation is often reversed.

With our jobs as physiotherapists, Bobath instructors, and scientists, we are first and foremost aiming to optimize the quality of life of adults with neurological dysfunction. We hope that readers will benefit from this book in developing their own practice, helping patients regain abilities to participate more in their own lives. Hopefully, this book will provide both undergraduate and postgraduate health professionals with more in-depth knowledge about the knowledge base and clinical reasoning used in the implementation of the Bobath Concept. As Karel Bobath himself pointed out, "the Bobath Concept is unfinished, we hope it will continue to grow and develop in years to come" (handed down personal communication).

We want to dedicate this book to all of our patients from whom we have learnt and are still learning, thank you.

Acknowledgments

The first edition in English was revised and updated from the first German edition. I did the revision and translation into English myself, with great help from English colleagues of the British Bobath Tutors Association (BBTA)—Lynne Fletcher, Janice Champion, and Linzi Smith—and I also received help and support from my German colleague Gerlinde Haase in updating some of the photos in the physiotherapy chapter.

My beloved husband, Olav Gjelsvik, who died in 2007, was a physiotherapist and Bobath Instructor as well as a close and critical colleague. He gave me valuable support, encouragement, and input throughout this process.

My great friend and mentor Mary Lynch-Ellerington is a Senior Bobath Instructor. She has, through many years, given me the basis for my conceptual understanding of the Bobath Concept. She is an extremely generous person, sharing her insight and knowledge with colleagues and course participants all over the world.

Last but not least, a special thank you to the patients and colleagues who were willing to participate in this book.

For the second edition of *The Bobath Concept in Adult Neurology,* my close friend and colleague Line Syre took on the task of updating the literature and revising the book during my time as a PhD candidate. Line has also contributed with an extensive case history on a patient with chronic stroke combined with updated literature to support the clinical reasoning process, as well as the use of standardized outcome measures. She, therefore, thoroughly deserves the title of coauthor, and this new edition would never have happened without her. Also in this edition, Carlos Martins Leite has contributed with a case history on the challenge of cerebellar ataxia and, as has Line, combined the assessment process with updated literature to support the clinical reasoning process and the use of standardized outcome measures.

Helge Haestad, specialist in neurorehabilitation at the University Hospital of Northern Norway and Bobath Instructor, contributed in the writing of Chapter 1, Applied Neurophysiology.

Thank you to my patients, both previous and new; to Line, Carlos, and Helge; as well as to colleagues, family, and friends, who have patiently supported the work, thereby making this second edition possible.

Bente E. Bassøe Gjelsvik

Introduction

The Bobaths: A Historical Overview

The following paragraphs are extracts from *The Bobaths. A Biography of Berta and Karel Bobath* by Jay Schleichkorn, PhD, PT (1992).

Karel Bobath and Berta Ottilie Busse were born in Berlin, Karel in 1906, and Berta in 1907. He studied medicine and qualified as a medical doctor in 1932. She graduated as a gymnastic teacher from the Anna Herrmann School where she learned about normal movements and different relaxation methods. Berta and Karel left for London before the 2nd World War.

The development of the Bobath Concept for adults started in 1943 when Berta was asked to treat Simon Elwes, a 43-year-old portrait painter who had suffered a stroke. "When I arrived I found him in bed, his arm and hand extremely stiff in flexion, his hand swollen, a bad shoulder–hand syndrome, and his leg covered up ..." [p. 20] "Instead of doing what I had been taught—exercises, I observed the patient. Slowly, by trial and error, by observation and deduction, I began relating things he was doing in response to what I was doing. It worked better than anything before." [s. xi] ... "I realised for the first time that the patient's pulling into flexion produced his spasticity, and that spasticity was not an unalterable state which could only be treated by stretching spastic muscles." [p. 20] Simon Elwes recovered well and started painting again. Berta treated Simon Elwes for 18 months, and discovered that this form of treatment was only a beginning. It took many years to develop the treatment from this simple way of reducing spasticity to the problem of making the patient active and participating without returning to a spastic state.

Berta graduated as a physiotherapist in 1950 and became a member of the Chartered Society for Physiotherapists. Karel and Berta's first Centre opened in 1951, and in 1957 "The Western Cerebral Palsy Centre" was established. Both children and adults with different neurological disorders were treated there, with the main emphasis on children with cerebral palsy. Berta educated the parents in handling of their children through daily activities like bathing, dressing, and how they should carry their children as living human beings and not lifeless dolls. She strongly advocated the importance of a multidisci-plinary approach, especially between physiotherapists, occupational therapists, and speech therapists. The physiotherapist Jenny Bryce, later to become the leader of the Centre for a long period, said that "the aspect which most impressed me was Berta's deep understanding of normal movement, and she applied that understanding in the treatment of both children and adults" [p. 35]. In 1990 she said that "The lasting fascination of the concept is that it is constantly under discussion and never in danger of standing still..." [p. 36]

Karel sought to explain the neurophysiological background for Berta's observations and treatment. About the Bobath Concept, they both stated in 1990: "It was based purely on empirical lines by Mrs. Bobath's observation of children and adults with neurological lesions and their response to treatment.... The concept is hypothetical in nature, although to some extent it has been confirmed and strengthened by recent research which we hope will continue in the future." [p. ix]

From 1958 Berta and Karel Bobath traveled widely over large parts of the USA, South-Africa, Canada, Europe, Asia, Australia, and Latin-America to teach, lecture, and demonstrate treatment. Berta Bobath was given an M.B.E. (Member of the Order of British Empire), a British honor, in 1978, and received many international honorary awards. Together, they have produced more than 70 publications and many unpublished congress articles from 1948 to 1990.

They both died on January 20, 1991.

The International Bobath Instructors Training Association—IBITA

There have been large and significant developments in the Bobath Concept since Berta and Karel's time. Assessment procedures have changed, and there are still many aspects of function, communication, and plasticity of the central nervous system (CNS) that remain unknown. The problems of patients whom professionals meet today are partly different from the problems patients formerly had: many patients survive due to improved acute care, they are treated in specialized units, and they are discharged earlier from hospitals and rehabilitation units. They are exposed to different demands and to many different treatment concepts or regimens. There is a continuous development of theory and clinical practice, and the demand for evidence-based practice is strong. Theoretical assumptions change as new knowledge becomes available, demonstrating that the profession is in a dynamic state of development. As Emerson Pugh stated in 1977, "If the brain were so simple that we could understand it, we would be so simple that we could not. Medical "truths" have short lives. As clinicians we need to be humble, accept that science changes, and develop our knowledge. At the same time, we have to be careful not to throw away clinical knowledge based on reasoning and experience, even if the effect of interventions has yet to be proven. Many of our interventions are not documented or researched. Changes witnessed by the therapist and experienced by the patient together in clinical practice may not show on the clinical scales that are used today due to the insensitivity of many of the outcome measures in existence.

The International Bobath Instructors Training Association (IBITA) was founded in 1984 and is a worldwide organization of qualified IBITA instructors. Today there are ~265 members of IBITA representing 31 countries.

The following was copied from the Website www.ibita.org in February 2015:

IBITA is the international organization of instructors, teaching the Bobath Concept applied to the assessment and treatment of adults with neurological conditions.

IBITA was formed in 1984 for the specific purposes of providing a forum for defining the continued interaction and education of its present instructors and the training of future instructors and for the formulation of the Bylaws and Rules & Regulations of the organization with respect to the teaching of the Bobath Concept worldwide.

Today **IBITA** unites instructors (physiotherapists and occupational therapists) worldwide.

IBITA is an association according to Article 60 ff. of the Swiss Civil Law Book.

The association is seated in Sankt Gallen, Switzerland.

The office is located in The Netherlands.

Vision
Throughout the world, adults with neurological dysfunction will be assured of the services of an interdisciplinary team trained in neurological rehabilitation, originating in the Bobath Concept and developed in accordance with current knowledge.

Mission
1. Members of IBITA plan, organize and run courses worldwide to train physical, occupational and speech therapists, medical doctors and registered nurses in the assessment and treatment of adults with lesions of the central nervous system.
2. Members of IBITA ensure that their teaching and clinical practice is founded upon and reflect current understanding of motor control, neural and muscle plasticity, motor learning and biomechanics, integrated within the Bobath Concept.
3. Members of IBITA recognize the importance of evidence-based practice and evaluate the research literature critically to implement such practice.
4. Members of IBITA strive constantly to improve their own standards of clinical expertise and to impart their knowledge and skills.
5. Members of IBITA play an active role in the training of new instructors.
6. Members of IBITA are aware of the need for research into the theoretical assumptions and clinical outcomes of treatment, and undertake to publish their findings.
7. Members of IBITA accept their role in education and empowerment of the patient, family and other caregivers.
8. Members of IBITA promote at all times the vision, mission and objectives of IBITA, in their clinical and teaching practice as well as in interaction with other professionals, with national and international organisations and with the public.

IBITA's Theoretical Assumptions and Clinical Practice

IBITA is continuously discussing its theoretical assumptions in the light of new knowledge, and seeks to bridge the gap between theory and clinical practice. Therefore, theoretical assumptions and statements regarding clinical practice are regularly reviewed and revised. The reader is recommended to read the current document on IBITA's Web site (www.ibita.org).

1 Applied Neurophysiology

Knowledge of central nervous system (CNS) functions has historically been drawn from experimental studies on animals. In recent years, developments in movement science have led to new studies, mostly of normal, healthy people. Advances in noninvasive neuroimaging techniques have made it possible to study local changes in the brain function of people with CNS lesions and also to follow changes in the CNS over time. Techniques such as functional magnetic resonance imaging (fMRI), positron emission tomography (PET), transcranial magnetic stimulation (TMS), electroencephalography (EEG), and magnetoencephalography (MEG) show changes in the structure of the brain and how these correlate with changes in the patient's physical functioning postlesion (Academy of Medical Sciences 2004; Ward & Cohen 2004).

Knowledge about neurophysiology, human movement, and deviation from optimal human movement forms the basis for clinical reasoning. This chapter therefore discusses movement and the postlesion alterations in movements and covers the following:

1.1 The organization of the central nervous system: an overview.
1.2 Systems control: Systems and structures concerned with movement and sensorimotor integration.
   – The somatosensory system and vision:
      • Sensory information and integration, and the formation of body schema.
   – Systems within the brain and spinal cord:
      • Systems important for production and control of movement.

   – The neuromuscular system:
      • The muscular system, communication with the spinal cord, and muscular plasticity.
1.3 Motor learning and plasticity:
   – How the brain is structurally and functionally modified by the information it receives.
1.4 Consequences of and reorganization after CNS Lesions:
   – Consequences of damage to the CNS.

This chapter provides an overview of CNS function as it relates to the production and development of sensorimotor function. The reader is advised to review other relevant publications for revision and more in-depth information (e.g., Brodal 2010; Kandel et al 2013).

1.1 The Organization of the Central Nervous System: An Overview

The nervous system can be divided into the central nervous system (CNS) and the peripheral nervous system (PNS). The CNS consists of the spinal cord and the brain, and the PNS connects the CNS with effectors and receptors throughout the body. The nervous system has two groups of cells: nerve cells (neurons) and glial cells. Neurons are responsible for functions that are unique to the nervous system, and glial cells are nonneuronal cells that mainly support and protect the neurons (Brodal 2010).

With regard to movement, the nervous system performs the following functions:

- Collects data.
- Records and processes data.
- Produces action.

The Building Blocks of the CNS

The CNS contains ~100 billion neurons (Brodal 2010), and there are ~10 times as many glial cells as there are neurons within the CNS. Glial cells are necessary for neurons to function normally.

Neurons

Neurons have a similar structure to all other cells of the body and are specialized to quickly receive and transmit information by chemical and electrical signals. They have a cell body (soma) that contains a nucleus and organelles. From the cell body two main types of processes extend: dendrites and axons. Dendrites receive and conduct signals to the cell body and are generally short, branched, and numerous. Each neuron has multiple dendrites, referred to collectively as dendritic trees. Structural differences in dendritic arborization are closely connected to functional differences between neurons.

Axons (or nerve fibers) lead signals away from the cell body. Each neuron has only one axon. An axon can range in length from 1 mm to more than 1 m. It usually ends with a number of ramifications, enabling its own cell to influence many other cells. The ending of an axon is termed the bouton or the axon terminal, by which the axon makes synaptic contact with another neuron. Within the CNS, a bundle of axons is referred to as a tract and within the PNS as a nerve.

Nervous tissues within the CNS are divided into gray and white matter. White matter receives its color from myelin surrounding the axons; the neuronal cell bodies (soma) and dendrites constitute the gray matter.

Neurons are classified into two major groups: projection neurons and interneurons. Projection neurons transmit information between different areas within the CNS, e.g., between groups of neurons in different parts of the cortex, between the brainstem and spinal cord or from the spinal cord to the muscles of the body. The interneurons are shorter and bring about cooperation among neurons that are grouped together (Brodal 2010).

Sensory neurons are specialized to receive signals from the internal and external environment (e.g., smell, light, taste, touch) and to distribute the information to the brain for processing. This process of transmitting information from the periphery to the CNS is referred to as afferent signaling.

Motor neurons send signals from the CNS to the muscle fibers (efferent signaling) and generate movement.

Glial Cells

There are three main kinds of glial cells: astrocytes (astroglia), oligodendrocytes (oligodendroglia), and microglia (Brodal 2010). In addition to these three main types, there are other specialized forms of glial cells.

A major type of glia is the star-shaped *astrocyte*. In the human brain, there are 10 times as many astrocytes as neurons. The astrocytes are located near the neurons and surround them closely. They resemble an octopus, with "hands" at the end of "arms." With the handlike structures they cling to neurons and adjacent capillaries and thus provide stability to both blood vessels and neurons. Due to their intimate contact with the neurons, capillaries, and cerebrospinal fluid, astrocytes (collectively referred to as astroglia) can control the environment of the neuron by removing excessive extracellular potassium ions (K+) and extracellular carbon dioxide (CO_2), hence controlling neuronal homeostasis. They also help with sealing the capillary walls so that no chemical substances in the blood may influence the neurons. The barrier created between blood and neurons is called the blood–brain barrier. It has recently been found that astrocytes have a greater impact than previously thought; in addition to supporting and nourishing the neurons, the astrocytes themselves seem to be involved in determining how neurons control their signals. They can produce brief electrical currents and affect the neurons directly, probably by synchronizing the activity in groups of neurons (Brodal 2010). Astrocytes also strengthen the contact point between neurons, causing increased efficiency of signal transmission in synapses.

Some axons are surrounded by a myelin sheath, formed by special glial cells (oligodendroglia in the CNS, Schwann cells in the PNS) wrapped around the nerve fiber. *Oligodendrocytes* are the myelinating cells of the CNS (Brodal 2010). Myelin, consisting of fat, serves as insulation and contributes to normal axonal function in the CNS. Myelin does not cover the whole axon; it forms small gaps, nodes, with 1 to

2 mm intervals (nodes of Ranvier), which facilitate rapid impulse conduction. Myelinated axons lead impulses faster than unmyelinated axons because the impulses jump from one node to the next. Thicker axons conduct impulses faster than thin axons. In very fast conducting axons, the conduction velocity can be up to 150 m/s. These axons can inform the brain quickly, such as when one steps on something sharp, or when a muscle is suddenly stretched due to an external event. Thin, unmyelinated axons can have a conduction velocity as low as 0.1 m/s.

Microglia serve to conserve homeostasis and are the "cleaning cells" of the CNS. They ingest and destroy worn-out cells and microorganisms through phagocytosis. After an injury, the number of cells with phagocytic activity increases in the CNS, and in certain diseases with particularly strong activation of microglia (and astrocytes) they can cause tissue damage rather than repair (Brodal 2010).

▨ Communication within the Nervous System

▪ Neural Conduction and Transmission

Communication within the nervous system requires transport of signals within and between neurons. Neurons have the special ability to produce and lead electrical signals (nerve conduction), and to chemically transmit these signals to receiving cells (neurotransmission). Information carried by the neuron is encoded into electrical signals that travel along its axon to a synapse, which is the point of contact between two neurons; between a neuron and a muscle cell; or between a neuron and a gland cell. When an electrical signal reaches the synapse, it sets off a cascade of reactions leading to the release of neurotransmitters into the synaptic cleft. A signal may have to travel through several neurons to reach its final destination.

The neurotransmitters are chemical messengers found in vesicles within the nerve terminal of the presynaptic cell. When released into the synaptic cleft, the neurotransmitters bind to receptors on the postsynaptic cell, giving rise to a brief (a few milliseconds) opening of the attached ion channel (**Fig 1.1**). As a consequence there is a change in the electrical membrane potential of the postsynaptic cell. If the influence on the postsynaptic cell is strong enough, this cell reaches the threshold for creation of a new signal to be conducted along its axon. In this way, an impulse can travel a long way through many neurons, either within the CNS or between the CNS and organs in other systems of the body.

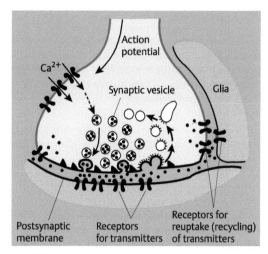

Fig. 1.1 Neurotransmission or synaptic transmissions are essential for the process of communication between two neurons. Neurotransmitter molecules are released into the synaptic cleft between two neurons. The molecules then bind to the receptor sites on the postsynaptic cell and consequently change the electrical states of the receiving neuron.

▪ Patterns of Neuronal Connections

One single neuron within the CNS can make contact with thousands of other neurons, and it can be contacted by thousands of other cells. Groups of neurons interconnect, and complex networks are formed.

When one neuronal axon branches and activates a large number of neurons, it is called *divergence*; for example, afferent information (from the periphery to the CNS) may spread sensory information to many areas in the spinal cord. Signals for postural activity will diverge from nuclei in the brain stem to several parts of the spinal cord (Brodal 2010).

Convergence is the opposite phenomenon, occurring when information from large areas (and numerous neurons) all reaches the same destination. For example, signals from cortical association areas, premotor areas, and limbic structures can converge onto neurons within the premotor cortex for selective hand function. On a spinal level, descending information from the cerebral cortex and the brain stem converge with primary afferents from a variety of peripheral receptors onto common motor-neuron pools. This normally ensures task-specific regulation of excitability of motor neurons, reflex gains, and gaiting of sensory information (Brodal 2010).

■ Summation

Summation of excitatory synaptic effects is necessary to depolarize the postsynaptic cell to threshold. Only when stimulated to threshold, a nerve cell will be activated to pass on information along its axon.

Spatial summation occurs when information from many different sources converges on one neuron (Brodal 2010). The depolarization of one synapse is almost never adequate to trigger an action potential at the postsynaptic cell. Inputs from many presynaptic neurons at different sites on the postsynaptic neuron must be added together to reach the threshold for depolarization.

Temporal summation occurs when many action potentials traveling at a fast frequency in an axon build upon each other (Brodal 2010), increasing the strength and duration of information. The repetition of impulses is regulated through presynaptic inhibition, and the repetition is stopped if needed. Thereby, the duration of the action potential bursts is controlled through temporal distribution.

■ Inhibition—Regulation of CNS Activity

The CNS regulates and modifies signal transmission through inhibition. The importance of inhibition for shaping neural activity was first demonstrated by Sherrington more than 100 years ago (Molnár & Brown 2010). Inhibitory synapses are present everywhere in the CNS and are of vital importance for its proper functioning (Brodal 2010). Inhibitory neurons in the spinal cord perform important roles in processing somatosensory information and shaping motor behaviors that range from simple protective reflexes to more complex motor tasks, such as locomotion, reaching, and grasping.

One motor neuron may receive input from as many as 50,000 synapses. Many inhibitory interneurons synapse directly with motor neurons to control their excitability. They also function indirectly through their actions on other interneurons, either to directly reduce excitability or to increase excitability via disynaptic disinhibition. It is the *sum of inputs to the motor neuron that decides the output*. A neuron may receive many inhibitory inputs and still reach threshold for firing.

Special neurotransmitters in the CNS are responsible for inhibition. γ-Aminobutyric acid (GABA) is the most common one. There are many forms of inhibition. The following seem to be especially important for movement:

- Presynaptic inhibition.
- Postsynaptic inhibition.
- Recurrent inhibition.
- Reciprocal inhibition.
- Nonreciprocal inhibition.
- Lateral inhibition.

Presynaptic Inhibition

Presynaptic inhibition is a mechanism by which neurotransmission from the presynaptic cell is reduced. Presynaptic inhibition is important for precise, focused, and graded muscular activity, and for regulation of sensory information (Brodal 2010). It is transmitted through axo-axonic synapses (an axon synapsing with the synaptic terminal bouton of another axon). The release of excitatory neurotransmitter substances from the presynaptic bouton is inhibited by presynaptic inhibition, and signal transmission is modulated and reduced, or stopped—irrelevant information is stopped, and the contrast between sensory information and awareness is increased (Brodal 2010) (**Fig.1.2**). This effect occurs in the presynaptic cell. The postsynaptic cell is unchanged (**Fig 1.3**).

In the clinical situation, somatosensory information may modify the activity of the CNS through presynaptic inhibition (Brodal 2010). Sensory input is often regulated at sensory axon terminals by presynaptic inhibition (Blitz & Nusbaum 2011). Reflex strength can be modified to the requirements of the specific task;

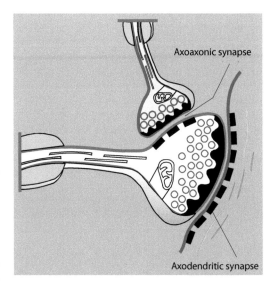

Fig.1.2 Presynaptic inhibition.

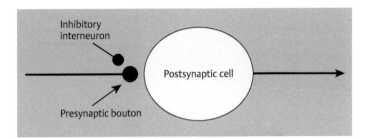

Fig. 1.3 Presynaptic inhibition. The inhibitory interneuron synapses on the presynaptic bouton of an axon, which in turn synapses with the postsynaptic cell.

different studies suggest that presynaptic inhibition on the Ia fibers from the muscle spindles is of particular importance for these changes (Kandel et al 2013). Presynaptic inhibition on Ia afferents reduces the release of neurotransmitters onto the motor neurons, thereby weakening the effects of Ia afferents on motor neurons. Consequently, a reduction of presynaptic inhibition increases the excitability of the reflex arc.

There is considerable axonal branching in the CNS. One axon may spread and influence many other neurons many times. Both spatial and temporal distribution of neural transmission can be regulated through presynaptic inhibition (e.g., to regulate the recruitment and modulation of motor units) (**Fig. 1.4**).

> Changes in afferent information may modify the activity of the CNS.

Presynaptic inhibition is important for movement: it is a very specific mechanism that is precisely modulated to different types of movement and aids the recruitment of muscles with appropriate timing in the right sequence (Rothwell 1994). The mechanism of presynaptic inhibition is used by several systems to modulate the activity between different muscles over different joints in an extremity; for instance, between the gastrocnemius and soleus in standing and walking. Also, Hayes and colleagues (Hayes et al 2012) demonstrated an interlimb coupling in walking by which loading on the stance leg strongly influenced the magnitude and timing of afferent presynaptic inhibition in the swinging limb, hence demonstrating that contralateral limb loading may be an important variable for reestablishing appropriate sensory regulation during locomotion.

Axonal branching from any one axon causes impulses to be spread to a large number of neurons (divergence). This leads to a *spatial distribution* of impulses. Presynaptic inhibition can be turned on or off where branching occurs (see **Fig. 1.4**, GABA$_a$)

to focus the distribution. The action potentials are thereby transmitted to where they are needed. In this way, the number of motor units required for an activity may be regulated. The CNS has the ability to modify or control the direction and spread of impulses to avoid a too diffuse activation of motor unit recruitment.

Presynaptic inhibition is often reduced after a stroke or spinal cord injury due to loss of descending control on the spinal cord (D'Amico et al 2014; Faist et al 1999), which may contribute to sensory dysfunction, such as increased tone (Hayes et al 2012).

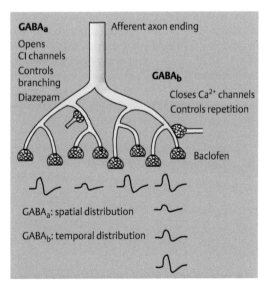

Fig. 1.4 Spatial and temporal distribution through presynaptic inhibition. Presynaptic inhibition may be activated or not at places where the axon branches (GABA$_a$) to select the spread of impulses (spatial distribution). The repetition of impulses (temporal distribution) is regulated through presynaptic inhibition (GABA$_b$), and repetition is stopped if needed (i.e., the strength of impulse transmission is modulated). Ca^{2+}, calcium; Cl, chloride ions; GABA, γ-aminobutyric acid.

Postsynaptic Inhibition

Postsynaptic inhibition occurs when one neuron inhibits another by increasing the threshold for postsynaptic depolarization. This may be in the form of the release of inhibitory neurotransmitters from the presynaptic cell, causing a brief (a few milliseconds) hyperpolarization of the postsynaptic cell membrane through a direct effect on the postsynaptic ion channels.

A different form of synaptic connection activates an intracellular second messenger system that, in turn, reduces the efficiency of the ion channels involved in fast synaptic transmission of precise information. The modulating effect of this system can last from seconds to minutes and is activated by motivation, emotions, and the like (Kandel et al 2013).

In both forms of postsynaptic inhibition, more facilitatory/excitatory impulses will be necessary to depolarize the postsynaptic cell (i.e., the threshold for depolarization has been increased).

Recurrent Inhibition

Recurrent inhibition occurs when a motor neuron inhibits its own activity. This is mediated through Renshaw cells, which are specialized inhibitory interneurons producing recurrent inhibition of *their own motor neurons*. The collaterals from the α-motor neurons connect with Renshaw cells (**Fig. 1.5**), which synapse back onto the same motor neuron. The Renshaw cells also distribute inhibition to synergic motor neurons, to their own agonist γ-motor neuron, synergic γ-motor neurons, other Renshaw cells, and Ia inhibitory interneurons (from the muscle spindle).

Renshaw cells are under supraspinal influence by the corticospinal system, but the precise functional role of recurrent inhibition to motor neurons and other forms of inhibition from the Renshaw cells is still not clear. Several studies have raised various suggestions as to their role (Brownstone & Bui 2010). There seems to be less recurrent inhibition in distal body segments where the movements are fast and mainly voluntary, whereas in the proximal areas, recurrent inhibition seems to be important for slow or tonic muscle contraction. Some of the following seem to be the effects of Renshaw cell activation:

- Reducing the number of motor neurons that fire as well as their rate of firing.
- Regulating motor neuron excitability and stabilizing firing rates.

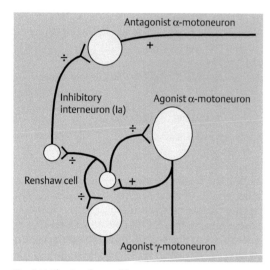

Fig. 1.5 The Renshaw cell loop.

- Increasing the contrast in motor neuron pools by making the motor neuron less sensitive to excitatory stimuli. This is best compared with lateral inhibition in the somatosensory system (see The Somatosensory System, Skin Receptors, The Sense of Touch).
- During walking, the Renshaw cell may contribute to the rhythm in the central pattern generators (CPGs) by shortening the impulse trains from active motor neurons and at the same time increasing the excitability of the antagonist motor neurons (Brodal 2010). In this way, unwanted oscillatory movements are prevented, and rhythmical changes may be facilitated.

The Renshaw cell distributes inhibition to the following:

- Own agonist α-motor neuron.
- Synergic motor neurons.
- Own agonist γ-motor neuron.
- Synergic γ-motor neurons.
- Other Renshaw cells and Ia inhibitory interneurons (from the muscle spindle).

Reciprocal Inhibition

Reciprocal inhibition is the automatic mechanism whereby the antagonist motor neuron is inhibited when the agonist muscle contracts (Knikou 2012). An increase in neural drive of a muscle or group of muscles reduces the neural activity of functional antagonists. This plays a significant role in improving the efficiency of the human movement system.

Ia inhibitory interneurons (IaINs) are responsible for *reciprocal inhibition.* IaINs are monosynaptically excited by muscle spindle primary (Ia) afferents, and project to and inhibit antagonist motor neuron pools. In addition, they inhibit IaINs that receive Ia afferent inputs from antagonist muscles. Activation of IaINs ensures that antagonist muscles remain relaxed during contraction of the agonist muscle, thereby preventing undesired co-contractions (D'Amico et al 2014). There is reciprocal inhibition between flexors and extensors normally (one inhibits the other), for instance, the tibialis anterior and soleus in the leg. In some pathological conditions this mechanism does not work: there is no reciprocal inhibition from the tibialis anterior on the soleus, whereas there is a strong reverse effect; increased pathological activation of the soleus may inhibit the tibialis anterior without the activity in the tibialis anterior being primarily affected by pathology. Several studies have shown decreased activity of the interneurons mediating reciprocal inhibition after loss of descending control (e.g., after stroke, multiple sclerosis, and spinal cord injuries) (Crone et al 2003; Nielsen et al 2007).

Nonreciprocal Inhibition

Nonreciprocal Ib inhibition is caused by activation of Ib afferents from Golgi tendon organs, and is mediated by segmental interneurons projecting to motor neurons of the same muscle. Similar to Renshaw cell and Ia inhibitory interneurons, Ib interneurons also receive diverse segmental and supraspinal inputs. Nonreciprocal Ib inhibition is part of a complex system regulating muscle tension to control posture and movement (Mukherjee & Chakravarty 2010).

Lateral Inhibition

Lateral inhibition will be discussed under The Somatosensory System, The Ability to Differentiate (Lateral Inhibition).

■ **Clinical Relevance of Inhibition**

Selective control of movement depends on musculature being recruited in the appropriate sequence at the appropriate time, and that the duration and strength of muscular contraction (eccentric/concentric) is appropriate to the goal activity. All the aforementioned mechanisms are used to achieve this. The importance of each mechanism and the interaction between them varies according to the task and within phases of a task. The peripheral inputs described under inhibition will, in some situations, have the opposite effect. For example, 1b stimulation of the Golgi tendon organ (GTO) of the triceps surae cause increased activity in this muscle during the stance phase and decreased activity during the swing phase of walking.

Patients with CNS lesions may have reduced control of movement for different reasons: there may be impairment of temporal and spatial distribution of activity; as the patient starts an activity, the recruitment of motor units and muscles in relation to grading of the duration, spread of involvement, and repetition is sometimes disrupted. The reaction or response may therefore be greater than normal (Cornall 1991).

When patients attempt to be functionally independent during a phase when the CNS is vulnerable and denervated, they may experience activation of muscles that normally would not be involved in the actual activity. Attempts at balancing in standing, transferring, or walking may lead to shortening of the patient's affected side, flexion of the arm or fingers, retraction of the pelvis, or push through the foot. Clinically, if the patient learns to control the movements more selectively, these pathological mass patterns may be disrupted. Improved selective control is a sign that the patient is learning to control the distribution and spread of impulses, as well as focusing the motor activity.

Regarding the somatosensory system, processing of sensory information in the CNS is also dependent on inhibitory synaptic transmission. It is now a firmly accepted theory that inhibitory interneurons in the spinal dorsal horn have important functions in the processing of sensory information (Goulding et al 2014). A deficiency in synaptic inhibition at this site will instantly cause changes in the sizes of receptive fields of dorsal horn neurons. In pathological and chronic pain states, it is a major factor contributing to central pain sensitization (Zeilhofer et al 2012).

> Improved selective control seems to stop the inappropriate spread of activity to other muscles. Pathological mass patterns may therefore be disrupted by the improvement of selective control of movement. After a CNS lesion the motor neurons may be hypersensitive to excitatory stimuli.

Summary

The nervous system has two groups of cells: nerve cells (neurons) and glial cells. See page 3.
Neurons are responsible for functions that are unique to the nervous system, and the glial cells are nonneuronal cells that mainly support and protect the neurons. See page 3.
In divergence of neural connections, one neuron contacts many other neurons, allowing the signal to spread from one neuron to many others. See page 5.
In convergence, each neuron receives synaptic contact from many other neurons. See page 5.
In spatial summation inputs from many presynaptic neurons at different sites on the postsynaptic neuron must be added together to reach the threshold for depolarization. See page 6.
In temporal summation many action potentials traveling at a fast frequency in an axon build upon each other, increasing the strength and duration of information. See page 6.
The CNS regulates and modifies signal transmission through inhibition, which slows down the excitation effect of the CNS. See page 6.
Changes in afferent information may modify the activity of the CNS. See page 7.
Improved selective control seems to stop the inappropriate spread of activity to other muscles. Pathological mass patterns may therefore be disrupted by the improvement of selective control of movement. See page 9.
After a CNS lesion the motor neurons may be hypersensitive to excitatory stimuli. See page 9.

1.2 Systems Control: Systems and Structures Concerned with Movement and Sensorimotor Integration

In the healthy brain, there is a highly organized relationship between sensory input from one part of the body and motor output to muscles acting on that same part. Precise motor activity depends on close integration between motor and sensory systems. Most movements require a constant flow of information from receptors in the skin, joints, and muscles to evaluate if the movement is proceeding as planned. Information from the ocular and the vestibular systems can be of vital importance for motor performance. Sensory information enables the CNS to update and correct outgoing commands to the musculature, either during ongoing movement or the next time it is being performed (Brodal 2010). Activity in ascending fibers may affect the activity in the descending fibers, and vice versa. Somatosensory and visual information is crucial for exploration of the environment. Human interaction with the environment forms the basis for muscular activity in movement and balance. Motor activity is context based.

| Movement is produced by multiple neural networks.

The integrated model of human movement, in which all systems—sensory, motor, perceptual, and cognitive—have important roles in making movement efficient. No system works in isolation; all systems network with other systems; they receive, integrate, and pass on information, and they influence and are influenced by other systems. "Movement is the output of a hybrid functional system interlinked with its environment in which sensory, cognitive and motor processes interact" (Mulder et al 1996). Motor behavior is the result of integration between the individual, the task, and the environment in which action is being performed. Different systems have different roles in different contexts to make behavior appropriate to the moment.

Localizing CNS function is a complex task and has undergone huge advancements, from the science of phrenology, in which "bumps" on a person's skull were thought to represent a specially developed brain area, to imaging techniques that permit us to see the human brain in action. Different regions of the brain are specialized for different functions, but it is the sum of activity in many interacting systems that produces motor behavior. The organization of the CNS is known as *parallel distributed processing*. Many sensory, motor, and cognitive functions are served by more than one pathway. To some degree, this helps regions or pathways to partially compensate for each other if damage occurs (Kandel et al 2013).

In the following text we will describe different systems and relate knowledge of their function to human movement and clinical reasoning.

The Somatosensory System

Our different senses enable us to perceive and act within the environment, and to perceive our body and ourselves. Inputs delivered by different sensory organs (receptors) provide us with information about our body and the environment. A major function of the perceptual system is to provide the sensory information necessary for our motor actions. A key issue in understanding how the CNS controls motor output is how sensory inputs direct and inform motor output (i.e., the sensorimotor process).

The term *somatosensory* is related to sensory experiences within the body (soma). In this chapter the discussion is limited to sensory information from the skin, joints, and muscles. The convergence of sensory input from Golgi tendon organs (GTOs) and cutaneous and joint receptors onto interneurons has a role in precision of motor action in, for example, hand function when grasping a delicate object.

There is a growing understanding that sensory information plays a fundamental role in motor control, which is consistent with a key understanding of movement within the Bobath Concept. For example, it is well established that movements made by patients with partial or complete sensory loss lack precision and coordination (Bard et al 1992; Stenneken et al 2006). Movements in deafferented patients (complete removal of all sensory input) with complete large-fiber sensory loss who have no cutaneous sensation or proprioception are imprecise and characterized by dysmetria (Forget & Lamarre 1995; Lavoie et al 1995), even in the presence of visual information (Bard et al 1999).

■ Skin Receptors

The skin covers our body and is our largest organ, providing us with information about our immediate environment. Many different afferent somatosensory fiber types innervate the skin. Mechanics of the skin and subcutaneous tissues are as central to the sense of touch as optics of the eye are to vision.

Functionally the skin receptors, just like receptors in other parts of the body, can be divided as follows:
- Mechanoreceptors.
- Thermoreceptors.
- Chemoreceptors.

Mechanoreceptors in the skin inform the brain about different qualities of touch, compression, and stretch of the skin. Touch receptors in our fingertips are important for fine tactile acuity, which allows us to manipulate objects with high precision.

There are four different types of mechanoreceptors, which are all highly sensitive, and their combined action gives us the sense of touch. The mechanoreceptors are located in different layers of the skin. There are two types of mechanoreceptors in the superficial layers of the skin (Meissner's corpuscles and Merkel's disks), and two within the deep tissue (Pacinian corpuscle and Ruffini's endings). Some of these receptors adapt quickly to stimuli (fast-adapting), others more slowly; some have a low threshold for firing, and others a high threshold. *Fast*-adapting means that the receptor responds quickly to stimulation and rapidly accommodates and stops firing if the stimulus remains constant. The fast-adapting receptors inform the CNS about the start and finish of impulse firing (i.e., variations). The other group of receptors are called slow adapting; for instance, pain receptors and receptors signaling about the body in space and the position of the parts of the body in relation to each other. These are slow adapting due to the need for continuous information with regard to balance (Brodal 2010).

The skin receptors inform the CNS of change. The *slow*-adapting receptors continue to send information as long as stimuli are present. In this way, the CNS is updated about the state of the body at all times. The most important functional feature of the slow-adapting receptors is the ability to detect skin deformation and pressure. We perceive an object as hard if it indents the skin, and an object will be perceived as soft if the skin deforms the object. Nevertheless, both slow- and fast-adapting receptors can be stimulated at the same time and provide information regarding the stimulation.

> The receptive field of the skin defines the tactile sensitivity of an area.

The mechanoreceptors have different receptive fields, which is relevant to the function of the receptors. The term *receptive field of a sensory neuron* is defined as the area from which the sensory unit receives its stimulation (Brodal 2010). In general, the density of sensory units is highest in the distal parts of the body (fingers, toes, and lips), and the receptive fields are smaller distally than proximally. Approximately 2,000 tactile afferents innervate each fingertip, and 10,000 afferent neurons innervate the remaining glabrous skin on the volar surface of the digits and the palm (Johansson & Flanagan 2009). As a result, it is easier to localize a stimulus more precisely in the hand than at the back (Brodal 2010).

The superficial layer of receptors detects fine spatial differences due to the restricted area from which they mediate their information; this gives rise to detection of fine tactile stimulation and enables humans to, for example, read Braille. The deeper layers of receptors inform from a broader area of skin. Most objects grasped by a hand are larger than the receptive field of any one receptor and will therefore stimulate a large population of sensory nerve fibers.

■ Lateral Inhibition

Lateral inhibition enables the brain to detect skin deformation from two stimuli given simultaneously (two-point discrimination), and is a form of presynaptic inhibition that exists only in the sensory system (Brodal 2010). When the skin is stimulated, information is sent to the CNS. Where the stimulus is at its strongest, for instance, at the edges of a book being held in the hand, the stimulated receptor organs transmit impulses to the spinal cord, where they give off collaterals that synapse with inhibitory interneurons in the dorsal horn (**Fig. 1.6**). The inhibitory interneurons inhibit sensory impulses from other sensory neurons arising from the periphery of the receptive field of the stimulated area (Brodal 2010). The CNS thus receives the strongest stimulation from sensory units at the center of the stimulated area. This improves the discriminative ability as compared with what

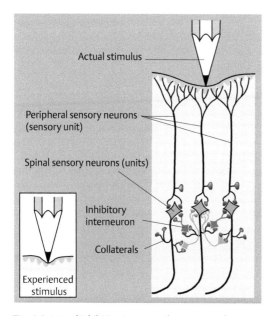

Fig. 1.6 Lateral inhibition increases the contrast of sensory impulses.

might have been found purely from the anatomical arrangement of the receptive field.

Thus the CNS is able to localize touch and is informed of changes (start/stop), edges, texture, and shapes (i.e., variations). If a person places her hand on another person's shoulder, she is informed of the shape and temperature of the area. If the hand is not moved, the receptors quickly adapt and stop sending impulses. So without moving the hand, the size, shape, texture, and temperature of an object cannot be evaluated. Movement is necessary to activate receptors and obtain information through variations, and therefore for sensation. Motor activity and sensation are closely linked, and motor activity is a tool of sensation. Brodal states that most movements need continuous information from specific receptors within muscles, tendons, joints, and skin to know if the movement is progressing as planned (Brodal 2010).

The Sense of Touch

Touch is a complex sense comprising a diversity of modalities. Among Aristotle's five primal senses, touch remains the least understood at the cellular level (Lumpkin et al 2010). Touch facilitates or makes almost every motor activity possible; without vision it permits the perception of objects and informs us of object properties (e.g., temperature)—information that is unreachable to the other senses. Touch can be active, as when you are moving your hand or other parts of your body against another person or a surface, or passive, as when something or someone touches you (Kandel et al 2013). Active touch and passive touch both stimulate the same receptors in the skin and evoke similar response in the afferent system (Kandel et al 2013).

The hand is often referred to as the third eye because touching an object creates a mental image of the object even without vision. Humans can recognize common objects on the basis of touch alone; this ability is called stereognostic sense. Klatzky et al found that blindfolded adults were able to identify each of 100 common objects with almost perfect accuracy within only a few seconds (Klatzky et al 1985). To discriminate between objects, we tend to move the item in stereotypical patterns referred to as exploratory movements. Humans use specific movements to create an optimal input from the receptors; for example, sweeping the hand on a silk scarf to feel its softness (these sweeping movements are referred to as lateral movements) (Lederman & Klatzky 1993). Stereognosis uses sensory information from cutaneous mechanoreceptors and thermoreceptors together with mechanoreceptors embedded in muscles, tendons, and joints. Stereognosis is also known as haptic perception and described as "the faculty of perceiving and understanding the form and nature of objects by the sense of touch"; that is, without the use of vision (Harris et al 2010). Stereognostic sense relates mainly to hand function. The stability, mobility, sensitivity, and adaptive ability of the hands are crucial for exploration of the environment and object manipulation.

Haptics (any form of interaction involving touch) is now commonly viewed as a perceptual system that is mediated by two afferent subsystems, *cutaneous* and *kinesthetic*, and involves active manual exploration (Lederman & Klatzky 2009).

> Stereognostic sense is based on somatosensory information, movement, the ability to recognize variations, and perception.

Recent studies suggest that, in addition to the sensory receptors contributing to the sense of touch, tissue mechanics shape responses to mechanical stimuli. This means that human tactile acuity is influenced by skin mechanical properties, such as fingertip size, epidermal stiffness, and the spacing of finger-print ridges (Lumpkin et al 2010).

During grasp, the safety margin (the ratio between grip force and load force) is precisely regulated (Johansson & Flanagan 2009). The grip forces are high enough to prevent the object from slipping while at the same time not too high. The regulation of grip force involves feedback from cutaneous afferents together with an internal model anticipating the grip force needed. The grip force output is modified ~100 ms after contact with the object and adjusted to the object properties (Johansson & Flanagan 2009).

The ability to manipulate different objects depends on anticipatory control that relies on experience about the relationship between the actual movement and the effect of the movement. The cutaneous receptors play an essential role in gaining this knowledge because information from tactile afferents provides direct information about mechanical interactions between the body and objects in the environment (Johansson & Flanagan 2009).

In addition to their important role of sensing size, shape, texture, and movement of objects, the mechanoreceptors provide important information for postural control. The cutaneous mechanoreceptors found in the feet play an important role in

controlling standing balance. A change in standing position is related to a change in the pressure areas under the feet. The receptors provide reliable and important information to the CNS about the direction and amplitude of motion of the center of pressure, foot placement, and loading. This information is part of the basis for the organization of anticipatory postural adjustments (APAs) for step initiation (read more about APAs in Chapter 2, under Postural Control). During walking, the sole of the foot is loaded during stance. Plantar cutaneous mechanoreceptors sense the local stress distribution and provide indirect information about movements of the body in relation to the base of support and stability limits. Both fast- and slow-adapting cutaneous mechanoreceptors are highly sensitive to the forces applied to the soles of the feet.

Different studies have investigated the importance of plantar skin receptors for postural control using different experimental designs to influence tactile afferent information (Kars et al 2009). In these experiments, postural stability was influenced negatively by different techniques used to reduce the sensitivity of the soles of the feet (cooling the mechanoreceptors, anesthetizing the receptors, or changing the characteristics of the supporting surface on which the subject was standing) (Kars et al 2009). The contribution of plantar cutaneous afferents to balance control is largely evidenced by these protocols.

Information from mechanoreceptors in the skin can also inform the CNS about joint position. Studies have demonstrated evidence of nonmuscular afferent contribution to position and movement (Collins et al 2005; Cordo et al 2011). The skin receptors have shown to fire reliably in relation to the position of nearby joints (Aimonetti et al 2007).

■ **Clinical Implications**

For humans, the active movement of the hand and fingers is vital to our tactile sense—we stroke a surface to detect texture, palpate gently or trace edges to judge shape, or press to define surface hardness (Lederman & Klatzky 1993). Brodal (2010) states that most movements need continuous information from specific receptors within muscles, tendons, joints, and skin to know if the movement is progressing as planned. This has important clinical implications: a patient who is unable to move receives little or no information from the receptors within skin, muscle, and joints, and the ability to recognize changes in joint position may be reduced as a result. Through formal testing of joint position sense, only the patient's *perception* and *cognitive awareness* are tested and *not* the patient's potential for detecting joint position through movement. Information from receptors is transmitted from the receptor areas in the body through to the spinal cord, modulated and passed on for further processing in the brain stem, the cerebellum, the thalamus, and the cerebral cortex. Decreased sensory awareness will, for most patients with CNS lesions, be linked either to dysfunction in perceptual processing or to lesions in the ascending pathways within the brain itself, for instance, at the level of the internal capsule. Therefore, somatosensory information will be integrated at many levels, even if the patient is unable to feel and perceive it. Only through observation of the patient in functional activity will the clinician be able to get a true picture of the patient's ability to receive and integrate sensory information.

If the patient is not able to move actively there is a danger of developing learned nonuse, and the therapist may have to consider delivering a "sensory stimulation package" to maintain and/or rebuild the body schema for the different body representations in the brain (see Motor Learning and Plasticity).

■ The Proprioceptors

Proprioception is the sense of position and movement of the body parts without vision, and plays an important role in human function. Although skin receptors contribute to joint position sense, the term *proprioceptors* is normally used to describe sensory receptors in the musculoskeletal system. There are two forms of specialized mechanoreceptors found in joints and in muscles; muscle spindles and GTOs.

The Muscle Spindle

Muscle spindles are unique sensory organs found in between and in parallel with the muscle fibers in skeletal muscles (**Fig. 1.7**). Both ends of each spindle are attached to the connective tissue within the muscle and therefore are indirectly attached to the tendon of the muscle. Due to this arrangement, the muscle spindles are stretched when the muscle

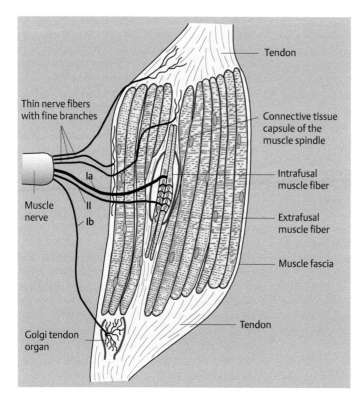

Fig. 1.7 The muscle spindle and the Golgi tendon organ. The muscle spindles are situated in between and in parallel with the extrafusal (skeletal) muscle fibers and are attached to the tendon through connective tissue.

is stretched; when the muscle contracts, the muscle spindles buckle unless their ends shorten. Their main function is to inform the CNS of the length of the muscle, length changes, and the speed of change.

The muscle fibers of a muscle spindle are called *intrafusal fibers*, whereas the muscle fibers of the muscle itself are called extrafusal fibers. Within a muscle spindle there are two types of specialized intrafusal muscle fibers: nuclear bag and nuclear chain. Due to the anatomy, the nuclear bag fibers are much more compliant and less resistant to being stretched and may contribute to the dynamic sensitivity of the spindle, whereas the nuclear chain fibers are much stiffer and probably contribute to the static sensitivity of the muscle spindle (Brodal 2010).

These intrafusal muscle fibers have contractile elements only at each end, leaving a midportion unable to actively contract. Each midportion is surrounded by sensory nerve endings that sense deformations induced by stretch of the fibers. Afferent information from muscle spindle stretch is conveyed to the CNS by primary (Ia) afferent fibers (thick myelin sheath and high conduction velocity) and secondary (group II) afferent fibers.

The muscle spindle is the only mechanoreceptor whose sensitivity can be changed by the CNS; the ends of each nuclear bag and nuclear chain fiber are innervated by a γ-motor neuron, by which the sensitivity of the muscle spindle is maintained during muscular activity (Kandel et al 2013). This enables the CNS to respond rapidly to any unwanted change in muscle length. The γ-motor neurons are also referred to as fusimotor, due to their innervation of the intrafusal fibers. Contraction of the ends of the intrafusal muscle fibers stretches the midportion, thereby changing the stiffness of the spindle and adjusting its sensitivity. There are more neurons in the motor cortex involved in the control of γ-motor neurons than those involved in control of α-motor neurons (Lan & He 2012).

To prevent buckling of the muscle spindle as the skeletal muscle fibers (the extrafusal fibers) contract, γ-motor neuron activity occurs in conjunction with α-motor neuron activity to the same muscle. A buckled muscle spindle is not sensitive to stretch. The simultaneous activity of α- and γ-motor neurons is called α-γ-*coactivation*. The CNS fine tunes the length of the muscle spindle to the anticipated length of the extrafusal muscle fibers. In this way the sensitivity of the muscle spindle is maintained during alterations in length of the muscle, and the CNS is enabled to respond rapidly to any unwanted change

in muscle length. Thus α-γ-coactivation seems to be important for the maintenance of tonic contractions, for example, keeping the knee stable during loading of the leg in the stance phase.

The Ia afferent nerve fibers monosynaptically connect to α-motor neurons of their own muscle. This forms the basis of the monosynaptic stretch reflex, expressed by tendon jerks in the patellar, Achilles, and other reflexes (read more in The Spinal Cord). The Ia afferents are also the primary sensory source of recurrent inhibition (see Recurrent Inhibition).

Information from the muscle spindles is used for our conscious and unconscious awareness of joint position sense. Together with information from cutaneous stretch receptors, joint positions can be encoded with high precision both for conscious use and as the basis for unconscious, automatic postural adjustments (Brodal 2010).

When the CNS plans and executes movements, the muscle spindles provide the CNS with continuous kinematic information about the initial state of the body and about ongoing changes in joint positions. Recent theories of motor control include "forward models," in which predicted sensory states are used to guide motor activity (see The Cerebellum). Information from the muscle spindles can contribute to the formation of these "forward sensory models," and fusimotor (γ) activity may carry centrally planned kinematic information of joint angles as the movement progresses. If the movement was not performed as anticipated, the CNS may correct the activity. In this way, the CNS may modulate and control motor activity accurately and increase the reaction to unexpected disturbances, for instance balance perturbations (Brodal 2010).

When a movement has ended, information from the muscle spindles contributes to the evaluation of the outcome of the performed motor actions by the brain. Thus the muscle spindle is involved in assessing the initial state of the body, to monitor movement progression, and to evaluate the outcome of executed motor actions.

The number of muscle spindles in different muscles varies, with greater numbers present where the need for precise grading of activity is necessary (e.g., in the small muscles of the hand or the deep postural muscles of the back).

The muscle spindles inform the CNS continuously of the state of the muscle (Dietz 1992). The CNS therefore knows at all times about the movement that is about to happen, is happening, or has happened, and compares these.

Golgi Tendon Organs

GTOs are specialized mechanoreceptors arranged in series with extrafusal muscle fibers, and located in the area in between the muscle and tendon (**Fig. 1.7**). The GTO has a much simpler structure than the muscle spindle; it consists of receptive endings that are interwoven between the collagen fiber bundles of the tendon. A small strand of muscle tendon destined to attach to muscle fibers passes through each receptor. This series arrangement, coupled with the very low threshold and high dynamic sensitivity exhibited by the sensory endings, enables GTOs to provide the CNS with feedback concerning muscle tension (Brodal 2010).

The muscle fibers connected to a GTO belong to *many different motor units*. The tendon organ is therefore able to detect tension changes and the distribution of activity in different motor units within the muscle at the same time, and is much more sensitive to tension produced by active muscle work than to passive stretch (Brodal 2010). The GTO has no efferent innervation from the CNS; therefore the CNS cannot adjust its sensitivity.

The GTO is innervated by a sensory nerve fiber called the Ib afferent, whose structure is identical to the Ia fiber (thick myelin sheath and high conduction velocity). When stimulated in a passive situation, the GTO causes inhibition of the corresponding muscle, elicited by the Ib interneurons in the spinal cord (see Nonreciprocal Inhibition). This was first thought to have only a purely protective role; preventing damage to the muscle. However, it is now known that these receptors detect small changes in muscle tension, and therefore inform the CNS about the state of muscle contraction. In a situation in which the muscle is supposed to be loaded (e.g., triceps surae in the stance phase of walking), information from the GTO will increase activity in the muscle and thereby aid in sustaining tension.

Generally, in walking, GTOs excite extensor motor neurons in the transition between swing phase to stance, thereby improving the stance phase (Brodal 2010).

Clinical Relevance

The foot is a key source of peripheral input in controlling and adjusting the muscle activation patterns of the lower limb, particularly during stance phase and standing. The foot represents an important receptive field, formed by numerous skin, joint, tendon, and muscular receptors (including intrinsic foot muscles), and it has long been recognized that damage to the foot, be it either by sensorineural loss or by physical damage to the muscles, bones, or supporting tissues, changes posture and gait stability (Wright et al 2012).

In humans, it is believed that both central commands and feedback from sensory receptors contribute to the control of locomotion. Afferent information plays a crucial role in adapting and modulating the activity of the central pattern generators (CPGs) to the environment (see Spinal Cord). More specifically, the contribution of load and/or length feedback, sensed by GTOs, muscle spindles, and joint and cutaneous receptors, is thought to give important feedback signals for motor control of walking (af Klint et al 2010). Data indicate that loading (heel strike) and unloading (heel-off) in locomotion provide the CNS with information from spatial and temporal parameters, proprioceptive information, pressure receptors, and recruitment patterns of the lower limbs (Trew & Everett 1998). Weight bearing regulates the step cycle by influencing stance duration, and sensitivity to loading has been observed in humans. Load information is provided by the GTOs from leg extensor muscles, and GTO activity from the leg extensor muscles during a stance phase inhibits flexor activity. This is functionally important because the load of the standing leg has to decrease before swing can be initiated (Hubli & Dietz 2013). The degree of leg extensor activation is highly correlated with the percentage of body loading and has been found to be functionally phase dependent (Mudge & Rochester 2001). As loading of the weight-bearing leg is reduced at the end of stance, the facilitatory activity of the GTOs is reduced, thereby assisting in phase transition toward swing. An important role of feedback from muscle afferent seems to be in timing of the step cycle by adjusting the duration of the various phases of the gait cycle and facilitating the switch between these phases (Rossignol et al 2006).

Patients with CNS lesions often have reduced control and mobility of the ankle and foot: at times hypertonicity or stiffness of the calf muscles prevents heel strike, the patient may show inactive ankle dorsiflexion, or activates patterns of inversion and plantar flexion during walking. An inability to place the heel on the floor as the first component of stance disrupts the ability to achieve a stable stance phase of locomotion as a prerequisite for an efficient swing phase.

> Heel strike is important for initiation of stance and therefore locomotion.
> Heel-off is an important signal for the termination of stance, and therefore for the swing phase.

Integration of Somatosensory Information at the Spinal Cord Level

Millions of sensory neurons deliver information to the CNS all the time (afferent neurons). Sensory information reaches the spinal cord through the spinal nerves. Integration of sensory input is considered to begin at the spinal level. *Integration* describes the mechanisms of *summation, gating, and modulation* that occur as a result of various combinations of excitatory and inhibitory synaptic activity by the afferent neurons.

The cell bodies of sensory neurons are located outside the brain and spinal cord in ganglia, located close to the spinal cord. The ganglia associated with spinal nerves are called dorsal (posterior) root ganglia, which is where the afferent fibers enter the CNS. The dorsal root ganglion neuron is the *primary sensory receptor cell* of the somatosensory system. Dorsal root ganglion cells are also known as *first-order neurons* because they initiate the sensory integration process (Kandel et al 2013). The afferent fibers from the receptors make synaptic contact with the first-order relay neurons in the dorsal root and carry impulses to the spinal cord to convey information not only to higher centers via the ascending pathways (also referred to as tracts) but also to *local neuronal networks* via the spinal interneurons. Local neuronal networks establish *reflex arcs for somatic and autonomic reflexes* (Brodal 2010). One of the mechanisms of sensorimotor integration is through the formation of reflexes. Both cutaneous and muscle afferents can give rise to reflexes. Reflex mechanisms allow sensory feedback to be rapidly integrated with central motor commands to modulate and refine motor control (see The Spinal Cord).

The majority of the spinal interneurons also make connections between neurons at different segmental levels via the *propriospinal fibers*; hence information entering the spinal cord can spread over several segmental levels. This extension of information is dependent on the synaptic influences these interneurons receive from the descending pathways. The first-order relay neurons represent one of the first stages at which peripheral input can be modulated.

The spinal cord has been extensively researched, especially in cats, and it is well documented that sensory afferents and descending motor pathways converge onto common spinal interneurons (Petersen et al 2003; Nielsen 2004; Brodal 2010). In humans, the integration of motor commands and sensory feedback signals has been shown to have a function in controlling muscle activity during movement. The convergence between descending supraspinal input and sensory feedback on common spinal interneurons is considered a cornerstone in the central control of movement (Nielsen 2004) (more detail under The Spinal Cord).

■ Ascending Systems

Overview

As we have already described, somatosensory information is received and carried through the peripheral nervous system from the different receptors in the body to the spinal cord. Now we will have a closer look at the transport of this information within the CNS. Somatosensory systems include the receptors and pathways for transmission of sensory information from the body to the portions of the brain that need to integrate this information and act upon it. *Tracts are communication pathways* within the CNS. *The ascending tracts are sensory pathways* and deliver information to the brain. The information from each type of somatosensory receptors is conveyed in separate pathways; the somatosensory submodalities remain segregated as they reach the cerebral cortex (Kandel et al 2013). Somatosensory tracts are named based on the origin and termination of the tracts. If the tract name begins with *spino* as in *spinocerebellar*, the tract is a sensory tract delivering information from the spinal cord to the cerebellum.

The transmission of *conscious somatosensory information* is through two major pathways: (**Fig. 1.8**) (Kandel et al 2013) *the dorsal column–medial lemniscus pathway* conveys touch, proprioception, and vibration, and the *anterolateral system* transmits pain and temperature. These two sensory pathways use three different neurons to bring information from sensory receptors at the periphery to the cerebral cortex (Brodal 2010). These neurons are named *primary* (where the sensory processing is initiated), *secondary*, and *tertiary* sensory neurons. In both pathways, primary sensory neuron cell bodies are found in the dorsal root ganglia, and their central axons project onto the spinal cord. The secondary sensory neuron

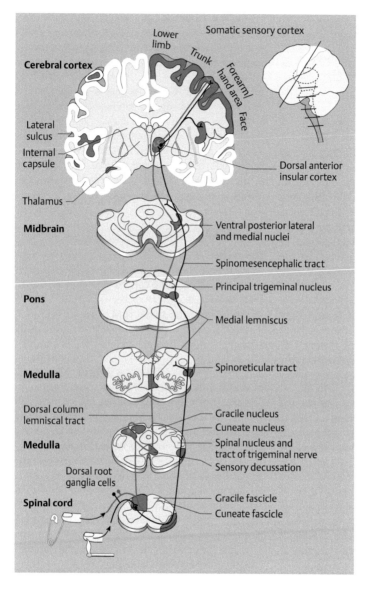

Lower limb **Trunk** **Forearm/hand area** **Face**

Somatic sensory cortex

Cerebral cortex

Lateral sulcus

Internal capsule

Dorsal anterior insular cortex

Thalamus

Midbrain

Ventral posterior lateral and medial nuclei

Spinomesencephalic tract

Principal trigeminal nucleus

Pons

Medial lemniscus

Spinoreticular tract

Medulla

Dorsal column lemniscal tract

Gracile nucleus

Cuneate nucleus

Medulla

Spinal nucleus and tract of trigeminal nerve

Sensory decussation

Dorsal root ganglia cells

Spinal cord

Gracile fascicle

Cuneate fascicle

Fig. 1.8 The figure illustrates the dorsal column–medial lemniscus system—the sensory nerve entering the spinal cord and the ipsilateral pathway to the nuclei cuneate and gracilis in the brain stem. Here, the nerves cross over to form the medial lemniscus. The spinoreticular and the spinothalamic tracts cross over as they enter the spinal cord to form the antero-lateral system. From the brain stem these two systems ascend together to the thalamus and to the cortex. (Redrawn with permission from Kandel et al 2000, p. 447.)

has its cell body in the gray matter of the spinal cord or in the brain stem; whereas the tertiary sensory neuron has its cell body in the thalamus. At each of these relay stations the sensory messages are subject to extensive filtering and processing before a conscious sensation is produced in the cortex.

In addition to the two pathways already mentioned there are somatosensory pathways to the cerebellum referred to as the *ventral* and *dorsal spinocerebellar tracts*.

Neurons in the sensory tracts are arranged according to three anatomical principles:

- Sensory modality: The information from each type of somatosensory receptor is kept separate within the pathways.
- Somatotopic: The fibers within the ascending tracts are arranged according to the site of origin.
- Medial-lateral rule: Sensory neurons that enter a low level of the spinal cord are anatomically more medial within the spinal cord, and sensory neurons that enter at a higher level of the spinal cord are more lateral.

The Dorsal Column—Medial Lemniscus Pathway

The main pathway of the somatosensory system from peripheral receptors to the cortex is the dorsal column–medial lemniscus pathway (Brodal 2010), and it mediates signals from low-threshold mechanoreceptors in the skin muscles and joints. The medial portion of the dorsal column of the spinal cord is called the gracilis fasciculus. The gracile fibers receive information from the lower part of the body, from areas inferior to T6. The more lateral aspect of the tract is called the cuneate fasciculus; these fibers receive information from areas superior to T6 (i.e., upper limbs, trunk, and neck (Brodal 2010). This pathway is a high-velocity system (highly myelinated) and conveys information about touch, pressure, vibration, and proprioception (Brodal 2010). The primary sensory neurons within this tract travel ipsilateral (uncrossed) to the cuneate and gracile nuclei (together referred to as the dorsal column nuclei) in the brain stem. Here, information is filtered and processed and transmitted to connecting secondary sensory neurons, which cross over to form the medial lemniscus system. The third-order sensory fibers from the thalamus ascend through the posterior limb of internal capsule. Eventually these fibers connect to the cerebral cortex in the postcentral gyrus, also referred to as the sensory cortex.

The Anterolateral System

The anterolateral system includes three pathways: the *spinothalamic tract*, the *spinoreticular tract*, and the *spinomesencephalic tract* (Kandel et al 2013). These tracts convey information related to crude touch, itch, tickling, pain, visceral information, and temperature. Crude touch refers to a poorly localized, poorly identified sense that is not precise enough to be carried by the dorsal column–medial lemniscus pathway.

- The spinothalamic tract is important for perception of noxious, thermal, and visceral information (Kandel et al 2013). The primary sensory neuron originates in the dorsal root ganglion (note that information about pain and temperature from the face follows a separate route to the thalamus), and the secondary sensory neuron from the dorsal horn in the spinal cord. The axons then cross midline and form the spinothalamic tract. These axons ascend uninterrupted to the thalamus. Third-order neurons from the thalamus project through the posterior limb of the internal capsule to terminate in the somatosensory cortex in the postcentral gyrus.
- The spinoreticular (or spinoreticulothalamic) pathway is important for the perception of dull, aching, or burning pain, and is also involved in the emotional aspects of pain. It originates in the dorsal root ganglion, and the second-order neurons project to the supraspinal levels and to other spinal laminae, and then bilaterally to the reticular formation. From the reticular formation the information goes on to the thalamus.

In the thalamus, these pathways are not precisely somatotopically organized; slow (dull) pain is not well localized. Projections from these thalamic areas reach multiple cortical areas, including the postcentral gyrus, insula, and anterior cingulate gyrus. Information about pain is carried in several pathways that distribute information to many areas of the nervous system; these tracts are referred to as spinothalamic, spinoreticular, spinomesencephalic, cervicothalamic, and spinohypothalamic pathways (Kandel et al 2013). Descending pathways that project to the dorsal horn can play an important role in modulating the transmission of nociceptive signals (Aziz & Ahmad 2006; Kandel et al 2013).

The Ventral and Dorsal Spinocerebellar Tracts

Although much sensory information reaches consciousness (synapsing in the cortex), vast amounts of sensory information do not reach consciousness. Two pathways originate among the interneurons within the spinal cord that terminate in the vermis or spinocerebellum as mossy fibers (see The Cerebellum) and are called the *ventral* and *dorsal spinocerebellar tracts*. Although they both originate from spinal interneurons, they transmit different modalities of information (Kandel et al 2013). The dorsal spinocerebellar tract conveys somatosensory information from muscle and joint receptors, both when a limb actively moves and when it is passively moved (Kandel et al 2013). The ventral spinocerebellar pathway solely transmits information when the limb actively moves. These inputs inform the cerebellum about different aspects of movement activity at the same moment in time, and permit comparison of signals.

The Thalamus

The thalamus is located deep within the brain and is a part of the diencephalon, which contains two major subdivisions: the thalamus and the hypothalamus. The thalamus is a large egg-shaped collection of 50 to 60 nuclei, which plays a crucial role in gating, processing, and transferring the majority of sensory information to and from the cerebral cortex (Kandel et al 2013; Cappe et al 2009). The thalamus is considered a core structure of the brain and contains highly specialized nuclei that are connected with distinct zones of the cerebral cortex, and it has a close relationship to motor and sensory areas of the brain. In addition to the thalamocortical connections, the thalamus has connections to the basal ganglia (BG), the red nucleus, and the cerebellum, and is thus able to process different types of information. The thalamus serves as an important center of integration of networks that underlie the ability to modulate behaviors (Haber & Calzavara 2009), and it influences the level of attention and consciousness (Brodal 2010).

The thalamic nuclei are classified into four groups: anterior, medial, ventrolateral, and posterior. The thalamus can be further organized into functional regions based on their connections with the cortex (Schmahmann 2003):

- Reticular and intralaminar nuclei subserve arousal and nociception.
- Effector nuclei are concerned with motor function and aspects of language.
- Associative nuclei are concerned with cognitive function.
- Limbic nuclei are concerned with mood and motivation.
- Sensory nuclei may play a role in multisensory and sensorimotor integration.

All pathways that carry sensory information from the receptors in the body to the cerebral cortex (except for olfactory) pass through the thalamus (Brodal 2010). In addition, the thalamus is also involved in descending inhibition to modulate nociceptive inputs at the dorsal horn of the spinal cord (Aziz & Ahmad 2006).

The sensory nuclei have a precise somatotopy, and lesions of the lateral ventroposterior nuclear group (VPL) and the medial ventroposterior nuclear group (VPM) result in focal sensory deficits in the affected regions (Schmahmann 2003). Somatosensory impulses leave the thalamus and are then forwarded to somatosensory areas of the cortex via the internal capsule. Furthermore, the cortex acts back on the thalamus via the corticothalamic connections. Hence the thalamic neurons receive a lot of input from the cortex by which the cortex influences the thalamus during sensory processing. Therefore, the cortex has the opportunity to influence thalamic processing and consequently shape the nature of its own input (Brodal 2010).

Vision, Visual Pathways, and Visual Processing

The visual system starts with the eyes and retina. The receptors for sight are called photoreceptors, of which there are two types: the rods and cones of the retina (Kandel et al 2013); each contributes to the information used by the visual system to form the representation of the visual world (Brodal 2010). Unlike other somatosensory receptors, the photoreceptors are not a part of the peripheral nervous system, but are included in the central nervous system. The area of the retina near the optical axis is called the fovea, and it is here that our vision is the sharpest (Kandel et al 2013).

The visual pathway begins in the retinal ganglion cells, and their axons leave the eyes in the optic nerve. About 90% of the axons in the optic nerve continue in the optic tract that passes through the lateral geniculate nucleus in the thalamus before terminating in the primary visual cortex. This pathway is referred to as the *primary* or the *geniculostriate pathway*. The last 10% of the tract passes through the mesencephalon, particularly the superior colliculus and the pretectal nuclei. This latter pathway conveys visual information to the nucleus superior colliculus in the midbrain, both directly from the optic nerve and indirectly through the visual cortex. This latter part of the pathway is primarily concerned with reflex movements of the eyes and head; humans are able to automatically turn the head toward something in the environment and to control eye movements at the same time.

Visual information is also transmitted to the cerebellum and has a role in coordination.

The Visual Cortex

The primary visual cortex is the first level of cortical processing of visual information (Kandel et al 2013). Several visual association areas surround the primary visual cortex and convert the basic signals from the eyes into meaningful information. According to Milner and Goodale (2008), visual information is transformed in different ways for different purposes. Visual information is segregated along two pathways, the ventral and dorsal streams, for further visual processing (Mishkin et al 1983; Kandel et al 2013). The ventral stream originates in the primary visual cortex and extends along the ventral surface into the temporal cortex; the dorsal stream also arises in the primary visual cortex but continues along the dorsal surface into the parietal cortex (Kandel et al 2013). The ventral pathway registers what the individual sees and information about "what" that object is used for; which is critical for object recognition. The dorsal stream conveys information about where the stimulus originates from, which is crucial for guiding movements. This pathway also registers "how to do" something: for example, how to grasp an object based on the visual information about shape and size (Koziol et al 2011). The dorsal stream pathway is also called the *vision-for-action pathway*. The two visual streams are heavily interconnected, but they also play complementary roles in the production of adaptive behavior (Kravitz et al 2011).

Eye–Hand Coordination

The act of reaching out to grasp an object is a basic visually guided task that is performed multiple times during the day. Optimal reach–grasp accuracy is obtained when hand movements are combined with eye movements. However, in planning goal-directed arm movements toward a seen target, vision and proprioception contribute differentially (Sarlegna & Mutha 2014). Research by Jeannerod and colleagues (1995) provided evidence for the idea that the reaching component is relatively independent from the formation of the grip itself: the *dual visuomotor channel theory* proposes that prehension (reach and grasp) consists of two movements; a *reach* that transports the hand with regard to an object's extrinsic properties (e.g., location) and a *grasp* that shapes the hand to an object's intrinsic properties (e.g., size and shape). Thus the control of manual prehension (reach and grasp) is controlled through two visuomotor channels: the reach component by which the hand is transported toward the object, and the grasp component where the fingers are preshaped according to the size and the center of mass of the object (Grol et al 2009).

To make the appropriate reach movement to the target, it is not enough to know the target location; knowledge of the initial hand position is also essential to make a movement plan. This knowledge is attained from either vision, proprioception, or both. Vision is the main source for encoding the location of the object (Khan et al 2007). Whereas the brain can either visually encode the position of the viewed hand or obtain information about the position of the hand through proprioceptive information from the arm (Vesia & Crawford 2012). Visual information

of hand position and localization of the target are mainly used in a first stage to define the kinematic plan of the reaching movement. Temporal integration of reach and grasp movements into a single prehensile act occurs in foveal vision (Karl & Whishaw 2013). However, hand movements can also be made, although less accurate, without eye movements, for example, when one reaches for a cup of coffee while continuing to read a book. This decreased accuracy when reaching for objects in the peripheral visual field may lie in the lower spatial resolution of peripheral vision.

Central and Peripheral Visual Fields

The visual field is the part of the environment the eyes perceive light from without moving the head or the eyes (Brodal 2010). The spatial design of the retina and the specificity of cortical networks to the central and peripheral retina produce visual-function differences between the central and peripheral parts of the retina. The central retina has high sensitivity to image contrast and displacement compared with the peripheral retina, whereas the peripheral visual field covers a larger spatial area than does the central visual field. These differences in visual function have counterparts in orientation and mobility performance; we see things best when we are looking directly at them, which is due to the density of photoreceptors in the fovea. Thus an object is perceived with greater clarity when the image falls directly in the fovea than when the image falls outside the fovea (Brown et al 2005). Several studies have demonstrated the importance of specific visual information for successfully completing a reach and grasp (Burbeck & Yap 1990; Levi & Klein 1996). In addition, peripheral viewing reduces our understanding of the hand's position relative to the target (Saunders & Knill 2004).

To move your hand accurately toward an object, you must process the location of both the glass and the hand. These two pieces of information can be combined to determine the exact location of the target relative to the hand. We use two types of information to determine the position of the hand: the felt position (proprioception) and the seen position (visual information). This results in a *visual–tactile representation*. When we see an interesting object, we are therefore able to automatically reach toward, grasp, and manipulate it. Seeing one's own hand improves tactile acuity of the hand. This is called the *visual enhancement of touch effect*. Viewing the body seems to establish a visual context, which enhances tactile processing (Cardini et al 2011). The strength of lateral inhibition in the somatosensory cortex appears to be modulated by visual context, specifically vision of the body. In addition to increasing tactile spatial acuity, vision of the body has other somatosensory effects: Longo and colleagues (2008) demonstrated that vision of the body also had an analgesic effect.

Clinical Implications

Trauma or different diseases of the CNS can disrupt vision at many points along the afferent visual pathway, from the retina to the visual centers in the brain; hence visual functions are frequently impaired in neurological diseases.

The occipital lobe processes, analyzes, and identifies visual information transmitted from the eyes. If the occipital lobes were destroyed, the result would be "cortical blindness," or cortical visual impairment (CVI). This is a condition that indicates that the visual systems of the brain do not understand or interpret what the eyes see even if the function of the eyes and the optic nerve remain unimpaired. The degree of vision impairment can range from severe visual impairment to total blindness. Cortical blindness is most commonly associated with stroke, but it may also appear due to traumatic or hypoxic lesions (Sand et al 2013).

Visual disturbances following a stroke are a result of the integrative nature of the brain and the fact that visual function involves considerable areas of the brain (**Fig. 1.9**).

Approximately 30 to 40% of patients with stroke and 50% with traumatic brain injury (TBI) suffer from poststroke visual impairments (Sand et al 2013; Kerty 2005). Hemianopia (defective vision or blindness in half of the visual field of one or both eyes) is the most common symptom, but also neglect, diplopia (double vision), reduced visual acuity, ptosis (drooping of upper or lower eyelid), anisocoria (unequal size of the eye pupils), and nystagmus (fast, uncontrollable movements of the eye) are frequent (Sand et al 2013). According to Rowe and colleagues (2013) gaze dysfunction occurs in 23% of stroke patients with suspected visual impairment. In neurologically intact subjects, walking and turning are accomplished by an anticipatory gaze and head shift preceding the changes in walking trajectory. Impairments in the coordination of gaze and posture have been demonstrated in stroke patients in altered coordination of anticipatory gaze and posture during walking and turning (Lamontagne et al 2007).

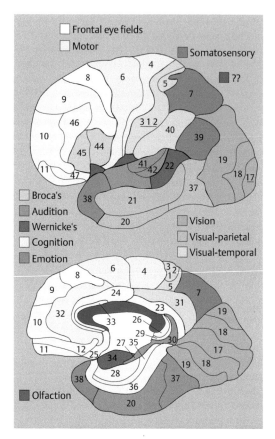

Fig. 1.9 Areas for vision, motor activity, speech, hearing, cognition, somatosensation, and emotion within the brain. Many of these areas receive or integrate information from the visual system. The numbers refer to Brodmann areas, which are the histologically defined regions. (Reproduced with permission from professor Mark W Dubin, MCD Biology, University of Colorado at Boulder, USA.)

Prehension (reach and grasp) is coordinated with activity of the eyes (i.e., we need to be able to turn our head and eyes toward an object to grasp it precisely). Anticipatory orientation and stability of the head and trunk are necessary for the control of gaze stability, and therefore for prehension.

The Use of Mirror Therapy in Treatment

In mirror therapy (MT), the patient sits in front of a mirror that is oriented parallel to the patient's midline and blocking the view of the (affected) limb, which is positioned behind the mirror. When looking into the mirror, the patient can see the mirror image of the unaffected limb, being positioned as the affected limb. This arrangement creates a visual illusion whereby movement of or touch to the intact limb may be visually perceived as affecting the paretic or painful limb. MT has been used in the treatment of stroke, phantom limb pain, and complex regional pain syndrome. The underlying mechanism of MT has been related mainly to the activation of "mirror neurons" (see The Secondary Somatosensory Cortex). In a recent systematic review article the conclusion was that "little is known about which patients are likely to benefit most from MT, and how MT should preferably be applied" (Rothgangel et al 2011). Nevertheless, important aspects to consider include the posture of the hand inside the mirror box with regard to the planned task; that the two hands have to be similarly positioned; and that the task has to be plausible for both hands. Therefore, the choice of task needs to consider both hands. The sitting posture will also be an issue, considering the possibility of a stable head on a stable body for orientation and gaze stability.

■ Brief Orientation of Various Areas of Cerebral Cortex

Before describing aspects of the cerebral cortex's role in somatic sensation, an orientation about the various areas of the cortex is in order.

The cerebral cortex is the outermost layer of gray substance that covers the cerebrum. It is divided into the left and right hemispheres, which constitute the largest part of the human brain (Kandel et al 2013). The surface of the cortex is folded, and these folds are called sulci. Between the sulci, gyri are formed. This anatomical arrangement increases the surface area of the cortex (i.e., more nerve cells are fitted into a limited space) (Kandel et al 2013). The most prominent gyri and sulci are named and form borders by which the cerebral cortex is divided into four lobes: frontal, parietal, occipital, and temporal. The lobes are named after the skull bones by which they are covered (Kandel et al 2013).

A *Brodmann area* is a region of the human cerebral cortex and was originally defined and numbered by the German anatomist Korbinian Brodmann (Kandel et al 2013). Brodmann divided the cortex into 52 anatomically and functionally distinct areas; *the cytoarchitectural maps of the brain* based on the organization and shapes of the neurons in the cerebrum. A cytoarchitectural map shows specialized functional areas of the cerebrum. Areas 1 through 3, for example, are the primary sensory cortices. Area 4 is the primary motor cortex, and area 17 is the primary

visual cortex (Kandel et al 2013). The lobes are richly interconnected and cooperate closely. The brain is a dynamic system where each part exists in broader neural networks that give rise to, for example, perception and action.

The frontal lobe consists of the front third of the cortex. This area includes the primary motor cortex, the MI, which is the most posterior part of the frontal lobe, and the motor association areas: the premotor area (PMA) and the supplementary motor area (SMA). In addition, the frontal lobe contains the prefrontal cortex, which is an association area important to executive functions. The parietal lobe is specialized for sensory and perceptual functions, the temporal lobe contains the primary auditory cortex, and the occipital lobe contains the primary visual cortex.

Somatosensory Areas of the Cortex

Many areas of the cortex are involved in processing sensory information (**Fig. 1.10**). The postcentral gyrus in the parietal lobe is the major receiving area for cutaneous, musculoskeletal and visceral sensory impulses (Brodal 2010). This area is referred to as the somatosensory cortex and has three major divisions: the primary somatosensory cortex (SI), the secondary somatosensory cortex (SII), and the posterior parietal cortex (also referred to as the posterior association area) (Kandel et al 2013). Sensory information is processed both in serial and in parallel.

The Primary Somatosensory Cortex (SI)

The SI area in the human cortex makes up four distinct fields or regions known as Brodmann areas 3a, 3b, 1, and 2.

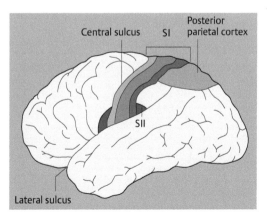

Fig. 1.10 Somatosensory areas of the cortex.

The human SI was mapped in the late 1940s by the Canadian neurosurgeon Wilder Graves Penfield who constructed the neural map of the human body also referred to as the sensory homunculus (**Fig. 1.11**), which is developed from information coming from the peripheral receptors (Brodal 2010). This representation gives a distorted picture of the body because the density of sensory receptors in that area and not the size of the actual area give the sizes of the different somatosensory areas. For example, more cortical space is devoted to the representation of the fingers and mouth than to the trunk. The primary somatosensory cortex receives information from tactile and proprioceptive receptors from the opposite side of the body because most of the ascending pathways cross over to the opposite side before eventually terminating in the cortex. Persons that use their tactile sense to an extraordinary degree in everyday life (e.g., violinists, readers of Braille) have an expanded representation of the trained part in the primary somatosensory cortex (greater detail on how these cortical maps can

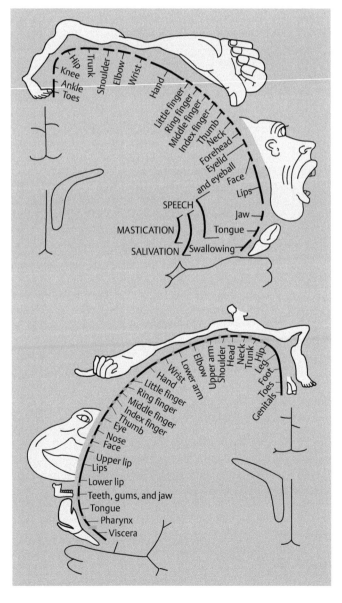

Fig. 1.11   The sensory and motor homunculi show the somatotopic organization of sensory and motor representation within the cortex.

change with experience or after injury is provided under Cortical Plasticity).

The Secondary Somatosensory Cortex

As the contralateral SI is considered to process and encode the type and intensity of a single modality of sensory input from the opposite body half, so the bilateral secondary somatosensory cortex (SII) is presumed to perform sensorimotor integration, especially integration of the two body halves. The SII is also involved in integration of pain stimuli and movement preparation (Beudel et al 2011). Like the SI, the SII contains maps of the body.

This region is included in the parietal-premotor circuitry and is active during motor activity, movement observation, and mental imaging of movements (Beudel et al 2011). The similarity between neural responses during movement execution and movement observation resulted in the involved regions being referred to as the mirror neuron system (MNS) (i.e., areas where mirror neurons have been found) (Rizzolatti & Craighero 2004). Activation during motor observation particularly occurs when the movements being observed belong to one's own motor repertoire, in other words, movement one is able to perform. According to a study done by Beudel and colleagues (2011), the SII may be of importance for matching sensory information with one's own body schema, to code the possibility of performing the same actions as those observed. The SII may therefore contain the neural substrates for storage of kinesthetic limb postures and map these representations onto the premotor and motor regions in which the corresponding motor programs are contained.

The Posterior Parietal Cortex: A Multimodal Association Area

Different pieces of information are held separate from the receptors when they reach the SI via the ascending pathways. To make a coherent representation of the body to enable interaction with external objects, the brain needs to integrate different kinds of somatosensory signals with visual and auditory information. The posterior parietal cortex (PPC) is generally considered to be a key region for this fusion of signals from different sensory modalities. In addition to integrating visual and somatosensory information, the posterior parietal cortex uses this information to issue commands to the premotor cortical areas, particularly with regard to visually guided movements (Kandel et al 2013).

The Prefrontal Cortex

On the lateral surface, the prefrontal cortex (PFC) may be further subdivided into ventrolateral, dorsolateral, and rostral regions (Gilbert & Burgess 2008). The prefrontal cortex receives a widespread variety of afferents from the sensory areas in the parietal, occipital, and temporal areas. In addition it is connected with the limbic association areas and the basal ganglia (Gilbert & Burgess 2008; Lundy-Ekman 2007). The PFC is thus well placed to integrate diverse, high-level representations and to exert control over various brain systems (Gilbert & Burgess 2008). The PFC subserves executive control, which is the ability to select actions on the basis of internal plans or goals (Lundy-Ekman 2007). Purposive behavior requires focused attention. The prefrontal cortex processes specific information in relation to the specific task at hand, hence it functions as an action-oriented area of the brain. Regions in the prefrontal cortex are important for selection of actions appropriate for the specific behavior (Brodal 2010).

Body Schema and Internal Models

Over a long period of time neuroscientists have been fascinated by how the brain represents the body. More than a century ago the neurologists distinguished three elements of bodily processing: (1) a postural schema for the appreciation of changes in position and movement of the body; (2) a surface schema for the localization of cutaneous stimuli on the body surface; and (3) more conscious visual images of the body (which may correspond to the concept of body image) (Holmes & Spence 2004; Kammers et al 2010; Dijkerman & de Haan 2007).

Several labels have been used in different books and different studies to try to define and explain the body schema after this original description. Currently it is believed that several types of body representations in the brain exist, but there is no consensus about what these representations are or how many there may be (de Vignemont 2010; Gallager 2005; Berlucchi & Aglioti 2010). In the literature, the terms *body schema* and *body image* have been used inconsistently. De Vignemont (2010) defines *body schema* as "a continuously updated sensorimotor map of the body that is important in the *context of action*, informing the brain about what parts belong to the body, and where those parts currently are located." Hence one can say that the body schema includes all information relevant for action (e.g., body posture as well as the size of the limbs, muscle strength, degrees of freedom of the joints)

(Kammers et al 2010), and that this body schema is continuously being updated through movement. The term *body image* concerns our conscious perception of the appearance of the body with regard to its size, shape, and other characteristics (Brodal 2010). In other words: body image is about perceptual identification and recognition and consciously knowing *where*, based on the judgment of one's own body properties. Although the body schema can be conceived as the representation the brain uses to plan and execute actions; it is about *how to get there*, based on information about the body that is necessary for movement, such as posture, size of the limbs, muscle strength, and so forth (Kammers et al 2010).

Historically there has been a strong emphasis on the contribution of the proprioceptive system to the multisensory body schema. However, the current belief is that the body schema incorporates all somatosensory information as well as visual, auditory, and, probably, vestibular information (Holmes & Spence 2004; Lopez et al 2012). There is evidence indicating that vestibular signals update the body schema during hand actions and that this information shapes the way we perform actions and interact with objects. This type of information attributed to the body schema takes into account the metric properties of the body that need to be included during grasping and reaching for objects (Lopez et al 2012).

Area 5 of the parietal cortex is particularly important for processing sensory information (Brodal 2010). It has been suggested that the body schema may be stored and maintained within this area (Buneo & Andersen 2006; Wolpert et al 1998). Area 5 projects to and receives information from MI, the premotor cortex, and the supplementary motor cortex, which indicates that it is closely connected to the motor system. The motor system uses the body schema at different stages during motor activity. In addition, the body schema is probably involved in motor imagery (de Vignemont 2010). (Motor imagery is further discussed under Clinical Relevance).

Body Schema and Peripersonal Space

The peripersonal space is the region immediately surrounding the body represented as neither purely bodily nor purely external; in other words a "gray" zone. This area is characterized by a high degree of multisensory integration between visual, tactile and auditory information, which is different from farther regions of space. The body schema and peripersonal space are intimately related. It has been claimed that bodily representations can extend to include prostheses, tools, rubber hands, and the like. The use of tools modifies the motor side of our body representation (i.e., our body schema), and therefore affects movement kinematics (de Vignemont 2010). An object is included in the body schema if it is perceived as a part to be included in the motor task. For example, when playing tennis, the racket will act as an extension of the arm and is integrated in the player's body schema; when trying to hit the ball with the racket, a practiced tennis player knows automatically where the ball will hit the racket. The same might happen when a person uses a walking stick; with prolonged use, the tool becomes an extension of the hand that uses it. It can therefore be difficult to unlearn to use the stick because it is a part of the body schema for that motor act.

Clinical Relevance

Control of movement and restoration of function depend not only on motor output but also on how sensory information required for this output is perceived, discriminated, and recognized for input and integration. For successful rehabilitation of the neurologically damaged patient it is important to understand how sensory information is processed and integrated.

Following a stroke, the normal balance of cortical excitability and the patterns of activation in the brain have been changed. Cortical plasticity has been associated with the recovery of function after a stroke or other neurological disorders. Recognition of the potential for sensory intervention to promote cortical plasticity is gaining ground. There is emerging evidence that interventions targeting the sensory systems can result in improvements in areas such as motor capacity, neglect, and spasticity (Rosenkranz & Rothwell 2012; Sullivan & Hedman 2008). Sensory intervention studies have reported positive functional outcomes for gait speed, amount and type of assistance required for gait, postural sway, balance, arm function, and swallowing effectiveness (Sullivan & Hedman 2008). In the Bobath Concept, the therapist aims to reeducate the individual's internal reference system using afferent information to give patients the possibility of more optimal and efficient movement or a bigger movement repertoire. This is discussed in more detail in Chapter 2.

◾ The Cortical Motor System

■ Sensorimotor Integration to Motor Actions—a General Overview

Sensory information is the framework by which the motor system plans, coordinates, and executes the motor programs responsible for purposeful movements (Kandel et al 2013) Many parts of the CNS contribute to motor control, the principal parts being the motor cortex, basal ganglia, thalamus, midbrain, cerebellum, and spinal cord (Kandel et al 2013).

Motor outputs are neural commands acting on the muscles, making them contract to generate movements. Voluntary movements are those under conscious control by the brain and thereby represent our least automatic movements; more automatic movements happen without our conscious involvement (Brodal 2010).

For quite some time, the role of the motor cortex was thought to be restricted to that of a simple map of muscles and muscle activity patterns by which the cerebral cortex controlled spinal motor neurons. However, several studies over the last 2 decades have shown that the cortical motor system is a thinking, active system involved in a vast amount of interrelated neural processes required to choose a plan of action, including contributions to cognitive processing that appear to be more perceptual and cognitive than motor (Kandel et al 2013). According to Kandel and colleagues (2013), the neural processes by which the brain controls voluntary behavior are divided into three stages: (1) the perceptual processes by which a unified sensory representation is made, (2) the cognitive processes to analyze and reflect on the internal reference frame to decide what to do with it, and (3) the voluntary motor behavior that results when the selected motor plan is put into action.

Voluntary movement thus depends on a contribution from many areas of the CNS, including areas that perform the following functions:
- Receive, integrate, modulate, and transmit impulses.
- Assist in the planning of movement.
- Link with motivation and affection.
- Link with motor execution.

The following sections take a closer look at the role of the cerebral cortex in movement production.

The cortical areas that today are viewed as strictly motor are the MI (area 4), the PMA, and the SMA (area 6) of the frontal lobe (Brodal 2010). However, recently both the human PMA and the SMA have been subdivided into several smaller functional zones: presupplementary motor area (pre-SMA); dorsal premotor cortex (PMd); predorsal premotor area (pre-PMd); and ventral premotor cortex (PMv) (Kandel et al 2013).

The Primary Motor Cortex

The MI is part of a distributed network of cortical areas, all with important roles in voluntary movement control. The executive role of the MI in the brain's motor network is strongly supported by the architecture of its outputs to the spinal cord: the MI is the final cortical processing site for voluntary motor commands before they descend to the spinal cord (Brodal 2010). The MI has been shown to play an important role in the accurate control of discrete voluntary movements of the fingers and face as well as for the modification of more rhythmical movements, such as locomotion. It is not known whether the MI stores memories of complete movements or whether it synthesizes a movement on a moment-to-moment basis by selecting muscle synergy modules (Capaday et al 2013). The MI contains a topographic map, *the motor homunculus* (**Fig. 1.11**), of motor output to different parts of the body. This motor map reflects the size of the representation of different body parts within the primary motor cortex: densely innervated areas like the hand and mouth occupy a relatively larger part of the map than more thinly innervated areas like the lower leg. Historically, finger movement representations in the MI were viewed as separate areas, controlling each digit. However, recent findings show that somatotopic maps of individual fingers in MI are overlapping, intermingled, and fractionated, suggesting that the MI is organized to control coordinated action of muscles and joints (movement patterns) rather than separate movements of muscles and joints (Kandel et al 2013). The motor maps are dynamic and adaptable and shaped by an individual's experiences, for example, reorganization of the map after learning a motor skill or after a focal lesion (see Cortical Plasticity). The MI has monosynaptic projections onto the spinal motor neurons through the corticospinal system (CSS); most dense for muscles in the distal arm, hand, and fingers (Kandel et al 2013). Hence the MI is able to control the activity of these muscles directly, leading to a possibility for selective control of the muscles in the hand and fingers.

The Premotor and Supplementary Motor Areas

The PMA includes the dorsal premotor cortex (PMd), predorsal premotor area (pre-PMd), and ventral premotor cortex (PMv).

The supplementary motor cortex is divided into an SMA and a pre-SMA; together referred to as the supplementary motor complex (SMC) (Nachev et al 2008).

Both the PMA and the SMA are also called *supramotor areas* (Brodal 2010). Premotor areas are thought to instruct the MI in what to do, which is supported by the fact that both areas are active before MI during voluntary movements (Brodal 2010).

The PMA is probably important for visually guided movements and to adjust goal- directed movements to altered external conditions. This area is especially active during learning of complex movement sequences. Interactions between the PMv and the MI are crucial for transforming visual observation about an object's geometrical properties, such as its size and shape, into a motor command suitable for grasping the object.

The PMv is included in the mirror neuron system because mirror neurons are also found here (Franceschini et al 2010). Recent work on these neurons suggests that the function of mirror neurons is related to intentional behavior and seems to be involved in understanding the actions of others because the observed action elicits a motor plan by which the outcome is known in the premotor cortex (Kandel et al 2013; Rizzolatti et al 2014). It has been shown that these mirror neurons also exist in humans, and many researchers believe they may also play a role in motor learning, although to date it is not entirely clear what exact role they play in these processes (Rizzolatti & Sinigaglia 2010).

The SMA participates in planning, generation, and control of sequential motor activity (Kandel et al 2013). In addition, the SMA contributes to complex movement control, such as bilateral tasks with the hands. This area makes a direct and substantial contribution to the corticospinal tract (CST): it comprises 10% of all corticospinal cells (Nachev et al 2008). The pre-SMA has a sparse projection in the corticospinal system. The SMA has reciprocal connections with the primary motor cortex; the pre-SMA does not. All parts of the SMC connect with the BG. Patients with Parkinson's disease (PD) consistently show reduced activity of the SMC, and these findings have led to growing interest in the contribution of SMC dysfunction to PD (Nachev et al 2008).

The Cortical Motor Areas Have Extensive and Complex Connections

Corticocortical association fibers connect ipsilateral cortical regions with each other and are essential for working memory, especially the fibers that connect the prefrontal cortex with parietal and certain temporal lobe regions. *The commissural fibers* are transverse fibers connecting the two halves of the brain, and pass to the contralateral cerebral hemisphere and allow the hemispheres to share information. *Corticostriatal tracts* connect the cortex to the BG, which have been shown to be important for the brain's intention programs. Cortical motor areas project in several parallel tracts to subcortical areas of the brain and to the spinal cord. Only the *corticospinal tract* goes directly; the other pathways are indirect, with synaptic connections in the brain stem. *The corticopontine tracts* descend from nearly all regions of the cerebral cortex to the pons (which in turn projects to the cerebellum and to the spinal cord) and to other brainstem structures (Brodal 2010; Jang 2014).

The corticospinal tract is described in further detail in the next section. Other descending pathways are discussed under The Brain Stem.

Descending Pathways from the Cerebral Cortex

The descending pathways have specific characteristics that target neurons in the spinal cord (Lemon 2008). Each descending pathway may execute several functional roles; however, due to the need to coordinate activity for functions such as balance, posture, walking, and reaching, the functions of the systems are linked together (Lemon 2008).

The CST consists of those fibers that leave the cerebral cortex and descend through the internal capsule to innervate interneurons and motor neurons in the spinal cord without synaptic interruption along the way (Brodal 2010) (**Fig. 1.12**). Most axons of the CST (75–90%) decussate from one side to the other in the lower brain stem (an area with a pyramid shape, hence the label *pyramidal tract*), and descend in the contralateral white matter of the spinal cord as the lateral CST. The lateral CST continues its descent on the contralateral side. A small percentage (10–25%) of axons do not decussate in the pyramid and descend as the ventral CST.

Improvements in tracking techniques have led to improved understanding of the origin and termination of the corticospinal (CS) neurons. Approximately 30 to 40% of the fibers arise in the MI; the rest of the fibers come from the SMA, PMA, somatosensory areas (SI and SII), and parts of the posterior parietal cortex (Kandel et al 2013; Lemon 2008). Although the CST is considered to be the principal motor system for controlling movements requiring the greatest skill and flexibility, it is increasingly clear that the CST originates from several cortical areas and has multiple targets in the spinal cord, and consequently plays different roles in

motor control (Lemon 2008). It is therefore argued that the CST is not only a "motor" system but also a system that has a large sensory role. This is discussed in greater detail following here.

The corticospinal fibers originating from the MI and PMA terminate on the motor regions of the spinal cord. Some of the CST fibers coming from the MI synapse with motor neurons and are referred to as cortico-motor-neuronal (CM) connections; this term is used to describe only the direct, monosynaptic excitatory inputs to motor neurons from the CST (Lemon & Griffiths 2005). This concerns mostly groups of motor neurons to the intrinsic muscles of the hand; therefore, the CM system probably provides the ability to fractionate movements and selectively control small groups of muscles (Lemon 2008). In particular, the appearance of CM connections correlates with the development of precision grip between the thumb and the index fingers in nonhuman primates and humans (Lemon 2008).

The corticospinal system also originates from the sensory cortex. These corticospinal fibers mostly terminate in the posterior (dorsal) horn of the spinal cord, where they synapse with interneurons receiving input from somatosensory receptors. According to Lemon and Brodal (Lemon 2008; Brodal 2010), these projections are probably involved in the regulation of afferent information from peripheral receptors to the spinal cord, and influence signal transmission from afferent somatosensory terminals in the muscle spindles, GTOs, and certain skin receptors transmitting pressure and touch. Through presynaptic inhibition, the corticospinal system may modulate or even inhibit excitatory impulses transmitted from peripheral receptors that otherwise would influence the CNS (Lemon 2008). In this way, the corticospinal system functions as a gate: it grades or filters incoming information, allows relevant and useful information to get through, and inhibits disturbing or unnecessary information. The CST contextualizes afferent information and is thereby able to preset (predict) the expected level of sensory information; this function is called *setting anticipatory contrast.*

In addition to the foregoing connections, fibers also descend from the cerebral cortex to innervate the cranial nerve nuclei and the red nucleus (Brodal 2010); the cortico-rubro-spinal pathway originates in the red nucleus in the midbrain. The cortical connections to the cranial nerves are referred to as the *corticobulbar tract.*

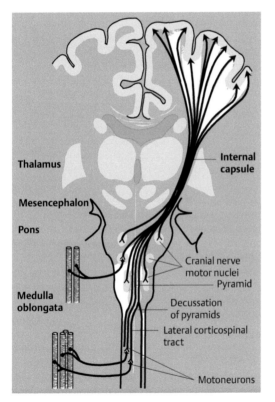

Thalamus

Internal capsule

Mesencephalon

Pons

Cranial nerve motor nuclei

Pyramid

Medulla oblongata

Decussation of pyramids

Lateral corticospinal tract

Motoneurons

Fig. 1.12 The fibers in the corticospinal tract originate from several areas in the cortex. The tract descends through the internal capsule, the pons and the medulla. In the lower part of the medulla most of its fibers cross over to the opposite side and continue downward to connect to spinal motor neurons. Some fibers leave the tract in the brain stem to make synaptic connection to motor neurons here, forming the corticobulbar tract. The corticospinal tract (CST) is mainly a crossed pathway, however a significant number of projections influence the ipsilateral spinal gray matter in the cervical and in the lumbosacral enlargement. These projections are significant for understanding the effect of cortical or spinal lesions.

Functions of the CST

The CST contributes considerably to the control of motor skilled movements (Lemon 2008). However, Lemon (2010) states the following: "It is probable that most corticospinal fibers terminate on spinal interneurons, providing the corticospinal tract with a range of functions, including the filtering afferent input, modulation of activity in central pattern generators and of reflex excitability." These are all functions united by a common feature: cortical modulation of spinal cord activity.

Corticospinal functions include the following:
- *Excitation and inhibition of motor neurons* (Porter & Lemon 1995; Lemon 2008).
    - The corticospinal system supplies mainly the distal musculature, partly monosynaptically and fast, partly via interneurons. It has an important role in the control and fractionation of movement. The cortex is therefore involved in voluntary movement (the least automatic), such as movement of the hand and individual fingers, as well the toes.
    - The corticospinal system also innervates the proximal, axial, abdominal, and thoracic musculature. Muscles involved in facial expression, eating, speech, and movements of the mouth are supplied through the same system.
- *Descending control of afferent inputs, including nociceptive inputs* (Wall & Lidierth 1997; Lemon & Griffiths 2005; Lemon 2008).
- *Selection, gating, and gain control of spinal reflexes* (Lemon & Griffiths 2005).
- *Long-term plasticity of spinal cord circuits* (Wolpaw 1997).

> The corticospinal system mainly supplies the distal musculature.
> Distal motor control (i.e., dexterity of finger movements and movements of the toes) is an example of voluntary (least automatic) activity.
> The corticospinal tract has several functions, including control of voluntary movement, gating sensory input, control of spinal reflex loops, and preparing the spinal cord for movements. It is assumed that the pyramidal fibers arising in the SI are as important for the signaling of impulses in sensory pathways as for the initiation of motor activity.

Clinical Relevance

Modern concepts view the CNS as working in distributed motor networks; this gives an understanding that movement alterations resulting from a lesion are a consequence of compensatory activity in the motor network as a whole, not solely due to the loss/reduction of signals through the affected area. However, studies on recovery of selective finger movements after subcortical stroke have shown the integrity of the CST to be of great importance (Lang & Schieber 2004; Ward 2011). Individual finger movements (and selective movements of the foot) require selective activation of particular sets of muscles. Such activation is controlled primarily by the motor cortex via the CST (Schieber et al 2009). Thus lesions of the CST cause a breakdown in fine sensorimotor control of the foot and hand causing deterioration not only in motor function but also in the ability to correctly interpret and explore sensory feedback from the hand (Lemon & Griffiths 2005). In healthy humans the CNS is able to decide and choose what information it needs in different situations by controlling sensory signal transmission; *setting anticipatory contrast*, for example, how hot it is supposed to feel when reaching for a mug with hot coffee, or how cold it is supposed to feel when reaching for a bag of frozen vegetables in the freezer. Loss or reduction of this function will lead to huge deficits in hand function.

Lesions to the cortex and/or internal capsule may affect all the descending pathways. The cortex provides a major input to the cells of origin of the brain stem pathways; thus these lesions affect not only the corticospinal and corticobulbar projections but also the corticostriatal, corticopontine, and other systems related to motor function.

Furthermore, there is an increasing body of evidence indicating that the functional consequences of a unilateral damage to the cortical motor areas are not only contralateral but also ipsilateral in the body (Suzuki et al 2011; Janowska & Edgley 2006; Mani et al 2013). The literature reports that about two-thirds of patients with stroke will have permanent problems with contralesional hand function. Some studies have suggested that contralesional deficits differ depending on which hemisphere is lesioned; for example, a study by Mani and colleagues (2013) indicated a role for the left hemisphere in intersegmental coordination and movement trajectory for both arms. However, Robertson and colleagues (2012) found bilateral reduction in postural control of the upper limbs, including the scapulae. Thus it is of great therapeutic importance to assess the whole body of the neurological patient.

■ **The Basal Ganglia**

Traditionally, the BG have been considered first and foremost to participate in motor control. However, the past 20 years have given us more knowledge of BG function, and, consequently, more functions are attributed to the BG (Haber & Calzavara 2009).

The BG are a collection of several interconnected nuclei: *the caudate nucleus, putamen, globus pallidus, subthalamic nucleus,* and *substantia nigra (SNr).* The caudate and putamen together are collectively known as the striatum (**Fig. 1.13**). The BG nuclei constitute one functional unit, also referred to as basal nuclei, and play a very important role in motor function.

The BG are interconnected with all lobes of the cortex and subcortical structures and are organized in several anatomically and functionally different networks. Cortical loops provide the BG with massive information that is processed before "replies" are sent back to the cortex. Different parts of the BG assist different areas of the cortex in specialized tasks. Four circuits are well established that originate from different parts of the CNS: the sensorimotor area, association areas, the limbic cortex, and the oculomotor cortical area (see **Fig. 1.14**). In addition to the cortical BG loops, two newly identified pathways provide a direct route for cerebellar activity to influence and be influenced by BG activity: a disynaptic projection from the cerebellum to the BG and a reciprocal projection from the BG to the cerebellum (Bostan et al 2010). The latter pathway provides the possibility for both normal and abnormal signals from the BG to influence cerebellar function (Bostan et al 2010).

Afferent Connections to the BG

* The striatum is the main receiving nucleus. The connections come from almost all parts of the cortex, the thalamus, and nuclei in the mesencephalon; the integration of information within

		Called the lentiform nucleus	
Caudate nucleus	**Putamen**	**Globus pallidus (pallidum)**	
Called the (neo-)striatum			
Called the corpus striatum			

Fig. 1.13 An overview of the different nuclei, both individually and grouped together.

the striatum determines the final output to other BG structures (Kishore et al 2014).

Efferent Connections from the BG

There are two main projections from the striatum: one to the substantia nigra reticulata (SNr) and one to the the globus pallidus (GPe).

Output from the dorsal striatum is organized into two primary projection pathways acting in antagonistic ways to control different functions. The coordinated activity of these two output streams is thought to be critical for learning and performing proper action sequences.

The pathway from the striatum to the thalamus is a *direct pathway that facilitates* movement (**Fig. 1.15**). Activation of this pathway removes inhibition of the thalamus, thus allowing activation of the cortical areas receiving thalamic input (Kandel et al 2013). This suggests that the BG serves as a "green light" that "allows" movement to happen, facilitating the change from one movement to another (Brodal 2010). This connection may be disrupted through a stroke affecting the internal capsule, explaining why some stroke patients can have parkinsonian symptoms.

The indirect pathway connects the striatum to the globus pallidus/substantia nigra/subthalamic nucleus (STN). Activation of *the indirect pathway* to the subthalamus *inhibits movement* (Kandel et al 2013), and thus prevents unnecessary movements (Takakusaki et al 2010).

In addition, the SNr has direct connection to the superior colliculus. The role of this connection is to aid in the control of coordinated head and eye movements (Brodal 2010).

In addition to the extensive connections from the BG to the thalamus, there are also BG connections to the reticular formation (BG–brain stem system). Important structures involved in the control of posture and locomotion and muscle tone are located in the brain stem (Takakusaki et al 2010), such as the pedunculopontine nucleus (PPN) and midbrain locomotor region (MLR). The BG connect with and probably control the MLR for locomotion and the connection with the PPN for muscle tone. Thus the BG can influence the regulation of muscle tone and posture–gait synergy (Takakusaki et al 2010; Brodal 2010).

Functions of the BG

The functions of the BG are not fully understood; however, they have been implicated in functions

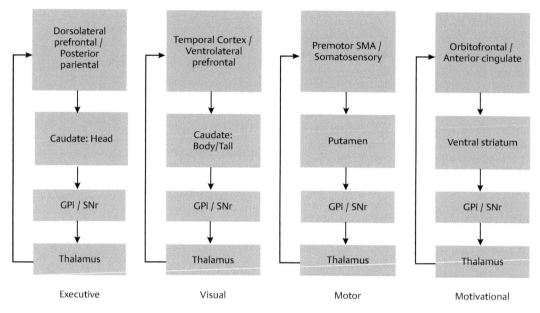

Fig. 1.14 Diagrammatic representation of four corticostriatal loops. Each loop connects cortical areas (top box) with striatal areas (second from top) and the output structures of the basal ganglia (bottom two boxes). For simplicity, only primary cortical projection sources are listed for each loop. SMA, supplementary motor area; GPi, globus pallidus, internal part; SNr, substantia nigra pars reticulata. (Reproduced with permission from Sage Publishers in Seger 2006, p. 286.)

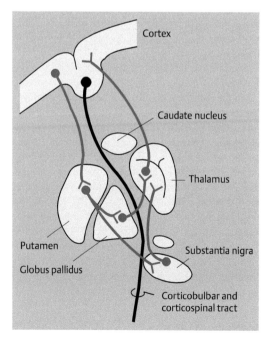

Fig. 1.15 A simple schematic model of the direct and indirect pathways.

as diverse as movement, learning, and motivation. The cortico-BG loops contribute in the control of movements that require volition, cognition, and attention (Takakusaki et al 2010; Wichmann & DeLong 2006). Basically, the BG integrates and processes massive information from all its connections. The adjusted information is conveyed to the thalamus (acting as a relay station, the thalamus also works closely with the cerebellum), and, after further modifications, the output is relayed to different specific areas in the cerebral cortex (**Fig. 1.16**).

The BG probably act as an intermediary between the cerebral cortex and brain stem for automating the selection and execution of context-specific postural responses (Grillner 2006; Grillner et al 2008; Takakusaki et al 2004), and is assumed to initiate locomotion as well as having a role in the control of posture (Takakusaki et al 2004; Jacobs & Horak 2007).

There is growing evidence that the BG connections to the brain stem can regulate muscle tone and posture–gait synergies by aiding in optimizing muscle tone for the ongoing gait or balance task (Takakusaki et al 2004; Takakusaki et al 2008).

The BG contribute not only to motor functions but also to higher-order aspects of behavior, linking emotion, reward, and executive functions (Kandel et al 2013). Disturbances in cognitive and psychological processes have been observed in patients with degenerative disorders that involve primarily the BG, such as PD. In addition to the functions described in the previous text, recent research has shown that the BG has a role in various aspects of learning (Brodal 2010; Seger 2006).

Clinical Relevance
Lesions to the BG produce three distinct types of motor disturbances: tremor and involuntary movements; changes in postural and muscle tone; and poverty and slowness of movement without paralysis.

Lesions do not cause paresis or paralysis, but they affect motor performance, such as by speed reduction.

BG disorders are manifested by an inability to initiate voluntary movements (akinesia) and to suppress involuntary movements; an abnormality in the velocity and amount of movement (bradykinesia); and abnormal muscle tone (rigidity) (de Lau & Breteler 2006).

Perhaps the best-known example of a lesion in the BG is PD, a disorder caused by degeneration of dopaminergic cells in the SNr (Wichmann & DeLong 2006). This is thought to result in hyperactivity of the indirect and underactivity of the direct BG pathways with increased inhibition of the thalamus, consequently reducing motor cortex activity (Kern & Kumar 2007). A major impediment of PD

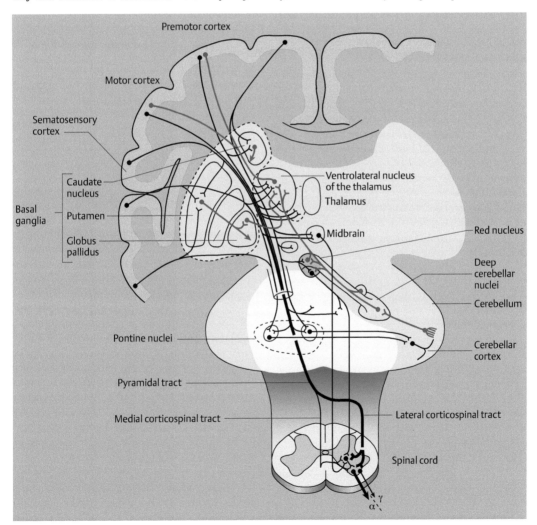

Fig. 1.16 Voluntary movement and the basal ganglia. (Redrawn with permission from Kandel et al, p. 347.)

is postural instability (Takakusaki et al 2008); people with PD often have difficulties modifying the magnitude and patterns of postural responses for changes in postural demand (Jacobs 2014). Damage to the BG affects primarily the timing and the magnitude of the APAs. (for more details see Chapter 2). Consequently, patients with PD frequently experience falling; up to 70% of patients fall at least once a year (Bloem et al 2004).

The BG seems to have an important role in the control of learned repetitive sequences of movement (Kandel et al 2013). During human movement, like walking, the automatic control exerted by the BG leaves attentional resources available for the performance of other simultaneous tasks. The consequence of loss of automatic movements is reduced balance; both anticipatory postural control and the ability to step and to produce protective arm reactions (Rothwell & Lennon 1994). Persons with PD have been shown to compensate for loss of more automatic motor skills by relying on other cortically controlled mechanisms. The added demand on attention, like thinking about how to walk, places further pressure on limited attentional resources in people with PD and may account for the difficulties in dual tasking. The use of cortical mechanisms to compensate for more automatic behavior may also be one reason for the reduction in speed that patients with PD experience. Furthermore the extensive communication with different areas of the cortex and the probability of its involvement in motor planning (Brodal 2010) may lead to other problems in motor performance. Compared with patients who have lesions to other parts of the CNS, patients with parkinsonian features may need treatment aimed at more cognitive strategies like external cueing with, for example, auditory impulses. PD patients can improve their motor performance (including balance and gait) by using external cues or by focusing attention on the task at hand (e.g., for bike riding), allowing the frontal cortex to compensate for the defective BG circuitry. However, these cognitive motor strategies could make PD patients vulnerable during performance of secondary tasks that distract their attention and render the patients more susceptible to falling.

Lesions to the BG may lead to increased muscle tone (rigidity) and may affect locomotion through their connections with the reticular formation in the brain stem (Visser & Bloem 2005).

The BG play an important part in integrating and weighting afferent sensory information from the visual system, the proprioceptive system, and the vestibular system. A lesion in the BG may cause an abnormal processing of sensory information (Visser & Bloem 2005). Jobst et al (1997) hypothesize that patients with PD experience movement problems due to decreased proprioceptive input. They refer to animal studies demonstrating that the putamen responds to somatosensory stimuli and to passive movement, especially rotational movements. Rotation gives more proprioceptive feedback than, for instance, palpation of muscle or tendon tapping. The authors suggest that the BG possibly influence movement by modulating sensory information or functions as a "sensory gate," and state that the sensory aspects of kinesia are defective in patients with PD because all the patients in this study had problems only when having to rely on their proprioceptive/kinesthetic sense alone. They say that the role of the BG is probably sensory modulation and integration of sensory input to motor tasks. Lesions to the BG would thereby lead to deficiency in the individual's ability to perform the following:

- Judge the position of the extremities in space, especially during movement.
- Control sequence and timing due to reduced or defective feedback from the movements of the extremities.

Jobst et al (1997) suggest that physiotherapy should focus on improving the patient's kinesthetic sense as well as other interventions oriented toward the improvement of the patient's motor function.

Dystonia is a condition characterized by repeated muscular contractions that cause uncontrolled, slow, writhing, repetitive movements as in *Huntington's chorea*, or abnormal stereotyped positions, such as cervical dystonia or *spastic torticollis*. Dystonic movements are triggered by voluntary movements, and also by mental and emotional stress. Most of the pathological conditions that give rise to dystonia are related to the BG–thalamocortical network (Brodal 2010). Dystonia is often classified according to whether it is primary or secondary to other neurological conditions, injuries, abnormalities, or drugs; whether it is of childhood or adult onset; and what body part(s) are affected (Jimenez-Shahed 2012).

One cause of dystonia may be *repetitive strain injury*. Movements that are performed repetitively may cause changes in the structure and function of the CNS (form–function). If a person pursues a profession or hobby requiring intensely repetitive movements of the hand (e.g., secretary or musician), an *occupational hand cramp* may develop (Blood 2013; Brodal 2010; Kaji et al 2005), which is a type of focal dystonia of the hand. Dystonia may also develop secondary to a stroke or head injury. Approximately half of the generalized dystonias are assumed to be secondary. For the focal dystonias, it is possible to diagnose a cause in only ~10% of those affected (Gjerstad et al 1991). If the disorder starts in childhood, it may be possible to find a cause in 40%; if it develops during youth, in 30%; and if it develops in adulthood, in 13% (Marsden & Quinn 1990; Borgmann 1997).

The Cerebellum

Introduction to Cerebellar Anatomy, Physiology, and Function

The cerebellum overlies the pons and the medulla and is relatively small in size, ~10 to 14% of the total brain size; at the same time it is a highly complex structure containing more neurons alone than the entire rest of the brain (Brodal 2010; Kandel et al 2013). The cerebellum is a major motor structure of the nervous system (Mottolese et al 2013) and can be considered as the area of the brain for behavioral refinement because it regulates the rate, rhythm, and force of behavior to coordinate and refine movement quality (Koziol et al 2010). The cerebellum is also linked to sensory processing, and recent research has unveiled that the cerebellum is also activated by a large number of cognitive tasks that do not involve movement (Koziol et al 2014).

The cerebellum receives 40 times more input than it sends out, and therefore has an important coordinating role in motor function. It receives information from virtually every sensory modality, including vision and proprioception. In addition, the cerebellum has high output to other parts of the brain; thus it is important for information processing and planning of sensorimotor activities (Manto et al 2012).

The Anatomical Organization of the Cerebellum

The cerebellum is composed of two main divisions, the *cerebellar cortex* and the *cerebellar nuclei* (**Fig. 1.17**).

Similar to the cerebral cortex, the cerebellum is covered by a layer of gray substance called the *cerebellar cortex*, which consists of five types of neurons organized into three layers:

1. The deepest layer, the *granular layer*, is the input layer with ~100 billion granule cells and a few Golgi cells. The axons of the granule cells are often called *parallel fibers* due to their long **T**-shape parallel to the surface of the cerebellar cortex. The parallel fibers are the only excitatory fibers within the cerebellar cortex.

2. The middle layer consists of Purkinje cells, which are specialized inhibitory neurons and the only cells that send their axons out of the cerebellar cortex. The middle layer is therefore also called the *output layer*. In humans, the number of Purkinje cells has been estimated to be ~15 million (Manto 2009).

3. The uppermost layer is a molecular layer containing cell bodies of the *inhibitory interneurons: the stellate* and *basket cells* as well as *dendrites of the Purkinje cells*, and has an important processing function.

The parallel fiber axons project to the middle layer and link many Purkinje cells together and are thought to tie together the activity of different cerebellar areas (Kandel et al 2013).

Each Purkinje cell receives ~80,000 to 200,000 synapses from an equal amount of parallel fibers (granule cells), and 150 to 200 synapses from *one* climbing fiber (climbing fibers are neuronal projections from the inferior olive, described in more details later) (Rothwell & Lennon 1994). Purkinje cells receive more synaptic input than any other type of cell in the brain. Thus enormous amounts of information converge and are modulated and integrated before the Purkinje cells transmit the "result" to the deep cerebellar neurons (relay stations in output/efferent connections of the cerebellar cortex).

The Output from the Cerebellum: The Cerebellar Nuclei

There are four nuclei on each side of the cerebellum and situated in the deep white matter: the fastigial nucleus, the dentate nucleus, and the globose and emboliform nuclei (called the anterior and posterior interposed nuclei in animals). These nuclei represent the sole output from cer-

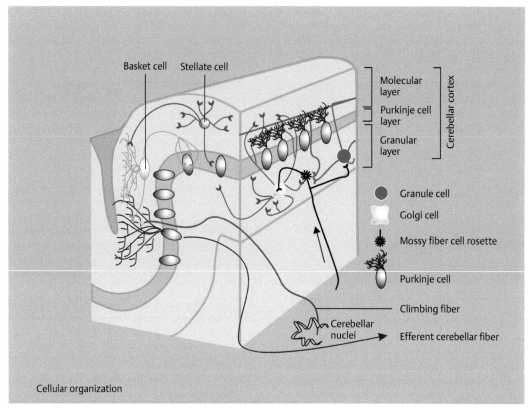

Basket cell   Stellate cell

Molecular
layer

Purkinje cell
layer

Granular
layer

Cerebellar cortex

● Granule cell

Golgi cell

✳ Mossy fiber cell rosette

Purkinje cell

Climbing fiber

Cerebellar
nuclei

→ Efferent cerebellar fiber

Cellular organization

Fig. 1.17 The anatomical organization of the cerebellum.

ebellar circuits, conveying signals, in particular to brain stem nuclei, thalamic nuclei, motor cortex, premotor cortex, and prefrontal association cortex (Manto 2009).

The *fastigial nucleus* is important for posture, automatic movements, and locomotion. The *dentate nucleus* is involved in voluntary (least automatic) movement, as well as locomotion and initiation and termination of movement. The *globose* and *emboliform* nuclei compare the central motor command with the actual movement. Connections from the cerebellar nuclei to the cerebral cortex are by way of the thalamus via the *cerebello-thalamo-cortical tracts* (**Fig. 1.18**). The majority of the cerebellar output is to ventral areas of the thalamus that project to the motor cortex. There is also a smaller projection to a region in the mediodorsal nucleus of the thalamus, which projects onto the prefrontal cortex. The dentate, globus and emboliform nuclei all project to the contralateral red nucleus. The motor cortex and the red nucleus are

crossed structures, hence this leads to an ipsilateral relationship between the cerebellum and limb movement.

■ The Input Pathways to the Cerebellar Cortex

The cerebellum receives extensive projections carrying cutaneo-kinesthetic information directly from the limbs via the spinocerebellar tracts and from the face and head via the trigemino-cerebellar tracts, in addition to information indirectly via the spino-olivary tracts (Stoodley & Schmahmann 2010) (Fig. **1.19**) There are two primary sources of input to the cerebellum: through the mossy fiber system and from the climbing fibers from the inferior olive. Both connect with cerebellar neurons but terminate in different layers of the cerebellar cortex, and probably mediate different functions (Kandel et al 2013).

Mossy fibers originate in the spinal cord and from a wide range of nuclei in the brain stem (the

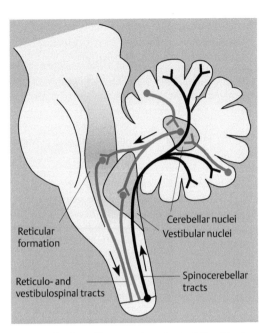

Fig. 1.18 The figure illustrates the output relationships from the fastigial nuclei of cerebellum with the vestibular nuclei and the reticular nuclei to the spinal cord. Outputs of the fastigial nuclei of the cerebellum to the reticular formation and vestibular nuclei are shown in grey. The figure also illustrates inputs to the cerebellum from the spinocerebellar tracts which are shown in black.

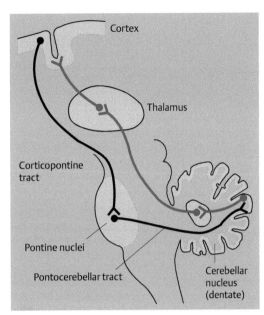

Fig. 1.19 The basic view of cerebrocerebellar interconnections. The cerebellum receives information from widespread cortical areas, including portions of the frontal, parietal, temporal, and occipital lobes. Efferents from the cerebellar nuclei project to multiple subdivisions of the thalamus, which, in turn, project to several cortical areas, including premotor, prefrontal, and posterior parietal areas of the cerebral cortex.

pontine, vestibular, trigeminal, and dorsal column nuclei) via the pons. From the pons, the fibers project to specific areas of the cerebellar cortex through the mossy fibers and from there to the deep cerebellar nuclei, in particular the dentate nucleus (Rondi-Reiget al 2014).

The climbing fibers originate in the inferior olive, a nucleus in the ventral part of the brain stem, and convey input from the spinal cord and nuclei in the mesencephalon. The information carried is somatosensory, visual, and cerebral cortical (Kandel et al 2013). The climbing fibers synapse with the Purkinje cells by twisting around the Purkinje cells and thereby forming many synapses with each cell. Each Purkinje cell receives input from only one climbing fiber, and each climbing fiber may contact between 1 and 10 Purkinje cells. The climbing fibers probably have a very unique role in informing about errors of movement (Kandel et al 2013) (for more details see The Role of the Cerebellum in Motor Learning).

■ Anatomical and Functional Connections between the Cerebellum and BG

The cerebellum and BG influence several aspects of behavior and make multiple synaptic loops with the cerebral cortex. Recent work from Bostan and Strick (2010) has shown that the BG and the cerebellum are interlinked. The pathway from the cerebellum to the BG originates in the dentate nucleus, goes via the thalamus, and connects to the striatum (the input part of the BG). The pathway from the BG to the cerebellum starts from the subthalamic nucleus and ends in the cerebellar cortex, passing through the pontine nuclei (Bostan & Strick 2010). The output of both the cerebellum and the BG can thus affect a larger area of the cortex than previously thought. One theory is that the BG may directly affect the function of the cerebellum and vice versa, which may have important implications for both motor and cognitive function; the direct connections between these two structures may cause abnormal activity at one structure to spread to the other.

Anatomical and Functional Connections between the Inferior Olive and the Cerebellum

The inferior olive is a nucleus within the brain stem medulla oblongata. It has three different sources of input:

- A connection linking the cerebral cortex, red nucleus, inferior olive, and cerebellar cortex together.
- A system that originates in the thalamus projects to the inferior olive and back to the cerebellum through climbing fiber inputs.
- The olivocerebellar pathway, which projects from the deep cerebellar nuclei to the olivary nucleus and then through the climbing fiber system to the cerebellar cortex.

The inferior olive provides all the climbing fibers to the Purkinje cells in the cerebellar cortex; hence it has a strong influence on cerebellar output. As a consequence, the processing of signals by the inferior olive is critical for cerebellar function.

As already mentioned, the inferior olive also receives projections from the cerebral cortex via the red nucleus. It has been suggested that these projections convey information from the cerebral cortex to the cerebellum modulating an ongoing process (Ausim Azizi 2007). Learning successful execution of new behaviors is dependent on correction of behavior from trial to trial. The inferior olive is thought to tune the cerebellar output such that the movements become more accurate with practice or are better adapted to new environmental conditions.

The Role of the Cerebellum in Different Functions

The cerebellum plays important roles in both motor and nonmotor functions (Koziol et al 2014). The following topics are covered in this section:

- The cerebellum and the control of accuracy and coordination in balance and voluntary movements.
  - Cerebellum and balance.
  - Cerebellum and locomotion.
  - Cerebellum and control of grip forces.
  - Cerebellum and movement timing.
  - Cerebellum and the control of single-joint and multijoint movements.
  - Cerebellum and sensorimotor synchronization.
- The role of the cerebellum in motor learning.
- Control of corticomotor excitability.

The Cerebellum and the Control of Accuracy and Coordination in Balance and Voluntary Movements

After the cerebellum has received, analyzed, and recognized a sensory or motor pattern, the predicted and actual movement patterns are compared and followed by appropriate corrections for the movement to be performed coordinated and without more effort than appropriate. To do this, the cerebellum presumably cooperates with the parietal cortex where information about the state of the body (body schema) and information about the spatial environment are stored (Frey et al 2011).

Cerebellum and Balance

The role of the cerebellum in balance control is due to the connections between the cerebellum, the brain stem reticular formation, and the vestibular system, which are the sources of the medial descending system providing the control of posture and balance. In addition, connections between the cerebellum and the cortex are also important for this task.

The cerebellum plays an important role in the control of posture by combining the appropriate anticipatory activity across several muscles and in response to changing demands, regulating muscle activity based on practice and knowledge of results.

The control of posture requires the ability to respond to external perturbations and to control posture during internally triggered voluntary movement, such as forces generated by voluntary movement and breathing. An individual prepares for upcoming and predictable perturbations even before they occur by use of APAs (for more details see Chapter 2). The ability to anticipate the effects of limb movements on postural control relies on knowing the static and dynamic properties of the limb (i.e., the body schema) (see The Role of the Cerebellum in Motor Learning). Signals from cortical motor areas during the period of motor preparation have been hypothesized to provide the cerebellum with information about upcoming movements essential for APA generation (Coffman et al 2011). Results from studies suggest that the cerebellar-cortical loop is responsible for adapting postural responses, appropriate scaling magnitude, and tuning the coordination of these responses based on prior experience (Thach & Bastian 2004).

The cerebellum may be involved in the cortico–brain stem circuit responsible for adapting postural responses with changes in the central set (Jacobs & Horak 2007). *A central set* is defined as a "neural state of readiness to receive a stimulus and generate a movement based on existing contextual factors, such as the predictability of impending postural perturbation characteristics" (Horak et al 1989). The magnitude of postural responses is based not only on sensory drive from the perturbation but also on this central set. The cortex can influence the central set for postural responses via two main loops: one including the cerebellum and one including the BG. The cerebellar–cortical loop is probably responsible for adapting postural responses based on prior experience, whereas the cortical–BG loop may be responsible for preselecting and optimizing postural responses based on the current context (de Lima-Pardini et al 2012).

Several studies have demonstrated that patients with cerebellar dysfunction show greater impairments in anticipatory balance control as compared with reactive balance control (Morton & Bastian 2004; Morton & Bastian 2006). Morton & Bastian (2006) demonstrated that cerebellar damage impairs the ability to adapt to predictable, but not sudden unpredictable, changes using split-belt treadmill walking. This does, however, not implicate that reactive balance reactions are normal. This is due to the fact that there is a relationship between proactive and reactive balance strategies where effective predictive balance (APAs) will reduce the need for large reactive balance strategies resulting in better balance control (Santos et al 2010). Thus poor predictive ability will immediately take a movement off course, and peripheral feedback processes would be scaled by the continuous need to guide the movement back to the intended goal.

Some authors claim that dystonia can be an expression of abnormal postural control mechanisms (Blood 2008). Although dystonias have been seen as dysfunction of the BG, there is increasing evidence that the cortical motor areas and the vermis of the cerebellum contribute to the source and maintenance of some forms of this disorder (Coffman et al 2011).

Cerebellum and Locomotion

The control of locomotion is complex and involves a network of areas. In addition to the CPGs in the spinal cord various subcortical and cortical control areas contribute. In this network, the cerebellum is regarded as crucial for avoiding obstacles and adapting walking to novel conditions (Takakusaki 2013).

However, the cerebellum may influence locomotion in several ways:
- Indirectly via vestibulospinal, rubrospinal, reticulospinal, and corticospinal pathways.
- By influencing extensor tone to maintain upright balance and stance on one leg.
- By intra- and interlimb coordination patterns required during locomotion.
- By exerting modulatory control over the rhythmic flexor and extensor muscle activations of the vestibular and reticular nuclei that generate parts of the locomotor pattern.

The cerebellum receives efferent copies of CPG output to motor neurons via ventral spinocerebellar and spinoreticulocerebellar pathways, as well as information about the activity of the peripheral motor apparatus via the dorsal spinocerebellar tract. This sensory feedback is used to provide adaptability to the locomotor pattern with regard to the control of timing, step length, tone, and coordination and "finetuning" of the output by adapting each step cycle to the environmental demands. In addition, the cerebellum contributes to gaze stability during head movements during walking by modulating the vestibulo-ocular reflex.

Cerebellum and Control of Grip Forces

When handling objects with the hands, the ability to control the grip forces is an essential part of this skill. When grasping and lifting an object, the rate of grip force generation and the balance between the grip and load forces are calculated by the CNS to meet the requirements of the object: such as weight, texture, or shape. Because the cerebellum has an important role in anticipatory tuning of muscle activity during voluntary motor actions, it appears to be important for predictive grip force modulation (Manto et al 2012). This fact has been supported by studies demonstrating that subjects with cerebellar disorders show impairments of predictive grip force control, whereas reactive control mechanisms are by comparison unimpaired (Manto et al 2012).

Normally, during self-produced manipulation of objects, grip–load force coupling occurs entirely automatically; we are not aware of constantly changing the force of our grip. This suggests that the prediction made by the cerebellum is a rapid process that occurs continuously during the activity and may be unavailable to conscious awareness.

The Cerebellum and Movement Timing

Many daily skills, such as walking, talking, and driving, require precise timing. When planning a complex motor action, the CNS executes an accurate integration of temporal and spatial information; thus timing is an essential part of movement control (Bastian 2011). Neurological disorders that interfere with motor timing lead to dysmetric or inaccurate movements (Bares et al 2011). According to Manto (2009), the cerebellum acts together with the BG and frontal cortex in the processing of timing function; the cerebellum is probably operating as an internal timing system delivering a precise temporal representation for both motor and nonmotor tasks (Ivry 2000; Ivry & Spencer 2004).

Motor coordination can be interpreted as the correct timing of muscle activity. Movements are normally generated through contraction of agonist muscles to move the limb toward a target, and contractions of the antagonist muscles control, decelerate, and eventually stop the movement. If, for example, the antagonist muscle is not working efficiently, then overshooting the target or tremor oscillations can occur.

Dysfunction in Cerebellar Timing Function

Lesions of the cerebellum can produce impairments in tasks where movements are time-locked to specific events (e.g., eye blink conditioning), where a response to an unconditioned stimulus is learned (Manto et al 2012).

Ataxia is both a neurological symptom that is manifested as uncoordinated movements of different parts of the body as well as a disorder as it refers to a family of neurological diseases. The ataxias are regarded as a heterogeneous group of diseases in which cerebellar dysfunction typically underlies the major neurological manifestations. Both environmental and hereditary factors can cause ataxia. *Ataxia* is a general term and may be manifested in different clinical signs, depending on the extent and areas involved. Ataxia may present itself as dysarthric speech, unstable gait and posture, and dysmetric limb movements. These impairments, seen in both timing and coordination, are often due to inadequate control of the interplay between agonist and antagonist muscles. Ataxic patients do not have the ability to specifically control the

timing critical for rapid movement productions and the coordination of multijoint movements. Clinically, it is important that ataxia be distinguished from weakness and loss of fractionated movement.

Cerebellum and the Control of Single-Joint and Multijoint Movements

Research findings indicate that cerebellar damage has a greater impact on multijoint than single-joint movements (Manto & Haines 2012). For movement to be efficient and functional, complex synergies of muscle recruitment across different joints are required which is biomechanically more complicated than single-joint movements. For example, when reaching for an object, shoulder movements will influence muscle activity around the elbow. This is referred to as *interaction torques in adjacent joints*. The cerebellum will normally integrate information from different sensory modalities to anticipate and adjust for the interaction torques to generate an optimal movement. This predictive ability is especially important in fast movements because the torque get bigger with movement speed and acceleration. Signs of ataxia in the upper limb are seen as dysmetria and intention tremor at the end of reaching or pointing movements, and become exacerbated during high-speed multijoint motion due to the inability of patients with cerebellar lesions to correctly predict the magnitude of the interaction torques (Bastian et al 1996). However, this impairment may also be seen as an impairment of APAs in proximal muscles leading to greater problems in multijoint movements than single-joint movements (Bruttini et al 2014).

Cerebellum and Sensorimotor Synchronization

A central issue in motor control theories is to find out how sensory information is used in the control of motor timing. Sensorimotor synchronization is the rhythmic synchronization between a timed sensory stimulus and a motor response (Molinari et al 2008). Synchronizing movements with events in the surrounding environment (i.e., the ability to recognize the next movement in a sequence and predicting what comes next) is an important aspect of human behavior and forms the basis of human adaptation to environmental change. The role of the cerebellum would seem to be involvement in the acquisition of the optimal internal model for sequencing movements for an optimal performance in a particular context. When learning a new motor activity, we must carry out the correct sequences of movements and at the same time optimize sensorimotor parameters, such as muscle force, velocity of movement trajectory, and movement timing. Research has shown that patients with cerebellar damage show impairment in the ability to detect sequences; patients with damage to the cerebellar hemispheres were unable to sequence pictures or words in the correct order (Manto & Haines 2012).

The Role of the Cerebellum in Motor Learning

Whereas the BG, via their many connections with the cerebral cortex, make decisions about *when* to act by allowing the thalamus to release the brake for behavior, the cerebellum teaches the brain *how* to act. It has long been known that the cerebellum plays important roles in the acquisition of motor skills (Koziol et al 2014). Classical knowledge of motor learning is based on the main role of feedback (afferent) control for error corrections. It is suggested that, during motor learning, the brain uses feedback error control to form *neural internal models* of the motor apparatus and the environment for planning and executing movements. An internal model is a stored model of the requirements for any specific activity, such as standing up from sitting, walking down stairs, or reaching, and includes all of the sensory and motor information required for performance of the specific activity (Brodal 2010). Currently, motor control theories suggest that internal models generate motor commands that are sent to the periphery to produce the desired movement, and that the internal models combine sensory inputs, prior knowledge, and volitional intention to produce motor commands (Genewein & Braun 2012). The motor system uses two types of internal models: the inverse model and the forward model (Imamizu & Kawato 2012). The forward model predicts the sensory consequences of the action based on the commands for action and information about the present state of the body. The inverse model is concerned with transforming a desired goal into a set of motor commands. Both of these models involve the body schema. The inverse model is responsible with regard to motor commands needed to achieve the desired goal based on current body status. The body schema feeds the inverse model with information such as the size of the limbs, joint angles, and the position of the hands or feet. At the same time, the motor system anticipates the sensorimotor consequences of the movement through the forward model. The anticipation of how body parts

will change through movement provides us with a predicted body schema allowing for anticipatory control of movement. As a result of movement there is a continuous flow of sensory feedback, which is used to update the body schema. Sensory feedback carries information only about the bodily parameters that have been altered (de Vignemont 2010).

It has been widely accepted that the cerebellum acquires and stores internal models (Wolpert et al 1998; Koziol et al 2014; Schlerf et al 2012). The cerebellum forms internal models that will be adjusted and refined as behavior is repeated through a learning process. Because of these internal models the motor cortex is able to perform an accurate movement using an internal feedback instead of the external feedback from actual behavior. Therefore, one can say that internal models are important for overcoming the time delays associated with sensory feedback (sensory feedback loops have delays that are too long and gains too low to control fast and coordinated movements).

Internal models may be taught via error signals originating in the inferior olive. The olive serves as an "error detection" mechanism within this process. When behavior does not fit the cerebellar model, the olive codes the error and sends a correction signal to the cerebellum through the climbing fiber system, which then modifies the internal model. The climbing fibers from the inferior olive can induce selective *long-term depression (LTD)*, which is one of two major forms of long-lasting synaptic plasticity in the mammalian brain (Kandel et al 2013). The cerebellum thus appears to be a "learning machine," and seems to be important for learning movement through trial-and-error practice. It is generally accepted that cerebellar damage leads to reduction of an error-driven motor learning process referred to as *adaptation* (Torres-Oviedo & Bastian 2012). Several studies have demonstrated that patients with cerebellar damage show impaired learning (Morton & Bastian 2006; Torres-Oviedo & Bastian 2012; Kitago & Krakauer 2013). Error reduction in learning of movement control is generally thought to occur via adaptation, and patients with cerebellar dysfunction are slow to adapt movement to novel contexts and often do not store the effect of short-term training. This has been demonstrated in visuomotor adaptation to prism glasses; adaptation to perturbations during standing; eye-blink conditioning; and adaptation to novel situations during walking (rotating treadmill, split belt treadmill). All of these examples need error-based learning and information from multiple parts of the body as well as the use of sensory inputs from one or more modality (Torres-Oviedo & Bastian 2012). Impairments of adaptation in patients with cerebellar dysfunction occur in most all types of movement (e.g., balance and walking, and movements of the arm and hand in reach and grasp). The patients are unable to maintain optimal calibrations for movement control, by which movements will be inaccurate and often frustrating (Bastian 2008). If cerebellar patients have difficulty learning movements through trial and error, then this could complicate improvement via rehabilitation training.

Learning seems to be implemented through different synaptic changes in the cerebellar cortex and deep nuclei (Kandel et al 2013). Changes in synaptic strength (synaptic plasticity) are one important mechanism of learning. The cerebellum exhibits a synaptic plasticity mechanism referred to as cerebellar LTD, which is defined as activity-dependent reduced synaptic efficiency that may last minutes to hours (Brodal 2010). This phenomenon happens in the Purkinje cell when two main excitatory inputs are activated in combination; during an inaccurate movement the climbing fibers respond to the errors and depress the synaptic strength of the parallel fibers involved in the error, resulting in a persistent decrease in the efficacy of the synapse between the parallel fiber and the Purkinje cell (Kandel et al 2013). Hence the Purkinje cells have a unique role in the control of movement and motor learning. Through their inhibitory activity they stop unwanted activity coming through. Plasticity related to motor learning is thought to be primarily due to LTD of parallel fiber–Purkinje cell synapses (Criscimagna-Hemminger et al 2010).

The cerebellum has been shown to be more active during a novel task (a different or unexpected input to the inferior olive), and shows less activity when actions are more automatic. The cerebellum would therefore seem to be important for making movement more automatic (i.e., for reducing the attentional demands on the details or specifics of a movement) (Ioffe et al 2007).

Even though several studies have shown that the cerebellum plays an important role in motor learning, other brain systems, such as the BG and the motor cortex-corticospinal system are also specifically involved in this process. However, the cerebellum seems to be one of the main structures involved in learning voluntary control of posture.

Neurorehabilitation aims for patients to gain skills through motor learning. The cerebellum learns from repeated experience. Through this learning process, an internal model is constructed. Internal models are not fixed entities, but are trained and updated by sensory experience (Nowak et al 2004); thus every time the behavior is repeated, the model will be refined. Internal models predict the posture or movements of body parts following a motor command and also predict the sensory consequences of actions, allowing the brain to perform the activity precisely, without the need to refer to direct sensory feedback from the moving body parts. However, to be accurate in all sensory predictions, the cerebellum needs continuous recalibration from the body at all times to match the changing properties of the environment and the sensorimotor system. Sensory feedback via the spinocerebellar tract plays an important role in this operation. An important clinical consideration is what happens with the cerebellar control of movement when the patient stops moving a body part (e.g., after a stroke) and the cerebellum stops getting the sensory information needed.

Apparently Einstein once said that "Insanity is doing the same thing over and over again and expecting different results." However, in neurorehabilitation, repetition of a task is necessary for training a motor skill. Task practice may work due to motor learning ensuring that repetition of the same motor task will lead to improvement of that specific action because errors are reduced and motor skill improves (i.e., refinement of the internal model). According to the error/novelty-detection function of the cerebellum, it is thought that the cerebellum is involved most when the movement or behavior is unusual and unexpected. For error feedback to be useful in predictive control, errors from past movements must be used to update subsequent movements. Hence varied repetition is essential for learning. When we stand up or sit down we do so to and from many different support bases: chairs, beds, benches, or the ground; from different heights, textures, sizes, and postural alignments (postural sets), and with goals that involve different tempos, timing, and direction. Through varied repetition we learn which components are essential to achieve the wanted activity and are therefore essential for the function. Other, irrelevant components are gradually filtered away for the sake of efficiency and ease of movement.

Clinical Relevance

A cerebellar lesion does not lead to movement loss but may instead cause movement dysfunction, such as *hypotonia, balance problems, ataxia* (meaning *loss of order*), *dysmetria* (meaning *abnormal measure,* characterized by impaired reaching, timing errors, and problems of direction and extent of movement), *terminal tremor* (irregular oscillation movements around a target), *visual problems*, and *incoordination*. These primary deficits often lead to secondary problems because the somatosensory, visual, or vestibular information is disturbed when the performance of movement is altered by pathology. The cerebellum receives misinformation, and the primary deficits may be enhanced.

Cerebellar damage can cause balance problems with sitting, standing, and walking as well as abnormal postural tone. Fear of falling affects how muscular coactivation is used as a postural strategy by, for example, inducing a stiffening strategy (Bakker et al 2006) associated with greater muscular coactivation during standing (Nagai et al 2013). Repeated falls or fear of falling causes patients to fixate different body parts to reduce ataxia and feel safer. This might result in more co-contraction of postural muscles (Asaka & Wang 2011). A rigid posture induced by strong muscle coactivation reduces flexibility and may compromise the ability to adjust to unexpected perturbations (Allum et al 2002). The Bobath Concept differentiates between fixation defined as static muscle activation strategies and dynamic stability defined as arrested mobility (Graham et al 2009), and movement based on postural stability rather than teaching fixation is encouraged (see Chapter 4).

Some patients with neurological deficits (e.g., stroke, multiple sclerosis, or head injury) seem to have reduced ability both to initiate necessary activity and to correct the movement if it is not appropriate. These patients do not seem to recruit the internal models as a basis for varied activity. There may be a spread of activity to muscles that normally would not be primarily involved, which sometimes starts even before the wanted activity. These "extra" movements may not be filtered away as the activity is practiced, but sometimes increase and get stronger in both range of motion and force production, often involving a whole limb. These unwanted and inefficient movement patterns may be established—learned—if they are practiced. If the cerebellum learns these movements as part of an activity, it would seem possible that a new internal model is established; a coarser, less refined, and less controlled form. The patient's CNS might include them as a part of the internal model in day-to-day activity. This would lead to increased stress and effort, disturb the patient's motor performance and—most importantly—negate the development of postural stability.

The cerebellum needs to receive direct and rapid information from sensory structures relevant to movement; cerebellar multisensory information processing is the mechanism that allows the state of the body that is needed for movement to be correctly established. It is therefore necessary to improve the proprioceptive awareness and contextualize the sensory input to improve motor control in patients with cerebellar dysfunction.

The Brain Stem

The brain stem is located at a lower part of the brain; it borders on the diencephalon; and, caudally, it is directly connected to the spinal cord. The brain stem consists of three parts: the midbrain (mesencephalon), the pons, and the medulla oblongata (Brodal 2010). The brain stem houses many of the centers for vital bodily functions (e.g., swallowing, breathing); nuclei that are important for sympathetic and parasympathetic autonomic functions. In addition, all of the cranial nerve nuclei except those associated with olfaction and vision, are located here. All efferent and afferent pathways travel through the brain stem, and several decussate (cross) here. Also, the reticular formation is located in the brain stem.

Having discussed both cortical and subcortical contributions to different functions, we are now going to consider the variety of ways in which motor commands from the brain stem reach the body. Descending pathways from the brain stem are mostly involved in the maintenance of posture and whole-limb movements.

The Reticular Formation

The core of the brain stem is called the *reticular formation* (**Fig. 1.20**) The word *reticular* means net-like. The reticular formation is a diffuse, but highly organized, collection of neurons with different connections and functions (Kandel et al 2013). For example, the reticular formation excites and inhibits activity, enhances flexion and extension, and regulates sleep and wakefulness (Brodal 2010). The reticular formation cooperates with most systems within the CNS and has a role in both proximal and distal movement. It activates both higher and lower levels, and it functions as an integration system.

Some neurons from the reticular formation project to motor neurons in the spinal cord and influence functions such as cardiovascular and respiratory control. Generally, the reticular formation is broadly

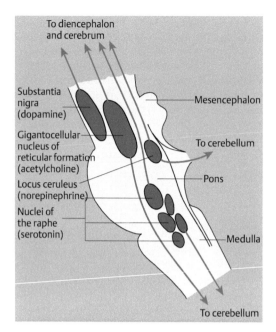

To diencephalon
and cerebrum

Substantia
nigra
(dopamine)

Mesencephalon

Gigantocellular
nucleus of
reticular formation
(acetylcholine)

To cerebellum

Locus ceruleus
(norepinephrine)

Pons

Nuclei of
the raphe
(serotonin)

Medulla

To cerebellum

Fig. 1.20 The reticular formation in the brain stem has some important specialized groups of cells.

divided into a lateral and a medial part. The *medial part* is located in the pons and medulla and is *mainly efferent*—it sends long projections to the thalamus and cortex, cerebellum, and spinal cord. The *lateral part* is smaller and receives many of the *afferent connections* to the reticular formation. Many secondary ascending fibers send off collaterals to the reticular formation, and the reticular formation therefore receives information from the:

- Most receptors, including pain and hearing.
- Cerebellum.
- Cortex.
- BG.
- Vestibular system.
- Limbic structures.

The reticular formation in the pons contains the *nucleus ceruleus*, which projects to every major region of the brain and spinal cord and maintains alertness to novel stimuli. It therefore has an important role in arousal as well as sensory perception and muscle tone. *The raphe nuclei* are located along the midline of the brain stem and project mainly to the forebrain where they help regulate sleep–wakefulness, affective behavior, temperature, and other functions. They also project to the spinal cord where they participate in the regulation of tone in motor systems and pain perception.

The sensitivity of the muscle spindle may be regulated from the reticular formation, and the cortex, cerebellum, and other higher centers via the reticular formation influence muscle tone. Psychological processes, such as motivation and happiness, may affect the reticular formation and seem to increase a person's initiative and thereby muscle tone. Depression seems to have the opposite effect and downregulates tone.

The midbrain contains neurons that are critical for the state of cortical arousal. These neurons project to the cerebral cortex, where they enhance cortical responses to incoming sensory stimuli. The ascending fibers of the reticular formation form a network—the *ascending reticular activating system* (ARAS). The ARAS is composed of several neuronal circuits connecting the brain stem to the cortex. These neuronal connections originate mainly in the reticular formation and project via the thalamus to the cerebral cortex (Yeo et al 2013). This system influences wakefulness and the overall degree of arousal and consciousness.

The upper brain stem contains neurons that control axial and proximal limb musculature for gait through their projections to the lower brain stem and spinal cord via bilateral, descending pathways. Locomotion is a rhythmic motor activity generated by neural networks in the spinal cord, referred to as CPGs (read more about CPG function under The Spinal Cord). The CPGs are initiated, modulated, and stopped by supraspinal structures. Several locomotor areas are located at various levels in the brain stem (Grabli et al 2012; Takakusaki 2013):

- The subthalamic locomotor region (SLR).
- The midbrain or mesencephalon locomotor region (MLR).
- The dorsal and ventral tegmental field of the caudal pons.

These are functionally defined areas of the brain stem within which it is possible to elicit controlled locomotion. The MLR is composed of the pedunculopontine nucleus (PPN) and cuneiform nucleus (CN). Both these structures are groups of neurons located in the reticular formation, have reciprocal connections with the BG, and have major outputs to the descending reticulospinal pathway and the ascending thalamocortical pathway. Several recent studies have shown that the MLR of the brain stem is implicated in the control of locomotion in humans and balance in mammals (Grabli et al 2013).

Because the function of BG structures is disrupted in PD, the brain stem motor areas the BG project to and control may also be dysfunctional. Gait and balance disorders are major problems in PD. In PD the PPN degenerates and probably contributes to the locomotor problems. Clinicians use knowledge about MLR function to stimulate these structures (deep brain stimulation) to alleviate locomotor symptoms of patients with PD (Ryczko & Dubuc 2013).

The *pontomedullary reticular formation* (PMRF) is a diffuse network of neurons distributed in the core of the brain stem. The PMRF is suggested to be an area of integration of various signals coming from cortical and subcortical structures whereby signals ensure that the postural responses are appropriately scaled in time and magnitude to the planned task (Yakovenko & Drew 2009). The PMRF receives signals related to *preparatory anticipatory postural adjustments* (pAPAs): postural adjustments that precede the movement; and *accompanying postural adjustments* (aAPAs): postural adjustments that accompany the movement (Yakovenko & Drew 2009), and integrate pAPAs and aAPAs into a unified descending command signal to control posture and movement.

Activity in the reticular formation is necessary for conscious perception and for a specific reaction to sensory information. The reticular formation receives input from the cortex via the *corticoreticular pathways*, which transmit information to both the excitatory and the inhibitory areas of the reticular formation and synapse in these areas before information is passed on to the spinal cord, forming the *corticoreticulospinal system* (CRS) (**Fig. 1.21**) (also called the extrapyramidal system).

Several motor pathways originate in the brainstem and project to the spinal cord. Two descending brain stem pathways (also called the *indirect pathways* due to their synaptically interrupted descent) have been identified: the *ventromedial brain stem pathways* and the *dorsolateral brain stem* (Kandel et al 2013). Functionally, these pathways effectuate the head–body–limb synergies by which locomotion and balance are promoted. In addition, these pathways are important for the necessary postural and attitudinal adjustments that allow skilled movements of the small muscles of the hands and feet to be executed as a product of CST activity (de Oliveira-Souza 2012).

The *ventromedial brainstem pathways* receive information from the cortex (corticoreticular fibers) and other subcortical areas (vestibular nuclei, BG, cerebellum) mainly for the control of posture and locomotion (Kandel et al 2013) and are as follows:

- The interstitiospinal and tectospinal tracts arising from the midbrain.
- The lateral and medial vestibulospinal tracts.
- The reticulospinal and bulbospinal projections arising from the pontine and medullary reticular formation.

The *dorsolateral brainstem pathways* consist mainly of the rubrospinal tract, which arises from the magnocellular red nucleus and descends contralaterally in the dorsolateral funiculus (Kandel et al 2013). The largest of the indirect pathways is the *reticulospinal tract (RST)* that arises in the pons and medulla (Kandel et al 2013). This pathway has two parts: the pontine and the medullary RSTs. *The pontine (or medial) RST* arises from the upper pontine reticular formation. Its principal projection is to *ipsilateral motor neurons*. According to Brodal (2010), this tract is probably more oriented toward axial musculature (neck, back, abdomen) due to its location in the spinal cord; facilitating spinal motor neurons that innervate axial musculature and extensors of the legs to maintain postural support (Brodal 2010) The medullary (or lateral) reticulospinal tract descends to the spinal cord and innervates motor neurons of extremity muscles.

There are extensive inputs to the RST from wide areas of the cerebral cortex, including the primary and all premotor areas of the cortex, in addition to other inputs from spinal afferents and the fastigial nucleus of the cerebellum. The RST is an important pathway communicating instructions for movement

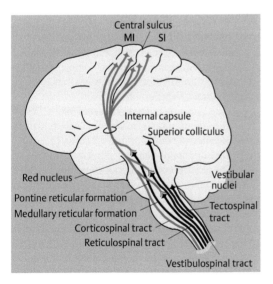

Fig. 1.21 Descending pathways to the spinal cord: the corticospinal tract and some pathways from the brain stem. Many of the pathways from the brain stem receive fibers from the cortex.

Labels in figure:
Central sulcus
MI / SI
Internal capsule
Superior colliculus
Red nucleus
Pontine reticular formation
Medullary reticular formation
Corticospinal tract
Reticulospinal tract
Vestibular nuclei
Tectospinal tract
Vestibulospinal tract

from the brain to the spinal cord. Several studies indicate that the RST is important for maintaining the upright position, for body orientation, and for reaching (Brodal 2010). Reticulospinal fibers synapse indirectly via interneurons or directly onto motor neurons (both α- and γ-motor neurons). These tracts are both crossed and uncrossed, and give off several collaterals on many levels within the spinal cord. Thus they simultaneously influence muscles in different parts of the body (Brodal 2010; Schepens & Drew 2004; Schepens & Drew 2006). In addition, reticulospinal axons also terminate on commissural interneurons; thus contralateral activity may also be mediated by this pathway (Jankowska et al 2003). This anatomical organization is used functionally to facilitate the coordination of interlimb activity and can produce the complex patterns of muscular activity for postural support in response to voluntary movements (i.e., APAs) (Schepens & Drew 2006; Yakovenko & Drew 2009). For example, the bilateral and unilateral innervations to the musculature enable contralateral stabilization of the body for arm reach or swing phase.

The *tectospinal tract* is a pathway that coordinates head and eye movements. The tract originates from a portion of the midbrain called the *superior colliculus*, crosses the midline, and descends contralaterally to terminate mostly on cervical motor neurons in the spinal cord (Brodal 2010). Hence the tectospinal tract is responsible for motor impulses arising from one side of the midbrain and activates muscles on the opposite side of the body. The function of the tectospinal tract is to mediate reflex postural movements of the head in response to visual and auditory stimuli.

Although the RST is usually associated with gross movements such as postural adjustments and walking, recent work has shown that it also connects to spinal centers involved in hand function (Baker 2011; Honeycutt et al 2013). Riddle and colleagues (2009) found that the RST provides input even to motor neurons projecting to intrinsic hand muscles. This knowledge has changed the view of distal hand control; it is possible that the reticulospinal and corticospinal pathways work in parallel to generate a large repertoire of diverse, coordinated movements in the hand. Reticulospinal pathways to the muscles of the hand may make this pathway a possible therapeutic target in patients where the CST is absent or injured as may occur in stroke or spinal cord injury (Riddle et al 2009; Honeycutt et al. 2013).

> Stability and balance are prerequisites for movement.
> Standing promotes awareness and arousal.

▇▇ The Vestibular System

The vestibular system processes information about head movement and orientation and plays a vital role in everyday life by giving us our subjective sense of self-motion and orientation, in addition to playing an important role in the stabilization of gaze and the control of balance (Cullen 2012). Furthermore, studies conducted in neurological patients even suggest that vestibular signals are also important for various aspects of one's body perception and awareness (Bottini et al 2001).

▇ Overview of the Vestibular System

The vestibular system is composed of a peripheral part: the vestibular sensory organs, and a central part: the vestibular nerve and the vestibular nuclei.

- The sensory organ of the vestibular apparatus: five receptor organs in the inner ear.
- The vestibular nerve, which transmits vestibular signals from the sensory organs of the inner ear to the vestibular nuclei.
  - The vestibular nuclei (**Fig. 1.22**): four main nuclei, which are a collection of neurons distributed in the brain stem and collectively referred to as the vestibular complex (Brodal 2010). Information from the vestibular system, cerebellum, spinal cord, and visual system is integrated in these nuclei:
  - *The lateral nucleus* (nucleus of Dieter).
  - *The medial vestibular nucleus* (MVN).
  - *The superior nucleus.*
  - *The descending* (or inferior) *nucleus.*

The vestibular sensory organs are located as a symmetric pair in the right and left inner ear. They consist of two types of sensors: the three semicircular canals, which sense angular acceleration in all three dimensions; and the two otolith organs (the saccule and utricle), which sense linear acceleration (i.e., gravity and translational movements) in all three dimensions (Cullen 2012). Thus the vestibular sensory organs can inform the CNS about the amount of body tilt with respect to gravity, in addition to body sway in all directions

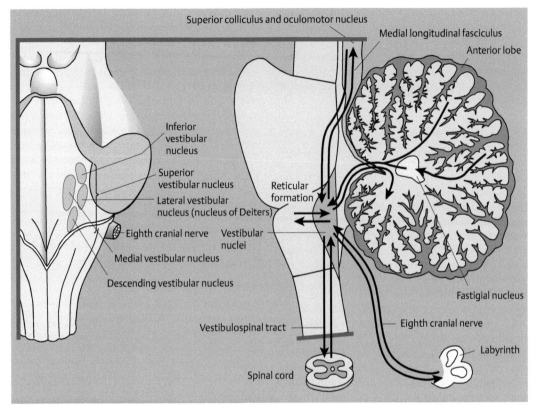

Fig. 1.22 The vestibular nuclei in the brain stem. The figure shows the most important afferent and efferent pathways.

(Kandel et al 2013). These receptors are active at all times; even at rest the otolith organs sense the force of gravity.

Vestibular signals transferred via the vestibular branch of the eighth cranial nerve to the vestibular nuclear complex for signal processing and rerouting. Here the vestibular signals are integrated with visual, proprioceptive, and other sensory information to estimate head and body orientation.

The vestibular complex receives information from the following:

- The vestibular sensory organs of the inner ear, signaling the position of the head and changes in movement, direction, and speed.
- The spinal cord (proprioceptive information), reticular formation, the cerebellum, and some nuclei in the mesencephalon (superior colliculus).
- The eyes.
- The cerebral cortex (mainly indirectly via the reticular formation but also via some direct fibers).

In the vestibular complex, information from muscles, joints, skin, and eyes is continuously integrated with input from vestibular sensory organs, hence the information processing in the vestibular system is multisensory and multimodal already at the level of the vestibular complex (Brodal 2010). In addition, the vestibular complex receives inputs from a wide range of cortical, cerebellar, and brain stem structures. The integration of vestibular information and extravestibular information is important for higher-order vestibular functions, such as perception of self-motion and spatial orientation (Angelaki & Cullen 2008).

■ Efferent Connections of the Vestibular Complex

Information from the vestibular system acts on three main regions:

- Motor neurons in the spinal cord via the *vestibulospinal pathways* giving us the vestibulospinal reflexes (VSRs).

- Motor neurons of the extraocular muscles: vestibulo-ocular reflex (VOR).
- Cerebellum.

The vestibular nuclear complex has reciprocal connections with the cerebellum for monitoring and modulating of vestibular reflex contributions to posture control.

Vestibulospinal Reflexes

VSRs play an important role in coordinating head and neck movement with the trunk and body to maintain the head in an upright position (Cullen 2012), and serve as a key to maintaining the position of the body in relation to gravity without conscious effort. Vestibular influences on postural control include modulation of the postural tone of the body, thus the vestibulospinal pathways can selectively adjust postural tone in response to unexpected head movements. The vestibular signals cannot differentiate between head movement or whole- body movement when the head moves on a stationary trunk; therefore neck-proprioceptive input provides important information about head movements relative to the trunk. Activation of proprioceptors in the neck musculature elicit the cervicocollic reflex, which works in combination with the vestibulocollic reflex for head stability and body posture (Pettorossi & Schieppati 2014).

Vestibulospinal Pathways

Most of the fibers to the spinal cord project from the lateral vestibular nuclei forming the lateral vestibulospinal tract, which extends the total length of the spinal cord and affects α- and γ-motor neurons monosynaptically (Brodal 2010; Markham 1987). Due to its monosynaptic connection it reacts quickly to restore balance.

The lateral vestibulospinal tract supplies axial muscles (the deep postural muscles of the trunk and neck) and proximal extremity muscles (Markham 1987). The lateral vestibulospinal tract sends collaterals to both cervical and lumbar regions of the spinal cord. The same message is therefore conveyed to both cervical and lumbar levels to allow coordination of the body and the extremities with the head and neck musculature. Vestibular system function is geared toward the here-and-now situation.

The lateral vestibulospinal tract affects the same side of the body; it is ipsilateral to the trunk and extremities. It promotes extensor and inhibits flexor motor neuron activity ipsilaterally and facilitates flexor activity on the contralateral body side at the

same moment in time (Dietz 1992). This view is supported by Kidd and colleagues (1992), who state that the lateral vestibulospinal tract is active during extension in standing and walking.

The *medial vestibular nucleus* innervates motor neurons in the cervical and the upper thoracic segments through the *medial vestibulospinal tract*. This pathway is smaller than the lateral and synapses with motor neurons ipsilaterally. Its function is to stabilize the head in relation to the body. The head is relatively free in standing and walking to allow visual scanning of the surroundings.

> The activity of the vestibular system is greatest when postural control is required.
> Head control and postural control affect each other reciprocally.

The VOR compensates for head movements by keeping the eyes still while the head moves (Kandel et al 2013). The vestibular sensory receptors signal how fast the head rotates, and this information is used by the oculomotor system to stabilize the eyes to steady visual images on the retina during movement; as the head rotates, the eyes rotate in the opposite direction. Visual processing is much slower and less efficient than vestibular processing for image stabilization. This reflex needs to be adapted through motor learning as body proportions change during growth.

Cortical Processing of Vestibular Signals

All vestibular nuclei project to the ventral posterior and the ventral lateral nuclei of the thalamus (Kandel et al 2013). The thalamus relays and modulates the flow of vestibular information to the cortex and plays an important function in *cortico-thalamo-cortical pathways*. From the thalamus the information is conveyed to the cortex. There is no single and well defined primary vestibular cortex (Lopez & Blanke 2011). Rather, a growing amount of data from neuroimaging studies have identified a highly distributed vestibular cortical network induced by vestibular stimulation, involving the posterior and anterior insula, the temporoparietal junction, the inferior parietal lobule, the somatosensory cortices, the primary motor cortex, and the premotor cortex (Brodal 2010).

There is increasing evidence that the vestibular system is involved in perception and oculomotor and postural control, and it also takes part in spatial cognition (Brodal 2010). Vestibular signals, and the neural structures involved in vestibular processing, are crucial for distinguishing self-motion and object-motion, for perceiving the world as upright, and for visual perception related to gravity (Cullen 2014). The CNS uses vestibular signals to work out an internal model of gravity, referencing arm movements and position. In addition, the vestibular signals to control muscle tone and contractions of limb muscles are fed back to the brain to update the current posture of the body. Thus the vestibular signals are involved in sensorimotor circuits between the brain and body parts contributing to perception of body segments (Lopez et al 2012).

Clinical Relevance

The vestibular apparatus plays a central role in balance and mediates key reflexes for the stabilization of posture and gaze. In standing, short-latency reflexes have an important role in countering unpredicted perturbations to balance. Short-latency reflexes in leg and trunk muscles have been shown to originate from vestibular receptors in response to head accelerations (Laube et al 2012). According to Forbes and colleagues (2015), the vestibular reflexes (VRs) vary across and within muscle groups and are modulated according to a muscle's contribution to the system dynamics, the different neural pathways innervating each muscle, and the consistency of sensory signals and motor commands for a given task . The task dependence on vestibular reflexes is especially important during locomotion because vestibular reflex responses are dynamically modulated in all locomotor muscles about the ankle, knee, and hip joints (Dakin et al 2013).

The activity of the vestibular system is greatest in standing and walking when the demands on postural control are greatest. Any displacement of position or posture, weight transference, or movements of the arm displace the center of gravity in relation to the feet and the base of support. Irrespective of how small the displacements are (breathing causes small, almost invisible alterations in the intersegmental alignment of the trunk, which are perceived as small perturbations to the center of gravity), muscle tone and activity will need to adapt to maintain equilibrium.

There are important functional consequences of the foregoing information. Through its ipsilateral innervation of extensor musculature, it may seem as if the activity in the vestibular nuclei is best facilitated when a person is standing on one leg. Dietz (1992) discusses this in relation to a "true" standing posture or position. Clinically, it is perceived that the align-

ment of the body needs to be optimized to facilitate balance. Bussel and colleagues (1996) refer to studies on paraplegic patients which seem to indicate that the flexor reflex may interfere with CPG activity during attempts to step or walk. Combining these different authors' findings with clinical experience, it may seem as if balance on one leg in standing is a prerequisite for free swing of the opposite leg. At the same time, if the swing is initiated actively too early in the swing, it may negate the stability of the standing leg.

> The ability to dynamically balance on one leg seems to be a prerequisite for a free swing. Active swing that is initiated too early may interfere with the stability of the standing leg.

Bringing the patient into a standing position to interact with gravity (placing or facilitating, depending on the patient's level of motor activity) could stimulate the vestibular system to facilitate more activity on the patient's most affected side. Weight transference to the affected side through optimized/normalized alignment would best facilitate activation of the vestibular system.

Both the reticular and the vestibular systems innervate body musculature on the same and the opposite side of the body (ipsi- and contralaterally). A lesion affecting motor pathways on one side of the brain may result in reduced motor control on both sides. Let us briefly consider the anatomical arrangement of the ventromedial system, which, although descending bilaterally, presents a primary ipsilateral projection. In a stroke located at a subcortical level (e.g., the internal capsule), it is very likely that the lesion will interfere with the neuronal connection between the motor cortex and the reticular formation. This may lead to an ipsilesional postural control dysfunction in the trunk (Schepens & Drew 2004; Schepens et al 2008; Silva et al 2014). Brain stem lesions may result in reduced balance and mobility problems as well as dysphagia and dysarthria because the nuclei of the cranial nerves are located in this region. Muscle tone may be increased or severely decreased depending on whether the inhibitory or the excitatory part of the reticular formation is lesioned. If the fibers innervating the excitatory area of the reticular formation are lesioned, there may be a loss of excitation to the spinal cord, and the patient may experience hypotonia; however, if the fibers synapsing in the inhibitory part are lesioned, there will be a loss of inhibitory influences to the spinal cord, and the patient may develop a problem with hypertonia.

The Spinal Cord

The spinal cord has often been referred to as a simple relay station between the brain and effector organs (muscles, skin, etc.). However, over the last 4 decades, researchers have found that the spinal cord is involved in far more complex functions than a simple conduit. The spinal cord receives information both from higher centers and from the periphery. It has a huge receptor area, and both receive and modulate information from the whole body (except the head), before the information is transmitted to other systems or translated into muscle activity. It has a gate control function, whereby information sent to the spinal cord is adapted to suit the needs of the organism and to protect the brain from overstimulation (Davidoff 1990; Kandel et al 2013). Because of its large receptor area and gate control function, the spinal cord influences activity in the higher centers. The spinal cord is involved in carrying signals between the brain and the rest of the body through several ascending and descending pathways. In addition, it contains both quite basic reflex arcs and more complex neuronal circuits controlling central pattern–generated motor behaviors. In several species, research has shown that the rhythmic muscle activation of some movements is programmed at the spinal level where it can be modulated according to the environment, for example, the well studied spinal network producing locomotion (CPG) or the cervical propriospinal system that has been shown to be involved in reaching and hand movements in cats and primates (Marchand-Pauvert & Iglesias 2008).

Internal Structure of the Spinal Cord

The internal structure of the spinal cord exhibits two types of tissue; *white and gray matter*. The white matter surrounds the gray matter throughout the spinal cord and serves as a relay for descending and ascending information. The white matter is divided into dorsal, lateral, and ventral columns (bundles of axons also referred to as tracts). The dorsal and lateral columns transmit sensory signals (see section on Integration of Somatosensory Information at the Spinal Cord Level) and the ventral columns are associated mainly with descending motor signals (Guertin 2013).

Gray matter, characterized by its butterfly or H-shape, consists of unmyelinated fibers. The lateral aspects of the gray matter are divided into regions also referred to as the dorsal, lateral, and ventral horns. The dorsal horn processes sensory information, whereas the ventral horn processes motor information. The lateral horns are present at only the thoracic level and contain the cell bodies of the preganglionic sympathetic neurons, and thereby process autonomic information (Lundy-Ekman 2007).

Within the spinal cord, interneurons may serve as processing centers as they relay nerve impulses and conduct impulses from the sensory neuron to a motor neuron (e.g., Renshaw cells, Ia and Ib inhibitory interneurons, interneurons in disynaptic pathways from group II afferents, and some of the interneurons in polysynaptic pathways from flexor reflex afferents [FRAs]). Interneurons of most spinal reflex pathways have been shown to mediate reflex responses evoked by a variety of peripheral stimuli and to contribute to several reactions, including voluntary movements.

Some of the neurons in the gray matter form local spinal reflex pathways (also referred to as reflex arcs), whereas others take part in more complex circuits involving specific functions. A reflex is defined as "a rapid, predictable, repeatable, stereotyped and involuntary motor response or movement induced by a specific stimulus" (Guertin 2013). For example, the Ia reflex pathway is considered the simplest reflex (also referred to as the monosynaptic stretch reflex or tendon jerk). It mediates primary afferent (Ia) inputs originating from the muscle spindles and is activated by muscle stretch. This reflex is generally considered to have a role in muscle tone and postural adjustments (Guertin 2013).

Although generally considered as stereotyped responses, the spinal reflexes can be modulated (e.g., by the level of anxiety or by training; the strength of the reflex can be enhanced or weakened depending on the need of the task) (Brodal 2010).

According to Alvarez and colleagues (2013) spinal cord motor function depends on the wiring and properties of the interneurons that modulate motor neuron firing and motor output. The spinal cord contains many types of interneurons that can be assigned into various types according to anatomical, physiological, and/or molecular criteria. Interneurons that spread their branches over several segments are called propriospinal neurons (PNs) and are found throughout the white matter of the spinal cord (Brodal 2010; Flynn et al 2011). Functionally, the propriospinal system participates in a variety of different tasks, including integration and modulation of inputs from descending supraspinal pathways (e.g., carrying motor commands from the brain) and peripheral afferents (carrying sensory information from the periphery). PNs are also important for synchronizing activity in motor circuits throughout the length of the spinal cord (Brodal 2010). In addition, locomotion is underpinned by coupling of cervical and lumbar spinal enlargements via a network involving PNs.

In recent years, PNs have been identified as an important substrate for functional recovery after incomplete spinal cord injury (SCI); PNs have the possibility of forming new spinal circuits, either with severed axons from descending pathways or by connections via their own sprouts or arborizations. The contribution of the propriospinal system to functional recovery in humans is uncertain; however, studies in animal models of SCI provide compelling evidence that PNs are promising targets for therapeutic interventions (Flynn et al 2011).

■ Central Pattern Generators and Locomotion

"The existence of networks of nerve cells producing specific, rhythmic movements, without conscious effort and without the aid of peripheral, afferent feedback, is indisputable in a large number of vertebrates" (Mackay-Lyons 2002). CPGs, neural networks in the spinal cord, are capable of producing rhythmical movements (Dietz 1992; Dietz 2003; Brodal 2010; Mackay-Lyons 2002) (**Fig. 1.23**). CPGs provide automatic, changing activity coordinating the two halves of the body, and have been mostly studied in vertebrates. CPGs for vital functions, such as breathing, chewing, and swallowing, have been located in the brain stem, whereas those for locomotive functions are contained in the spinal cord. The probability of their existence in humans is high (Kandel et al 2013). The early stepping reactions of babies demonstrate rhythmical spinal activity and suggest that these networks are innate, and may be an expression of pattern generation (Kandel et al 2013). In humans, findings are consistent, with separate CPGs controlling each limb, and these CPGs are located in the spinal cord of both cats and humans (Dietz et al 1994; Mackay-Lyons 2002; Zehr & Duysens 2004). The CPGs for each side are linked together through complex interneuronal networks. The dorsal root fibers from peripheral receptors terminate on in-

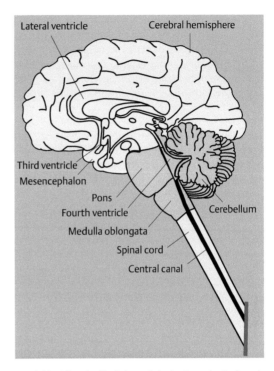

Fig. 1.23 A longitudinal view of the brain and spinal cord. The spinal cord and brain stem contain specialized groups of cells—neuronal pools called central pattern generators. Long propriospinal fibers (from the cervical to the lumbar areas) are necessary for coordination between the right and left side of the body during walking, and this rhythmical interchange of activity between the two sides is thought to be caused by cells with pacemaker properties.

terneurons that branch within the spinal cord. The impulses from one dorsal root fiber may therefore spread over several segments, both up and down.

There is a neural coupling between arms and legs in humans. This is a task-dependent neuronal coupling of upper and lower limbs, which allows us to involve the arms during gait but to disconnect this coupling during voluntarily guided arm/hand movements. During walking, our arms move rhythmically out of phase with the corresponding leg. This is not a passive mechanical effect; several arm muscles, especially at the shoulder joint, show rhythmic alternating activity during the gait cycle.

It has been proposed that this may be comparable with quadrupedal locomotion in four-legged animals and that this activity is reflective of spinal CPG (Zehr et al 2009). Propriospinal pathways contained within the spine are thought to be critical for quadrupedal coordination by coupling cervical and lumbar CPGs.

The CPGs are, in their original form, independent of somatosensory information. Studies in humans and monkeys have shown that voluntary motor tasks, such as reaching and grasping, and other rhythmical movements, including swimming and walking, can be performed following deafferentation (Knapp et al 1963; Mackay-Lyons 2002). However, the interplay between central and sensory influences is critical in the production of adaptive behavior, and recent research on locomotor control has highlighted the role of afferent input in shaping motor output during walking (Dietz et al 2009). According to Juvin and colleagues (2012) the crucial role played by limb sensory feedback in regulating locomotor CPG network operation in the mammalian spinal cord is now widely recognized.

Somatosensory feedback is an integral part of the overall motor control system and is essential in modifying CPG-generated motor programs to facilitate constant adaptations to the environment during walking (Mackay-Lyons 2002; Zehr & Duysens 2004; Dietz 2010). The CPGs use afferent information from several sources in the visual, vestibular, and somatosensory systems. CPGs and motor neurons receive extensive feedback from various sensory receptors for the control of balance and the direction and speed of locomotion (Grillner 2006). In addition, sensory feedback provides information ensuring that motor activity is adapted to the biomechanical state of the moving body parts for position, direction, and strength (i.e., facilitation of phase changes).

Three important sensory sources for locomotion have been identified (Duysens & Van de Crommert1998):

- Information on loading from force-sensitive GTOs in extensor muscles.
- Loading feedback from mechanoreceptors in the sole of the foot.
- Positional information from stretch-sensitive muscle spindles in the hip musculature.

Extensor reinforcing feedback, the information from force-sensitive GTOs in extensor muscles and loading feedback from mechanoreceptors in the sole of the foot, is believed to increase stance-phase muscle activity and duration of the stance phase of gait. Positional information from muscle spindles in the hip musculature facilitates the onset of the swing phase (Duysens et al 2000), the functional consequence being that the swing phase is not initiated until the extensor muscles are unloaded and that the forces exerted by these muscles are low. In other words, when limb loading decreases at the end of the stance phase, the extensor reinforcing feedback is reduced,

and the onset of swing is facilitated (Takakusaki 2013).

Dietz and Duysens (2000) state that afferent information is necessary to strengthen CPG activity of antigravity muscles. Information about unloading, heel strike, and weight transference is critical for the control of stepping (Maki & McIlroy 1997). Kavounoudias and colleagues (1998) researched the role of cutaneous receptors in the soles of the feet for balance. They anesthetized the feet and found that subjects were unable to balance on one leg after the loss of foot sensitivity. A specific distribution of mechanoreceptors in the feet codes the spatial origin, the amplitude, and the rate of changes in the amplitude of pressure exerted on the skin. Thereby the CNS is continuously receiving information regarding the spatial and sequential distribution of pressure from the soles of the feet.

In addition to CPG activity in the spinal cord for locomotion, there are many other networks in the CNS that have key roles in achieving successful walking. The higher centers involved in the initiation, modulation, and control of locomotion are as follows (Takakusaki 2013; Guertin 2012):

- The MLRs.
- The vestibular system.
- The reticular formation.
- The cerebellum.
- The BG.
- The cortex.

Nuclei in the mesencephalon, referred to as the MLRs, initiate locomotion through activation of the lower brain stem reticulospinal neurons (Mackay-Lyons 2002; Takakusaki 2013). Three different zonal areas have been identified, all of which have different roles in the initiation of locomotion:

- The lateral hypothalamus initiates gait in relation to hunger, thirst, or the need for the bathroom.
- The zona incerta initiates tourist-type walking (i.e., visually directed walking).
- Periventricular zone initiates anger and fear (fight and flight) responses.

The reticular formation and vestibular system in the brain stem are both involved in activating antigravity musculature. The reticulospinal tract activates the spinal rhythm–generating system and in addition increases postural muscle tone (Takakusaki 2013). The BG integrate posture and movement, thus modifying muscle tone and adapting locomotion. Further modification is through the cerebellum, which is thought to coordinate CPG activity for the right and the left side of the body. Connections from the motor cortical areas to the BG and the cerebellum may contribute to accurate and adaptive movement control that requires volition, cognition, attention, and prediction (Takakusaki 2013). The cerebellum is also active in motor learning and error correction. The cortex exerts little influence on simple unobstructed walking, but it has a role in visual scanning, perception, and navigation, and in modifying the activity of the CPGs to make the activity appropriate to the moment; as walking becomes more complex, the cortex becomes more active. The CPGs cannot see the ground; therefore, when locomotion becomes complex, especially where footfall is narrowly specified and the need for visual input increases, the cortex fires more rhythmically to guide the placement of the foot (Lacquaniti et al 2012).

> Walking on a flat, even surface is probably controlled by CPGs in the spinal cord and brain stem and coordinated by the cerebellum (i.e., it is mainly an automatic activity).

■ Clinical Relevance

Pattern generation may have an important role in the early activation of postural activity and coordination in the acute/subacute stage in patients with a CNS lesion because facilitation of stepping in a simple, noncomplex environment does not require cognitive problem solving by the patient:

- A pattern-generated step is a result of selective displacement and is different in its motor activity from a reactive step resulting from overdisplacement.
- Pattern generation may be facilitated automatically, even in patients with severe motor, sensory, or perceptual dysfunctions.
- Pattern generation may enhance motor activity in the body as a whole by facilitating the interplay and coordination between the different segments and the two halves of the body, thereby promoting balance control.
- Early facilitation of stepping activates the CNS and neuromuscular system and motivates the patient.
- A good stance phase resulting from heel strike facilitates the swing phase on the same side (release of kinetic energy).
- A good stance phase provides stability to the postural system and therefore also frees the opposite leg for swing. Thus the better the control of posture the better the gait initiation.

- Pattern generation depends on appropriate afferent information to adapt the activity to the environment.
- Tempo must be at an appropriate level for the individual to facilitate phase changes because individuals seem to have different inherent speeds.
- Early facilitation of stepping may enhance the patient's awareness of the environment and improve perception.
- Focused attention by the patient on the gait pattern may disrupt the natural CPG rhythm by taking priority away from the peripheral input.

For optimal rehabilitation of locomotion of patients with spinal or cerebral lesions, the appropriate afferent input has to be provided to activate and strengthen the CPGs, in addition to guiding the postlesional plasticity mechanisms (Molinari 2009). The role of afferent activity in this regard is to shape the locomotor pattern, to control phase transitions, and to reinforce ongoing activity. According to Rossignol and colleagues (2007), "it is likely that active sensory stimulation and various forms of training with enhanced sensory stimulation will lead to better recovery of locomotion after spinal lesions."

■■ The Neuromuscular System

The end result of CNS processing in movement production is the action of skeletal muscles. The muscular system and the CNS exchange information and requirements continuously. The muscular system is specialized in its structure and function to meet the needs of a variety of movements in different settings to perform a multitude of tasks. The neuromuscular system has an adaptive capacity: changes in information sent by the CNS to the muscular system may alter the structure and function of the musculature and vice versa (i.e., altered use of the muscles due to CNS lesions may result in changes in the structure and function of the CNS).

■ Structure and Function of Skeletal Muscles

The human body has more than 300 bilateral pairs of skeletal muscles (Kanning et al 2010).

Skeletal muscle contains *contractile and noncontractile elements* and *specialized sense organs* or receptors. The contractile elements are the extrafusal muscle fibers and ends of muscle spindles. The noncontractile elements are the connective tissue and sense organs (GTOs and muscle spindles).

All skeletal muscles are composed of multinucleated cells called *fibers*. Each fiber constitutes contractile proteins, *myosin* and *actin*. The interaction of these proteins allows muscles to contract. The myosin protein has specialized projections called cross-bridges ending in myosin heads that are capable of binding with actin. A muscle contraction occurs when the actin slides relative to myosin (Lundy-Ekman 2007).

The myosin and actin filaments are arranged in regular bands within structures called *sarcomeres*. A repeated sequence of sarcomeres forms structures called *myofibrils*. Each muscle fiber contains a large number of parallel myofibrils, and the force generated by a muscle fiber is proportional to the number of myofibrils it contains.

Motor Neurons and Motor Units

Motor neurons share the same function: they drive the contraction of muscle fibers and are the final common pathway (i.e., the area of convergence of all the central and peripheral pathways involved in motor actions) (Manuel & Zytnicki 2011). Motor neurons are the only central neurons with axons that leave the CNS to innervate nonneuronal tissue and link the nervous and muscular systems together. Their cell bodies are located in the anterior horn of the gray matter of the spinal cord (Floeter 2010). In mammals, there are three kinds of motor neurons; alpha (α), gamma (γ), and beta (β) (Floeter 2010). The α motor neurons innervate skeletal (striped or striated) muscles, and the gamma

motor neurons innervate the intrafusal muscle fibers. The β motor neurons innervate both intra- and extrafusal fibers (Kanning et al 2010). *The motor unit is the functional unit of the motor system. It is composed of a motor neuron and several muscle fibers.* Each motor unit supplies muscle fibers with the same structural and functional properties. A muscle is composed of a mixture of several motor units containing different muscle fiber types (Schiaffino & Reggiani 2011) (**Fig. 1.24**). The size of a motor unit varies; in the case of small muscles used for fine motor control, motor neurons may innervate only a few small motor units. In larger force-producing muscles with less demand for delicate control, a motor neuron may innervate many motor units. For a muscle to effectively contribute to smooth, coordinated movement, motor neurons must selectively activate an appropriate number and combination of motor units to generate the required activity.

Skeletal Muscle Fibers

Skeletal muscle fibers can be divided into two generalized groups: the "red" muscle fibers with slow contraction times and the "white" muscle fibers with fast contraction times (Brodal 2010; Floeter 2010). These two are again divided into three main groups and several subgroups. The three main groups are as follows:

- Type 1, also called slow twitch (ST) (Brodal 2010) or slow oxidative (SO) (Rothwell & Lennon 1994; Floeter 2010). This fiber type is often described as red due to its high content

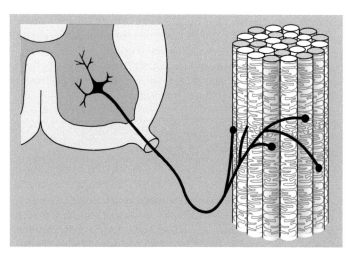

Fig. 1.24 A motor unit comprises several muscle fibers with the same muscle fiber type, the α-motor neuron that innervates it, and the axonal branches of the α-motor neuron to the individual muscle fibers. Muscle fibers belonging to different motor units are dispersed within the muscle.

of myoglobin. Type 1 fibers have a high level of endurance, are precise in their action, and produce a moderate amount of power. The action of these fibers is often referred to as tonic due to the ability of the fibers to maintain dynamic contraction over time; they are mostly found in areas of the body where maintenance of activity against gravity is the main function. They have a stabilizing function through their precise grading of activity. Tonic activity is dynamic, and the word *tonicity* refers to something that is "characterized by tension or contraction, esp. muscular tension" (Thomas 1997). The motor units containing type 1 fibers are characterized as S (slow to fatigue) (Rothwell & Lennon 1994).

Examples

The soleus muscle is continuously active during standing and walking requiring high endurance, and it therefore consists mainly of tonic/type 1 motor units. The soleus muscle is characterized as a postural muscle.
The small muscles of the hand, the interossei, and the lumbricals also have mostly type 1 fiber (Rothwell & Lennon 1994). The small muscles of the hand stabilize the palm and the metacarpophalangeal joints and provide the hand with a postural background for individual finger movement and precise fine motor control.
The small muscles of the foot have a stabilizing function for the maintenance of body equilibrium.
The small muscles of the back are important for postural control of the trunk and therefore core stability.

- Type 2 fibers are also called fast twitch (FT) because they have a faster contraction speed than type 1 fibers. These muscle fiber types are described as white and have a low oxidative capacity with little endurance but increased tempo and force production. They are phasic by nature, and their main function is the production of movement. The motor units are classified as FF (fast, fatigable). Type 2 fibers are further subdivided as follows:
  - Type 2A or fast oxidative glycolytic (FOG) (Rothwell & Lennon 1994; Floeter 2010). The motor units are classified as fatigue resistant (FR) because they have more endurance.

Example

The gastrocnemius muscle has an important role in force production during locomotion, running, jumping, moving on uneven ground, and climbing steps, all of which require both endurance and force. The muscle therefore has a larger proportion of FOG muscle fibers.

- Type 2B are the truly white fibers (Brodal 2010). The motor units are classified as fast glycolytic (FG) (Rothwell & Lennon 1994) and have low endurance and produce a lot of force.

Example

The tibialis anterior muscle works intermittently during locomotion and in standing. Its use therefore is mainly aimed at phasic activity and low demands of endurance.

The Ability of the CNS to Control the Level of Activity of the Motor Neurons

The force of muscle contraction may be graded in two ways (Brodal 2010):
1. *The number of motor units that are recruited.* If the number increases, so does the force production.
2. *The impulse frequency of the motor neuron.* If the frequency increases, it leads to increased force production.

Motor activity of a muscle is recruited sequentially through the Henneman recruitment principle (Henneman 1985; Mendell 2005) whereby small, slow motor units (containing type 1 muscle fibers) are activated before the larger and faster motor units containing phasic muscle fibers. The recruitment principle has been called the size principle of recruitment by Brodal (2010) and recruitment order by Rothwell (Brodal 2010; Rothwell & Lennon 1994).

Functional Relevance

Small motor units that demonstrate the greatest ability for endurance are to be found in maximum numbers in muscles whose main function is postural activity (i.e., sustained activity against gravity). Several authors have described postural activity as the basis for function of the extremities (Dietz 1992; Massion et al 2004; Shumway-Cook 2011).

Motor units in a muscle are recruited sequentially, whereby the smaller motor units are activated before the larger motor units.
Postural stability is the basis for selective movement control and function.

Most muscles have a mixture of different motor units. The musculature is therefore able to function in relation to different activities: a muscle may have a stabilizing function in cooperation with some muscles or more of a mobility function when working with others. Motor units are recruited sequentially to enable the musculature to grade its activity in relation to strength, synergistic musculature, and required function (Massion 1992). Muscles can vary their activity and function as agonists, antagonists, or synergists depending on how they are being used.

Most muscles have internal selectivity based on the distribution of motor units and muscle fiber type and size. Motor units may be activated differentially; some may work eccentrically at the same time as others are working concentrically to varying degrees. Anatomically defined muscles that cross two joints or more may eccentrically lengthen over one joint while shortening over the other. This ability is called *compartmentalization* (van Ingen Schenau et al 1990).

Example

The quadriceps muscle continuously varies its activity during locomotion; in the stance phase, the proximal part has to contract eccentrically to allow for hip extension, whereas at the same time the distal part has to work concentrically to stabilize the knee for weight bearing. During the initial swing, the activity of the quadriceps is reversed; the proximal part undergoes more concentric contraction to assist in swinging the leg forward, whereas the distal part works more eccentrically to allow knee flexion.

Compartmentalization describes the ability of a muscle that crosses more than one joint to perform different functions simultaneously.

Motor Unit and Muscle Fiber Plasticity

A remarkable feature of the skeletal muscle fiber is its ability to change in response to various environmental and physiological demands (Matsakas & Patel 2009; Brodal 2010). There is strong evidence that muscle fibers, and therefore motor units, not only change in size in response to demands but may also change from one fiber type to another (Scott et al 2001). This ability to change in response to stimuli, which is also referred to as muscle plasticity (e.g., in training and rehabilitation), enables adaptation to different functional requirements.

At birth, most muscles are composed of slow (type 1) muscles, and only as the body matures does the final proportion of slow and fast muscles

emerge (Rubinstein & Kelly 1981). Athletes have different distributions of muscle fiber types depending on their preferred sport; long-distance runners, cyclists, and cross-country skiers have a larger percentage of type 1 red fibers, whereas weight lifters and short-distance runners (i.e., sports that require rapid production of force), have a larger percentage of white type 2 fibers. This is probably due, in part, to individual genetic profiles, but muscle plasticity forms a major basis for physiological adaptation to the external environment.

Examples of muscle plasticity are adapting to exercise, effects of a microgravity environment, aging, and different pathophysiological conditions. Muscle plasticity can be both beneficial and maladaptive. Changes in muscle fiber types are also responsible for some of the loss of function associated with deconditioning (Scott et al 2001).

Muscle cells display a tremendous ability to adapt to new levels of gene expression in response to a wide range of environmental demands and clinical conditions (Sieck 2001). *Gene expression* is the process by which a gene's information is converted into the structures and functions of a cell (Flavell & Greenberg 2008). Alteration of muscle fiber types is a result of changed gene expression. This may be termed *use-dependent plastic adaptation*.

Trials using electrostimulation have demonstrated that muscle fibers may change with changes in the information to and functional demand on the muscle fibers (Kidd 1986; Doucet et al 2012).

> Muscles are able to alter their fiber type to some degree in relation to use.

The number of sarcomeres determines the length of a muscle fiber: the more sarcomeres, the longer the muscle. In the human body, the number of sarcomeres and therefore the length of the muscle are normally optimal for the function of the muscle. The force of contraction is therefore at its best within the range of movement where it is most needed. The sarcomeres are able to produce very little force if the fiber is overstretched or kept in a much-shortened position. The length of the muscle fibers is affected by the way the muscle is being used. If a muscle is kept in a much-shortened position over time, this will lead to an anatomical shortening of the muscle due to the loss of sarcomeres (Lundy-Ekman 2007). Sahrmann (1992) states that a shortened muscle is more easily recruited than its antagonists that are in a lengthened position, and that, as a result of this, the shortened muscle is stronger. Sahrmann calls this *biased recruitment.*

If a muscle is kept stretched over time, it may "grow"; that is, the number of sarcomeres may increase, which may render the muscle incapable of producing the force required for an activity. Sahrmann (1992) calls this *stretch weakness.*

Functional Relevance

An important issue in rehabilitating the neurological patient is reducing the effects of immobilization on skeletal muscles, especially muscles immobilized in the shortened position. The length of a muscle affects its ability to create tension (Gray et al 2012). The *force–length relationship* shows how muscle tension varies at different muscle lengths. Muscle fibers lengthen as the joint angle increases and shorten as the joint angle decreases. There is a certain position that generates an optimal force for each joint, and this depends on the relative position of the tendon insertion on the bone and internal and external forces. This position depends on the optimal number of cross-bridges being formed by the actin and myosin filaments.

For example, if the ankle is positioned in plantar flexion for longer periods, the plantar flexors will adapt to this new length by reducing the number of sarcomeres, thereby maintaining the resting position of the ankle in plantar flexion. Also, the position in which peak force in the plantar flexors is obtained will be changed, and as a result will contribute to muscle weakness and limit functional ability as the peak force of the plantar flexors is now created in a position no longer optimal for functional purposes (Gray et al 2012).

> The length of a muscle is important for movement and function.

Muscle Balance

Muscle balance is the result of cooperation within and between many muscles or muscle groups surrounding a joint: agonists, antagonists, and synergists. In humans with an intact CNS and musculoskeletal system, the grading of activity in the different muscle groups is finely tuned and adapted to the relevant function and situation. Maintenance of muscle balance depends on neurological, mus-

cular, and biomechanical factors (Sahrmann 1992; Sahrmann 2002; Stokes 1998):

- Muscular factors—such as the length–tension relationship of the muscle and its ability to produce force appropriately.
- Neurological factors—the sequence of recruitment of motor units within the muscle and the sequence of activation of different muscles or muscle groups.
- Biomechanical factors—alignment, structure, and function of the joints.

Muscle imbalance may result if any of the aforementioned factors are disturbed, as in some neurological disorders, and lead to malalignment.

> Muscle balance depends on muscular, neurological, and biomechanical factors. Alterations in recruitment and the distribution of motor activity affect alignment. Altered alignment affects muscle function.

Zackowski and colleagues (2004) describe *impaired joint individuation* as the inability to stabilize a joint during movement of another joint, a phenomenon they refer to as impairment in motor control. The authors point to other studies providing further evidence for reduced capacity of an impaired limb to generate certain muscle coactivation patterns, which may be due to abnormal spatial tuning (distribution) of muscle activity.

Noncontractile Elements in Muscle

Bundles of muscle fibers are held together by connective tissue, and the muscle is fully enclosed in connective tissue, called fascia. The connective tissue in muscle and fascia is continuous with the muscle tendon (Brodal 2010), and it unites, supports, and holds the structures of the body together. Fibrous tissue is elastic and supports muscles and joints as well as allowing movement. Changes in the properties of the tendon are also an important component, considering the muscle forces transmitted through it. With increasing age, fibrous tissue loses its strength and elasticity. If fibrous tissue is kept shortened, contractures may result (Tyldesley & Grieve 1996). A more compliant tendon reduces stored energy, contractile speed, and amount of power generated (Gray et al 2012). Clinically, it is important to maintain the integrity of the tendon and minimize compliance to prevent overshortening of the muscle fibers (Gray et al 2012).

Muscle Tone

Tone is related to the state of the muscle fibers, the activity within sense organs, muscle viscosity, and connective tissue. *Muscle tone* is an expression of the stiffness of the tissue. The relationship between muscle length and tension is called *stiffness* (Brodal 2010). The control of this relationship is called *stiffness control*.

Muscle tone is usually the term used to describe tension in relaxed muscle, and is also called *resting tone*. Brodal (2010) states that muscular contraction is the most important factor in changing the level of tone. The viscoelastic properties of the muscle fibers, connective tissue in the muscle, and the muscle tendon add to this to a lesser degree (Simons & Mense 1998). Shumway-Cook and Woollacott (2006) define *postural tone* as activity in muscles that counteracts the force of gravity in the upright position. They state that "muscles throughout the body, not only those of the trunk, are tonically active to maintain the body in a narrowly confined vertical position during quiet stance." They use the term *ideal alignment* to describe the increase of muscle work needed when the body moves outside a narrowly confined vertical position (i.e., even small ranges of movement increase the demands on muscular activity). To maintain normal function, tone needs to be high enough to allow the body to be *dynamically active* in relation to gravity. Postural tone is influenced by information from somatosensory receptors (skin receptors in the soles of the feet and neck receptors, among others) as well as visual and vestibular inputs. Other factors that influence tone are pain, fear, emotion, and inputs from other areas of the brain and spinal cord.

> Tone is related to the state of the muscle fibers, the activity within the sense organs, muscle viscosity, and connective tissue. The most important cause of alteration of tone is muscular contraction.

Information to the spinal cord comes from all somatosensory receptors in the body, for instance skin, joints, connective tissue, muscles, and tendons, as well as from other sensory (vision, hearing, equilibrium) and motor systems within the CNS. On any one motor neuron there may be as many as 50,000 synapses from sense organs and receptors, and from all levels and pathways within the brain and spinal cord (**Fig. 1.25**). Information is modulated continuously and may result in motor activity. Muscle length, tension, and activity will, in most situations, be appropriate for the function or activity to be per-

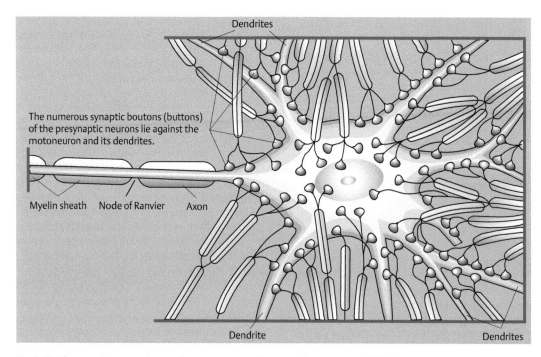

Dendrites

The numerous synaptic boutons (buttons) of the presynaptic neurons lie against the motoneuron and its dendrites.

Myelin sheath   Node of Ranvier   Axon

Dendrite

Dendrites

Fig. 1.25 The synaptic connections to the motor neuron. There may be as many as 50,000 synapses on one motor neuron.

formed because of this integration of information (Brodal 2010).

Clinical Relevance

Many people who have suffered a CNS lesion experience a reduction in balance, selective control of movement, and strength. The lesion itself, how the person is being positioned (how he sits, lies), demands for independence, stimulation, training, and the person's ability to activate and control his own body, will influence the neuromuscular adaptations that occur over time. The neuromuscular system adapts to the new situation and how the body is being used. This may lead to any of the following:

- Changes in the length–tension relationship, alteration of tone.
- Altered recruitment pattern of motor units, which may disrupt the ability to stabilize the body/body part as a background for movement.
- Muscle imbalance (reduced interplay between different muscle groups).
- Muscle fiber type changes and the level and constitution of connective/fibrous tissue; increased or decreased length of muscles; increases in muscle stiffness or stretch that preclude functional and efficient activation.
- Changes in the way the patient moves and uses her body; the need for new movement strategies to achieve goals. Patients who lack the ability to initiate the appropriate activity for a required function may use and develop compensatory strategies. Patients use the available movement strategies to enable them to be functional here and now. Inappropriate activity may strengthen the above factors and complicate and limit the patient's choice of movement in both the short and the long term
- Alignment problems as a result of tonal factors, use, and changes in contractile and noncontractile tissue will affect muscle function.
- Altered somatosensory information or perception may affect the patient's ability to move.

Hypotonia and *hypertonia* are terms used to describe tonic changes within muscle. Brodal (2010) describes hypotonia as reduced tone in the musculature. In a clinical situation, this is perceived as reduced ability to activate muscles appropriately, and as a lower muscular tension or stiffness than expected in the same situation when compared with people without a CNS lesion. Hypertonia is described as a continuous increase in tension or stiffness, even if the person attempts to relax. Clinically, this is perceived as an inability to grade and modulate tone, or as a higher muscular tension or stiffness than expected in the same situation when compared with healthy people.

In the early stages of an acute brain lesion, such as with stroke, patients may display a more generalized paresis, and in acute traumatic brain injury patients may have severe hypertonia throughout the body (opisthotonus). Lesions of certain parts of the brain stem may give a clinical picture of severe low tone/paralysis, often bilaterally. However, the therapist rarely encounters patients who are either totally hypo- or hypertonic. In most patients there is a mixture of muscles and muscle groups presenting with high and low tone and some areas with more normalized activity. Increased tone causes more stiffness of muscle and less pliability and flexibility, whereas low tone may result in instability, when the precise grading of activity is inappropriate.

The musculature seems to lose its variability and flexibility after CNS lesions. Altered distribution of motor unit activity and changes in alignment may affect muscle function negatively because the muscles have new working conditions. The patient may therefore be unable to align and recruit the neuromuscular activity necessary to reach the desired goal efficiently. *Efficient* in this context means that the patient does not need to use more force or exertion than would be normal for a healthy person.

The latissimus dorsi is anatomically described as one muscle, but it comprises many segments working together to create function. When the whole muscle contracts it brings about extension of the spine, increased lumbar lordosis combined with internal rotation, adduction, and extension of the arm. During normal conditions, the latissimus dorsi is able to activate differentially by increasing lumbar extension at the same time as the arms are stretched above the head as a jumper is pulled over the neck and head during undressing (**Fig. 1.26**) (i.e., it contracts concentrically distally and eccentrically in relation to arm function proximally at the same moment in time. In the author's clinical experience with CNS lesions, it seems as if the ability of the muscle to perform differential actions is disturbed. The patient's ability to compartmentalize muscle activity may be reduced, and the muscles seem to contract in their total range of movement when activated. In the case of the latissimus dorsi, the arm tends to rotate internally, adduct, and extend, together with lumbar extension when activated. If this total pattern of movement is learned, the patient's functional ability and independence may be reduced.

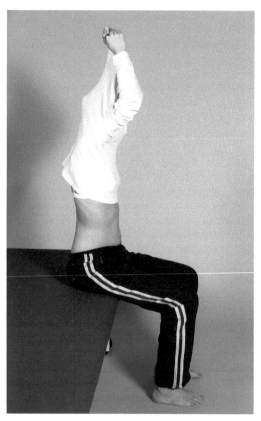

Fig. 1.26 Activation of the latissimus dorsi.

Muscle fiber changes have been shown in CNS lesions (Ada & Canning 1990; Gray et al 2012). Inactivity due to immobilization, denervation, or reduced activation makes the musculature prone to atrophy. Muscle fiber type changes may also be present: Hufschmidt and Mauritz (1985) state that a tonic transformation of muscle fibers may be one reason for the increased resistance to stretch experienced in spastic muscles. The function of phasic muscle fibers may be transformed toward more tonic activation.

In many neurological conditions it seems as if the patient's postural control is the most affected function. Clinical experience suggests that the patient uses the available strategies to maintain balance, for instance, by fixing with the arms, increasing arm support, or flexing and adducting the hips. When the arms are used for balance, they are being recruited to support the body and are not free for functional use. Normally, phasic activity dominates in the arms due to the need for rapid movement in a variety of contexts. When arm muscles are recruited to maintain stability, the functional demands on arm musculature change and a gradual transformation of muscle fiber type may ensue, contributing to the increased stiffness of the muscles of the arm experienced by some patients.

Muscle length changes occur in pathological conditions of the CNS (Goldspink & Williams 1991; Gray et al 2012). When patients are kept sitting for many hours each day, the hip flexors are kept in a shortened position. The muscle fibers shorten and adapt to the position in which they are being held. This may lead to a reduction of sarcomeres causing the hip flexors to become anatomically shortened. When the patient attempts to stand up or is being transferred through standing by helpers, the shortened muscles experience stretch. The muscle spindles and GTOs inform the spinal cord of the stretch and tension, the α-motor neurons are activated to contract the hip flexors to take the tension off the spindles, and the hip flexors contract too early due to predisposed recruitment. So the patient either lifts the leg off the floor and is thereby destabilized, or is pulled down in the hips and pelvis and is not able to reach a standing position.

Conversely, the patient's hip extensors are in a lengthened position while sitting. As the patients may sit for many hours each day, the hip extensors are passively stretched and are stimulated to "grow" in length. As a result, the number of sarcomeres may increase, which renders the muscle unable to produce an appropriate amount of force to allow the patient to stand up, maintain standing, or stabilize the hip during the stance phase of walking. This is due to overstretch weakness. As a result, the patient may have to use the arms for support during transfers, in standing, and walking. The use of arm support increases the patient's flexor activity (pressing down) through the arms and trunk—the patient therefore attempts to maintain standing through flexor activity and negate extension.

If a patient's arm is kept positioned on a table in front of him or in his lap for long periods every day, there is a danger of the biceps shortening distally. Proximally, the length changes will depend on the position of the shoulder. Triceps will experience prolonged stretch distally and usually shortening proximally. Both ends of the muscle lose their ability to be activated functionally (Ada & Canning 1990).

Inactivity causes the amount of fibrous tissue within the muscle to increase, and the muscle becomes stiffer (Goldspink & Williams 1991; Gray et al 2012). The opposing muscle groups, joint capsule, and ligaments may become stretched, and the stiffness decreases in the stretched muscle. As a result, there may be an imbalance in the supporting tissues and therefore loss of stability. This may negatively affect the patient's ability to move.

Summary

The organization of the CNS is known as parallel distributed processing. See page 10.

Motor activity is the result of a complex interaction between sensory, motor, and cognitive systems. See page 10.

A major function of the perceptual system is to provide the sensory information necessary for our motor actions. See page 11.

Sensory information plays a fundamental role in motor control. See page 11.

Motor activity and sensation are closely linked, and motor activity is a tool of sensation. See page 12.

Somatosensory systems include the receptors and pathways for transmission of sensory information from the body to the portions of the brain that need to integrate this information and act upon it. See page 17.

Stereognosis is also known as haptic perception, and is based on somatosensory information, movement, the ability to recognize variations and perception. See page 13.

In addition to their important role of sensing size, shape, texture, and movement of objects, the mechanoreceptors provide important information for postural control. See page 13.

The muscle spindles inform the CNS continuously of the state of the muscle. The CNS therefore knows at all times about the movement that is about to happen, is happening, or has happened, and compare these. See page 15.

The GTOs detect small changes in muscle tension, and therefore inform the CNS about the state of muscle contraction. See page 16.

The contribution of load and/or length feedback, sensed by GTOs, muscle spindles, joint- and cutaneous receptors, is thought to give important feedback signals for motor control of walking. Heel strike is important for initiation of stance and therefore locomotion. See page 17.

Heel-off is an important signal for the termination of stance, and therefore for the swing phase in locomotion. See page 17.

The transmission of conscious somatosensory information is through two major pathways; the dorsal column–medial lemniscus pathway and the anterolateral system. In addition there are somatosensory pathways to the cerebellum referred to as the ventral and dorsal spinocerebellar tracts. See pages 17-18.

The visual pathways start with the cells in the retina, sending their axons to the thalamus, and end in the visual cortex. See page 20.

Seeing one's own hand improves tactile acuity of the hand—the visual enhancement of touch effect. See page 21.

Prehension (reach and grasp) is coordinated with activity of the eyes. See page 22.

The body schema is a continuously updated sensorimotor map of the body that is important in the context of action. See page 26.

Voluntary movement thus depends on a contribution from many areas of the CNS. See page 27.

The corticospinal tract (CST) is a name given collectively to those fibers that leave the cerebral cortex and descend through the internal capsule to innervate interneurons and motor neurons in the spinal cord without synaptic interruption along the way. See page 28.

The corticospinal system mainly supplies distal musculature. Distal motor control (i.e., dexterity of finger movements and movements of the toes) is an example of voluntary (least automatic) activity. See page 30.

The CST has several functions, including control of voluntary movement, gating sensory input, control of spinal reflex loops, and preparing the spinal cord for movements. It is assumed that the pyramidal fibers arising in SI are as important for the signaling of impulses in sensory pathways as for the initiation of motor activity. See page 30.

The BG are interconnected with all lobes of the cortex and subcortical structures and are organized in several anatomically and functionally different networks. See page 31.

The cerebellum is a major motor structure of the nervous system and can be considered as the area of the brain for behavioral refinement because it regulates the rate, rhythm, and force of behavior to coordinate and refine movement quality. The cerebellum is also linked to sensory processing, and recent research has shown that the cerebellum is also activated by a large number of cognitive tasks that do not involve movement. See page 35.

The reticular formation cooperates with most systems within the CNS and has a role in both proximal and distal movement. It activates both higher and lower levels and functions as an integration system. See page 43.

The PMRF is suggested to be an area of integration of various signals coming from cortical and subcortical structures whereby signals ensure that the postural responses are appropriately scaled in time and magnitude to the planned task. See page 45.

Two descending brain stem pathways have been identified: the ventromedial brain stem pathways and the dorsolateral brain stem pathways. These pathways effectuate the head–body–limb synergies by which locomotion and balance are promoted and are important for the necessary postural and attitudinal adjustments that allow skilled movements of the small muscles of the hands and feet to be executed. See page 45.

The vestibular system processes information about head movement and orientation and plays a vital role in everyday life by giving us our subjective sense of self-motion and orientation, in addition to playing an important role in the stabilization of gaze and the control of balance. See page 46.

The spinal cord is involved in carrying signals between the brain and the rest of the body through several ascending and descending pathways. In addition, it contains both quite basic reflex arcs and more complex neuronal circuits controlling central pattern-generated motor behaviors. See page 50.

Neural networks in the spinal cord, called CPGs are capable of producing rhythmical movements. See page 51.

The limb sensory feedback in regulating the locomotor CPG network is crucial in human locomotion. See page 52.

Muscle fibers are able to alter their fiber type to some degree in relation to use. See page 56.

The length of a muscle is important for movement and function. See page 57.

Motor units are recruited in a sequence, whereby the smaller units are activated before larger motor units. See page 56.

Compartmentalization describes the ability of a muscle that crosses more than one joint to perform different functions simultaneously. See page 56.

Muscle balance depends on muscular, neurological, and biomechanical factors. Alterations in recruitment and the distribution of motor activity affect alignment. Altered alignment affects motor function. See page 57.

Tone is related to the state of the muscle fibers, the activity in the sense organs, muscle viscosity, and connective tissue. The most important cause of tone is muscular contraction. See page 58.

1.3   Motor Learning and Plasticity

▆ Introduction

In 2004, the Academy of Medical Sciences (2004) stated the importance of science for neurorehabilitation: "The last two decades have seen unprecedented advances in neuroscience that have transformed our understanding of the extent to which functional recovery is possible following neural damage, how this recovery takes place and how it may be promoted." The milestone discovery of adult brain plasticity in animals and humans has hugely influenced the theories and concepts applied in neurorehabilitation research and their translation into practice. It is now clear that, rather than being fixed and unalterable, the human brain has the ability for persistent plasticity across the lifespan. The goal of physiotherapy in neurological rehabilitation is to minimize functional disability and optimize functional motor recovery. This is suggested to be achieved by modulation of *plastic changes in the brain*, which is an inherent ability for lifelong skills learning and relearning (Cai et al 2014). Neuroplasticity has been defined as "the ability of the nervous system to respond to intrinsic and extrinsic stimuli by reorganizing its structure, function and connections" (Cramer et al 2011).

Hypotheses about the structure and function of the brain, and its ability for restructuring and repair, were originally based on studies on starfish and frogs. Until relatively recently, the general view was that there was no possibility for repair or change within the CNS after a lesion. Clinically, however, therapists found that many patients improved and learned how to move again, either as they had done before or by using other strategies (Bobath 1990). Scientific research has now shown that the structure of the brain changes and adapts to how it is being used by patients who have suffered a stroke, and that there is a connection between behavior and brain structure after lesions to the CNS (Ward & Cohen 2004). The human brain has a great ability to learn, and learning leads to structural and functional changes, both in a healthy and in a lesioned CNS. Evidence of repetitive behavior producing motor skill acquisition as a result of changes in neural structure and function is now convincing (Richards et al 2008). Functional improvement after CNS lesions is a *relearning process;* during therapy, patients are facilitated through practice to try and reacquire the ability to produce behaviors lost after the damage to their CNS. The human brain will depend on the same neurobiological processes it used to acquire those behaviors initially. One might question whether a CNS with damage to crucial motor networks can respond to motor learning as well as an intact brain. In the immediate weeks after stroke or a lesion to the CNS, the brain's readiness to respond is increased because brain remodeling mechanisms are upregulated (Richards et al 2008). Knowledge of learning-dependent neural plasticity in the intact brain provides us with valuable insight into how the injured brain may adapt during rehabilitation. This is discussed in greater detail later on in this chapter.

The advances in technologies enabling noninvasive exploration of the human brain have increased our understanding of brain reorganization after a CNS lesion. These imaging modalities can be divided into two global categories: functional and structural imaging (Fantini & Aggarwal 2001).

Functional imaging represents a range of measurement techniques in which the aim is to extract quantitative information about physiological function from image-based data, such as fMRI, PET, TMS, EEG, and MEG. Functional imaging techniques make it possible to show different aspects of brain activity as specific images of the changes in the structure of the CNS, which can be correlated with changes in the patient's functional ability after a CNS lesion (Ward & Cohen 2004). This kind of research does have its limitations because the patients need to keep their head still while the image is being taken, but new methods are developing all the time, such as functional near-infrared spectroscopy (fNIRS).

Structural imaging represents a range of measurement modalities that can provide anatomical information. These modalities include X-ray, computed tomography (CT), magnetic resonance imaging (MRI), and diffusion tensor imaging tractography. Diffusion tensor imaging tractography is a recent technique that enables noninvasive visualization of fiber tracts in the human brain in vivo (**Fig. 1.27**).

The fact that we have an ability to learn demonstrates that the function of the nervous system at the synaptic level can be altered by external influences. Plasticity is present on all levels of the CNS, in the peripheral nervous system, and in the musculature (See Motor Unit and Muscle Fiber Plasticity). Plastic adaptation occurs throughout life; on a local, cellular level this may cause substantial transformation of axons, dendrites, the internal environment, synapses, and transmitters. Learning probably causes synaptic changes in many parts of the CNS, with a distribution that is specific to what is being learned (Brodal 2010). For example, motor skill learning is associated with synaptogenesis and dendritic spine plasticity in the motor cortex and the cerebellum, as well as motor map plasticity (Kleim et al 2003; Adkins et al 2006). Experience seems to change neuronal structures and synaptic efficacy, remodels vasculature and glial processes, and alters the rate of neurogenesis (Kleim & Jones 2008).

Neuroplasticity cannot be explained without first understanding the ways in which learning occurs in the noninjured brain. Neurorehabilitation is based on the assumption that principles of motor learning can be applied to motor recovery after injury, and that training can lead to permanent improvements in motor function in patients with motor deficits. Some basic principles of motor learning derived from laboratory studies in healthy subjects are discussed next.

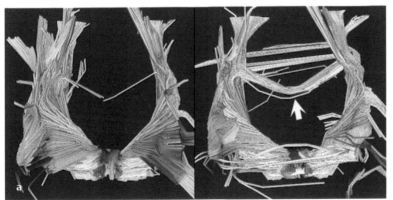

Fig. 1.27 Noninvasive imaging techniques. **(a)** Diffusion tensor imaging (tractography) is an example of a non-invasive brain monitoring technique whereby the anatomy of the brain is being studied. Both the figures demonstrate the same part of brain anatomy with the arrow showing the difference in the size of the fibre paths (tracts) between the two figures. (*Continued*)

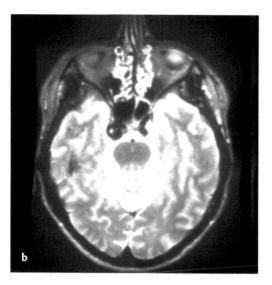

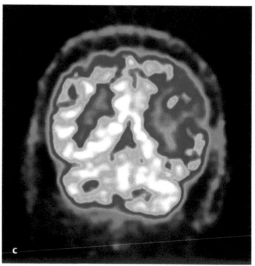

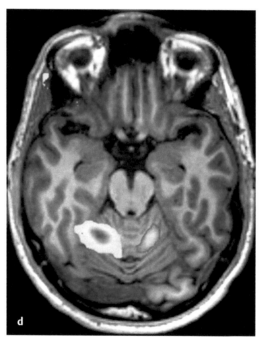

Fig. 1.27 *(continued)* **(b)** Magnetoencephalography. **(c)** Positron emission tomography. **(d)** Functional magnetic resonance imaging.

Motor Learning

The human motor system has the capacity to learn through practice and experience. When the brain learns to perform a movement, it constructs an association between motor commands and sensory feedback. The result of such learning is a (new) internal model of a particular task, which is used to predict the sensory consequences of self-generated action. Motor learning can be regarded as the development of internal models representing an exact match between perceived sensory and motor information (Wolpert et al 1995). The movement pattern will be stored after being learned, and it will be brought back and used in the appropriate context (Bastian 2008). Learning and construction of these internal models are thought to rely on error signals based on feedback from prior performance. Experiments indicate that internal models learned for one type of movement can be transferred to other movements: According to Krakauer (2006), "The importance of the concept of internal models to rehabilitation is that the model can be updated as the state of the limb changes. Thus rehabilitation needs to emphasize techniques that promote formation of appropriate internal models and not just repetition of movements."

Motor learning is a term without a universally accepted definition. However, Lee and Schmidt (2008) describe motor learning as "the process by which the capability for skilled motor control becomes represented in memory. Motor memory is the product of learning." Motor learning includes two distinct types of motor learning (Kitago & Krakauer 2013):

- Motor adaptation.
- Skill acquisition.

Motor adaption is one specific component of motor skill learning (Kitago & Krakauer 2013; Reisman et al 2010). According to Bastian (2008), adaptation can be defined as "the process of adjusting a movement to new demands through trial-and-error practice." A key feature of adaptation is that more practice without the new demand is required to return the movement to its original state. Thus motor adaptation is a "short-term motor learning process" (Bastian 2008). Efficient movement relies largely on the process of adaptation and seems to be important for human behavior and for rehabilitation. Adaptation provides the nervous system with an important flexible control by which predictable changes in the demands of the task can be accounted for. Thus "learned" motor patterns can be adapted to many different situations (Bastian 2008).

The ability to predict error (i.e., the difference between the predicted movement outcome and the actual outcome of the movement) is believed to be the driving force behind adaptation. Adaptive learning is mediated by the cerebellum, and damage to the cerebellum has been found to impair the process of adaptation (Shadmehr et al 2010). This has been shown across many types of movements, including eye movements, arm movements, walking, and balancing (Bastian 2008) (See The Role of the Cerebellum in Motor Learning).

The specific characteristics of errors (e.g., the size of the error) may influence how the learning process occurs (Criscimagna-Hemminger et al 2010). Studies have shown that the bigger the errors during the process of adaptation, the less transfer of learning to natural movements (Orban de Xivry et al 2011). This is supported by Reisman and colleagues (Reisman et al 2007), who used a split-belt treadmill task (one belt is running faster than the other) and demonstrated that a gradual introduction to changes in belt speeds was important in promoting adaptation. Suggesting that learning from small gradual errors is how we mostly learn as adults, not from big errors.

Skill learning relates to the changes that lead to improvements in performance over time (e.g., learning to ride a bicycle) (Shmuelof et al 2012). Adkins and colleagues (Adkins et al 2006) define *skill training* as "the acquisition and subsequent refinement of novel combinations of movement sequences." Motor skill acquisition refers to the process by which movements produced alone or in a sequence are performed effortlessly through repeated practice and interactions with the environment (Doyon & Benali 2005).

Kandel and coworkers (2013) state that behavior is shaped by learning, and that long-term memory, which is the outcome of learning, has at least two forms (**Fig. 1.28**).

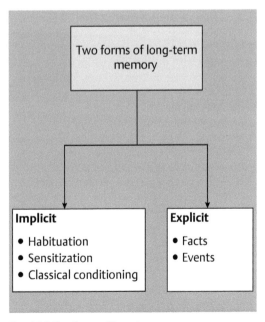

Fig. 1.28 Two forms of long-term memory.

Implicit (nondeclarative or procedural) *memory* is the unconscious memory for perceptual and motor skills (i.e., the memory that cannot be recalled consciously, such as riding a bike); it is inadvertent. Implicit memory demands less attention, is fundamental to relearning most everyday skills, and occurs when the patient is not consciously aware of the components of the task. Implicit learning and memory systems engage areas in the medial temporal lobe, dorsolateral prefrontal cortex, cerebellum, basal ganglia, and sensorimotor cortex. Because of its widespread distribution, the ability to learn implicitly is usually not completely lost following stroke (Levin et al 2009). Implicit memory has many forms—*habituation, sensitization, and classical conditioning*—which have been studied mostly in vertebrates and invertebrates but which are much more complex in humans:

- *Habituation* is a learning process in which the response to a stimulus decreases after repeated exposure to it. This demonstrates that an animal or a human can learn to ignore a stimulus as a result of repeated exposure to it. Habituation involves presynaptic depression of synaptic transmission. There is a decrease in synaptic strength resulting from a decrease in the number of transmitter vesicles released from presynaptic terminals of sensory neurons. The plastic changes in the functional strength of synaptic connections constitute the cellular mechanisms mediating the short-term memory for habituation. Learning can lead to changes in synaptic strength. There is both a short-term and a long-term form, and the duration of the short-term memory storage is determined by the duration of the synaptic change.
- *Sensitization* involves presynaptic enhancement of synaptic transmission and thereby of reflex responses caused by the application of harmful stimuli. It is more complex than habituation because stimuli to one pathway produce a change in another pathway. Repetition of the stimulus decides whether this is a short-term or a long-term change.
- *Classical conditioning* is learning through the association of ideas—associative learning—and involves the pairing of two stimuli. It is a means by which an animal learns to predict events in the environment (Kandel et al 2013). This is dependent on activity in both the pre- and the postsynaptic cell and involves presynaptic facilitation of synaptic transmission. The postsynaptic

component is a retrograde signal from the sensory neuron. Three signals in a sensory neuron must converge to produce the large increase in neurotransmitter release that occurs with classical conditioning; two of which are caused by action potentials to activate chemical processes for the conditioned and unconditioned stimuli. The third is a retrograde signal from the sensory neuron indicating that the postsynaptic cell has been adequately activated by the unconditioned stimulus. These different forms of implicit memory interact and may strengthen each other for longer-lasting enhancement.

Explicit (declarative) *memory* involves conscious recollection of previous experiences and is the acquisition of declarative knowledge of components of a motor action. Explicit learning occurs when the patient is aware of the components of the skill being learned. Explicit instruction can be given prior to practicing a task, for example, when the therapist informs a patient of the steps vital to be able to stand up from sitting. Conversely, a patient can gain explicit awareness during practice of a task through practice without instruction, such as when the patient becomes consciously aware of the steps required to stand up from sitting. Explicit learning and memory are distributed over the medial temporal lobe and the dorsolateral prefrontal cortex (Levin et al 2009; Kandel et al 2013).

Traditionally, therapists often use rational arguments and many verbal instructions to engage patients in motor learning (i.e., they use explicit forms of motor learning). In patients with brain damage this approach is often not feasible.

During learning, reversible physiological changes in synaptic transmission take place in the nervous system; in order for learning to take place these changes must be stabilized or consolidated (Lamprecht & LeDoux 2004). Memory is the *capacity to retain learned information,* and can be divided into *short-* and *long-term* memory on the basis of its duration. The temporary, reversible changes are referred to as short-term memory (STM), or working memory (Kandel et al 2013), and the persistent changes as long-term memory (LTM) (Lamprecht & LeDoux 2004).

Unlike adaptation, which may occur within a single session, motor skill acquisition can be obtained only through extended practice, perhaps after several days, weeks, or even years, depending on the complexity of the task (Kitago & Krakauer 2013). The brain must first process and store short-term memories, which is associated with plastic changes lasting from seconds to minutes and caused by changes in the presynaptic membrane. Long-term memory, however, may last for as long as many weeks and is caused by changes in the postsynaptic membrane. Both these pre- and postsynaptic changes are called *short-term potentiation* (STP) (Kandel et al 2013). Changes lasting as long as months and years are associated with changes in the gene expression in the cell nucleus and are called *long-term potentiation* (LTP) (Kandel et al 2013). Cortical LTP is vital to the enhancement of sensory input, formation of memory, and learning (Carmichael 2010).

Memory consolidation refers to either the stabilization or the enhancement of a motor skill, referred to as off-line learning. Consolidation is the neurological process that involves the gradual transition from short-term memory to long-term memory; this process begins at the synaptic level as the CNS begins to form new pathways, and can occur over a period of days to years. Sleep following motor skill practice has been found to provide an environment in the CNS that promotes several cellular and molecular mechanisms by which the consolidation of memory is enhanced (Siengsukon & Boyd 2009). In young, healthy adults it has been shown that explicit learning and memory are enhanced by sleep. Emerging evidence has demonstrated that people with brain injury also benefit from sleep to enhance off-line consolidation of implicit and explicit motor skill learning (Siengsukon & Boyd 2009).

A basic principle in motor learning is that the degree of performance improvement is dependent on the amount of practice (Krakauer 2006). However, studies on motor learning in neurorehabilitation have shown that, rather than blocked massed practice (repetition of one task), varied repetition (i.e., "repetition without repetition") is more effective for retaining motor learning over time. Variable practice has also been shown to increase generalization of learning to new tasks (Kitago & Krakauer 2013).

Understanding the relevance of the task to be practiced to reach the overall goal may enhance motivation. Selecting relevant treatment goals and including the client in the target-selection process can be expected to increase motivation. The individual's role with regard to society, family, social relations, possibilities, limitations, goals, demands, and needs is important for how an individual develops and learns. How individuals use their body and mind shapes their CNS. Movement, activities, strategies, and patterns of movement determine the connections in the CNS.

▮ Neuroplasticity

Kidd and coworkers (1992) stated that "neuroplasticity is a concept based on the ability of the central nervous system to adapt, rebuild and reorganize itself in relation to its molecular form and function." Kidd introduced the concept *form–function* to reinforce the interdependence between form (structure) and function. The interaction between form and function allows humans the opportunity to develop and meet functional needs. Plastic adaptation is use dependent and the result of our interaction with the environment.

Neuroplasticity has several ways of expressing itself in both the intact and the lesioned CNS, and it occurs at many levels from molecules to cortical reorganization (Johansson 2011). Brodal (2010) describes how experimental data suggest that *use-dependent synaptic plasticity* is the basis for learning and memory. *Synaptic plasticity* implies that the presynaptic action potential leads to an increased release of neurotransmitters, and that the postsynaptic cell changes its response to the same amount of transmitter, or both. A prerequisite for change of the postsynaptic cell is that precise sensory information and modulating transmitters (e.g., those transmitting information about motivation and awareness) hit the synapse at the same moment in time. This explains why motivation is important for structural changes to occur (i.e., for learning). Synaptic activity is based on several factors, and sculpturing of synaptic connections occurs throughout life (Benowitz & Routtenberg 1997). Cellular plasticity may eventually cause system reorganization.

▮ Structural Basis of Neuroplasticity in the Adult Brain

The structural elements that express plasticity in the mature brain include the following (Jellinger & Attems 2013):

- Synaptic efficacy and remodeling.
  - Mechanisms that cause changes in the efficacy and strength of a single synapse.
- Synaptogenesis.
  - Formation of synapses in the CNS.
- Collateral axonal sprouting and dendritic remodeling.
- Neurogenesis and recruitment from neural progenitor cells.

The following processes manifest plasticity:
- Anterograde and retrograde transport.
- Cell interactions (neuron–glia).
- Neuronal networks and related activities.

■ Factors That Determine Plasticity in the Human Brain

Neuroplasticity depends on *gene expression, neurotrophic factors, axonal transport, collateral sprouting, neurogenesis, glial cells,* and probably many more factors.

Gene Expression

All cells of the body have a complete set of genes. The different genes have different functions expressing skin, hair, nails, eyes, different types of muscle fibers, different types of nerve cells, and so on. The fact that nails become nails is a result of expression of the nail gene only—the other genes in the nail cells are silent. This is called gene expression (Martin & Magistretti 1998; Brodal 2010).

The term *genotype* refers to the complete genetic constitution of an organism as decided by the specific combination and localization of the genes on the chromosomes. Organisms with the same genetic makeup belong to the same genotype. The human race, *Homo sapiens,* constitutes a genotype (Harris et al 2010). As humans, we have a common inheritance that allows us to balance and walk on two legs and at the same time use our arms and hands for functional activities. Humans are the only genotype to have developed these fundamental abilities, which are the basis for the intellectual development of the human race (Eccles 1990). Individuals inherit a unique combination of genes from their parents, and each person develops through the interaction of nature and nurture to a unique phenotype.

The *phenotype* is defined as the complete observable characteristics of an organism, and includes anatomical, physiological, biochemical, and behavioral aspects, formed by the interaction between the genetic makeup of the individual and the environment (Harris et al 2010). Each individual has an inherent ability to develop and express genes in his or her own, unique way. Therefore, as individuals we move differently, behave differently, and have different talents that we develop in our own ways—each person is unique. We do, however, have a common repertoire of movement that is expressed individually. The ability to learn is the basis for individual and specific characteristics of physical and intellectual abilities. Lasting plastic changes are a result of altered gene expression.

Several scientists describe changes in the CNS as activity dependent (Seil 1997; Martin & Magistretti 1998; Brodal 2010; Ward & Cohen 2004).

> Environmental influences and stimuli direct plasticity and thereby learning.

Neurotrophic Factors

There are many proteins responsible for growth, development, and programmed cell death (apoptosis) in the CNS. Together these are called the *neurotrophic factors* (also referred to as neurotrophins). There are many different types of neurotrophic factors; for instance, nerve growth factor (NGF), growth-associated protein (GAP-43/B-50), brain-derived neurotrophic factor (BDNF), and more are being discovered all the time. The production of these proteins is guided through gene expression; they are present at all times in the nervous system, but levels are higher during development and when the need for regeneration and reorganization is at its greatest.

Neurotrophic factors influence and guide (Stein et al 1997; Butz et al 2009) the following:
- Collateral sprouting and regeneration.
- Survival of damaged neurons.
- Neuronal death (apoptosis).
- New terminals and growth cones of axons.
- Formation, maintenance, and transmission across new synapses.
- Inhibition of the named processes.

Neurotrophic factors are necessary for the process of learning. Physiological activity in the form of training, exercise, and daily activity stimulates the release of neurotrophic substances; activity maintains the production, and inactivity reduces production (Agnati et al 1992; Bailey & Kandel 1993; Olson 1996). These factors stimulate nerve cell metabolism, nerve fiber growth, and activity-driven changes in synaptic efficacy. They depend on retrograde signals from the postsynaptic to the presynaptic cell. The CNS is influenced by motor activity; how movement is performed, i.e. how our body moves and is used, as well as activity in general.

Neurotrophins promote recovery after a lesion in the CNS by enhancing (Ergul et al 2012) the following:
- Angiogenesis (the formation of new blood vessels from preexisting vessels).

- Neurogenesis (generation of neurons).
- Synaptogenesis (the formation of synapses between neurons).
- Neuronal plasticity.

The beneficial effects of angiogenesis after a lesion to the CNS may be negatively impacted by premorbid disease, as is seen in diabetes and hypertension (Ergul et al 2012). Patients with Alzheimer's disease and Parkinson's disease have reduced neuroplasticity as a result of diminished growth factor expression (Jellinger & Attems 2013).

> Activity and movement facilitate plastic changes in the CNS, both positively **and** negatively.

■ Axonal Transport

Nerve fibers, or axons, contain axoplasm. The axoplasm moves at various speeds in the axon by a process called *axoplasmic flow* in two directions and carries particles with it (Olson 1996; Benowitz & Routtenberg 1997):

- *Anterograde axonal transport*—from the cell body to the synapses.
- *Retrograde axonal transport*—from the synapse and back to the cell body.

These axonal transport mechanisms represent adaptations of mechanisms that facilitate the intracellular transport of organelles in all secretory cells (Kandel et al 2013). Particles are actively transported in a start-and-stop (salutary) fashion along linear tracks aligned with the main axis of the axon. Axonal transport is a type of information transmission between neurons in addition to *action potentials* (Kidd et al 1992). Retrograde transport is also used to deliver signals back to the cell body (Kandel et al 2013). Action potentials may influence the speed of transport of the particles that the CNS needs for development, learning, and reorganization.

> Motor activity may facilitate axonal transport.

Axonal transport has an important role in regeneration and reorganization of the CNS and the neuromuscular system. All plastic changes in the nervous system depend on trophic processes. Axonal transport is responsible for moving proteins and other particles to and from the cell bodies to the synapses.

Activated growth factor receptors are thought to be carried along the axon by retrograde transport to their site of action in the nucleus, and, for instance, cytoskeletal matrix is transported anterograde. *Synthesis* is the production of complex substances from simple ones through chemical processes. Protein synthesis in the CNS is essential for gene expression and learning.

Through retrograde transport the cell bodies are informed of activity at the synapses and the postsynaptic cells and about the effect caused by the presynaptic cells. The presynaptic cell may then, based on this form of feedback, alter its synaptic effect if necessary (Brodal 2010). The effector cells thereby have an important influence on the neurons innervating them and may inform the CNS about what information they need. The state of the muscles is, therefore, important for the function of the CNS, and the activity of motor neurons is essential for the maintenance of the structure of the motor end plate and the metabolism of the muscle. The motor end plate, the density and distribution of specific receptors within the muscle, and the functional characteristics of the muscle fiber types may be changed through direct stimulation (Troen & Edgar 1982).

> Muscular activity enhances the transport and production of neurotrophic substances. Stimulation may cause changes in the metabolism, structure, and function of muscle.

■ Collateral (Axonal) Sprouting

Axons may sprout as buds on a tree (**Fig. 1.29**). This is called *axonal* or *collateral sprouting* and is present in both intact and lesioned nervous systems. If a nerve cell is damaged through a CNS lesion, its axon degenerates from distal to proximal and leaves behind empty synaptic sites where they previously made contact. This happens on all levels in the nervous system. Undamaged axons nearby are stimulated to sprout through reactive synaptogenesis or reactive reinnervation by neurotrophic substances that are released as a response to damage. Retrograde axonal transport carries information about activated growth factor receptors that may stimulate the formation of a growth cone on the axon. GAP-43/B-50 is a protein released by nerve cells with empty synaptic sites. The ensuing branches, or

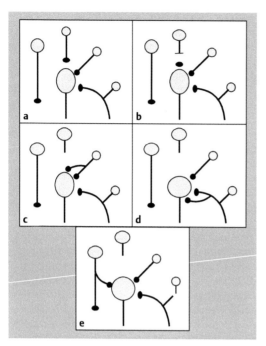

Fig. 1.29 Simplified illustration of the formation of new synapses through collateral sprouting. **(a)** Normal situation. **(b)** Damage leads to degeneration of axons from distal to proximal. **(c)** Sprouting from an interneuron. **(d)** Sprouting from an afferent (sensory) fiber. **(e)** Sprouting from a descending fiber.

the collaterals, seek new contact sites to form new synapses where the old ones have been lost (Hallett 1995; Lee & van Donkelaar 1995). The new connections will not restore the original pattern of innervation (Brodal 2010); they may use other neurotransmitters, and may therefore be unable to fully reestablish lost function.

The effect of collateral sprouting may not always be positive; it may not lead to normalization of control of movement or other lost functions (Brodal 2010). If the collateral sprouts arise from sensory neurons, the patient may become hypersensitive to peripheral stimuli. Collateral sprouting is not necessarily a result of learning; experimentally, collateral sprouts from nearby axons may form new synapses due to the release of local trophic factors. Whether they are retained would seem to depend on whether they are being used (i.e., stimulated) and whether the organism experiences them as appropriate. If the patient attempts to move appropriately, a secondary change of the first random contacts may result. These may

become more permanent and contribute to more—or less—appropriate patterns of movement.

> Both appropriate and inappropriate movement may be learned.

■ Neurogenesis

Until the early 1990s, it was believed that there was no regeneration of nerve cells in the adult brain. Since then, new regenerated nerve cells—stem cells—have been found in the hippocampus, which is the memory center of the brain (Eriksson et al 1998; Kempermann et al. 1998; Jellinger & Attems 2013). Neuroplasticity in the adult brain is therefore not restricted to structural modifications at the level of axons, dendrites, and synapses, but also includes generation, differentiation, and maturation of new neurons in limited brain regions (Faralli et al 2013; Cayre et al 2009).

All damage to the CNS initiates an endogenous neuroprotective response by which neuroplasticity and neurogenesis are combined. This response is initiated and modulated by neurotrophic factors (Jellinger & Attems 2013). Several studies have shown that an ischemic CNS lesion leads to an increase in proliferation of neural stem cells, and is followed by an increase in the generation of new neurons in the subgranular zone of the dentate gyrus (regions in the hippocampal formation) and in the subventricular zone (Greenberg 2007; Chen et al 2010; Komitova et al 2006). Neurogenesis continues throughout life but declines with increasing age due to a reduction of the proportion of neuronal stem cells that may become mature neurons. Exercise has been shown to increase neurogenesis in the dentate gyrus of the hippocampus (van Praag 2009).

Neural progenitor stem cells give rise to neurons, astrocytes, and oligodendrocytes, and have an inherent plasticity providing self-renewal and differentiation. Indeed, studies of animal models have shown that neural stem cells can specifically replace populations of diseased or damaged cells, in some cases leading to behavioral recovery (Hori et al 2003).

■ The Contribution of Glial Cells to Postlesion Plasticity and Repair

Plasticity is not exclusively a function of neurons but a shared function by which the astrocytes contribute. Astrocytes participate in several functions that are central to development, function, and repair of the CNS (see The Building Blocks of the CNS). Nearly half of the cells in the human brain are astrocytes that have an intimate association with synapses throughout the adult CNS, where they help regulate ion and neurotransmitter concentrations. Recent studies have found that astrocytes also exert powerful control over the number of synapses that forms within the CNS; that they are essential for postsynaptic function; and that they are required for synaptic stability and maintenance (Faralli et al 2013). Moreover, astrocytes are participants in activity-dependent structural and functional synaptic changes throughout the nervous system (Ullian et al 2004; Faralli et al 2013). It has been proposed that astrocytes should not be viewed primarily as support cells, but rather as cells that actively control the structural and functional plasticity of synapses in developing and mature organisms. In addition, they might promote neuronal survival, synaptic remodeling, and synaptogenesis (Faralli et al 2013). Glial cells are excitable and communicate with other cells (Diniz et al 2014).

Cortical Plasticity

A cortical response to sensory input, experience, and training as well as to brain lesions, is reorganization of the cortical representation areas (cortical maps) (Johansson 2004). A variety of neurological phenomena underlie the modification (i.e., plasticity) of cortical maps, including recovery of function after brain or peripheral nerve injury but also phantom pain and sensation after amputation (Johansson 2004). Reorganization of cortical maps and behavioral abilities appear to be interrelated, and the study of these mechanisms is of vital importance for our understanding of the process of recovery after central and peripheral nervous system injury (Dancause & Nudo 2011).

There has been extensive research into cortical plasticity. A seminal study by Nudo and colleagues (1996b) has received intense attention because it demonstrated that the elbow and shoulder areas of the motor cortex learned to take over the control of hand movements after intensive training in monkeys who were inflicted by a stroke in the hand area of the motor cortex. Many later studies have shown that the cortex has a significant ability for functional and structural plasticity, and the notion that input and output properties in cor-

tical sensory and motor areas are plastic throughout life is now widely accepted and is generalizable across all cortical regions (Dancause & Nudo 2011). MRI studies have demonstrated activity-dependent responses in brain structure; for instance, London taxi drivers have developed an increased volume in the hippocampus, which is thought to be related to spatial navigation, which was found to be correlated with the amount of time that the drivers spent in navigating the streets of London (Chen et al 2010). Moreover, piano players and Braille readers have larger representations in the motor areas of the cortex representing manipulative skills (dexterity, fine motor activity) than the average population (see **Fig. 1.11**). Lack of sensory input leads to cortical remodeling, in turn leading to a distorted cortical representation with enlarged and overlapping cortical receptive fields. For example, people with an amputation have larger representation areas for body parts proximal to the amputation than the average population. Altered somatosensory perception causes changes in the functional architecture in the brain, and activity is needed to sculpt the connections that form the neural representations (Bailey & Kandel 1993). Reorganization of cortical areas can occur rapidly after changes in peripheral input (Johansson 2004). Huber and colleagues (2006) demonstrated that only a short period of immobilization is needed to bring about cortical plastic changes. In their study, immobilization of the upper limb for 12 hours induced significant changes in somatosensory-evoked potentials (SEPs) (a noninvasive method of assessing the functioning of the somatosensory system) and the amplitude of motor-evoked potentials (MEPs) (recorded from muscles following direct stimulation of the exposed motor cortex, or transcranial stimulation of the motor cortex). Today it is well known that both limb nonuse and immobilization induce corticomotor depression, which is reflected by a decrease of excitability of motor areas (Huber et al 2006; Avanzino et al 2011), and clearly indicates the importance of early onset of sensory-relearning and stimulation for a patient with a CNS lesion.

Cortical reorganization is not simply due to increased or decreased use; repetitive motor activity alone is not sufficient to produce plastic changes in cortical motor maps. Several studies demonstrate that the type of training matters for cortical plasticity. For example, motor skill learning in animals has been shown to alter the topography of representations in the motor cortex, demonstrating that movements which are used in a newly learned task are represented over larger cortical territories (Adkins et al 2006). The cortical areas associated with the sensorimotor function of the body parts that are most active in the skill training have an increase in the number of connections and/or size because of new learning (Nudo 2003; Ward & Cohen 2004). Skill training is associated with an increased area of representation, increased synaptic density, increased number of synapses, as well as increased thickness of the cortical motor areas, probably due also to angiogenesis (more blood vessels, increased blood flow) (Nudo 2003). TMS has been used to show learning-dependent neural plasticity in the human motor cortex associated with skill training; subjects who trained on a piano-playing task with five fingers demonstrated an increase in the motor cortical area representing the trained hand muscles as well as increased MEP amplitudes; human subjects trained in a skilled ankle movement demonstrated an increase in movement representation areas and increased MEP amplitude of the trained muscles in comparison to untrained controls (Kleim 2011); and fMRI studies have shown that subjects learning skilled finger movements demonstrate changes in the motor cortex, cerebellum, and BG (Chen et al 2010).

The sensory and motor cortices have a significant ability for reorganization throughout life, both in an intact CNS and after damage (as long as degenerative disease does not disrupt the ability to change). Therefore, there are considerable possibilities for functional plasticity in the human adult neuromuscular system. Nudo (2011) describes several mechanisms for the reorganization in both somatosensory and motor cortices:

- Unmasking of existing but functionally inactive pathways: This process depends on neurons or neural pathways having a much larger region of anatomical connectivity than their usual territory of functional influence. Some zones may be kept in check by tonic inhibition. If the inhibition is removed (e.g., after a stroke), the region of influence can be quickly increased or unmasked.
- Collateral sprouting and the formation of new synapses: Collateral dendritic sprouting plays a role in long-term cortical remodeling.
- Reorganization of adult cortical areas, which is thought to involve LTP and LTD: LTP and LTD are permanent changes in synaptic strength. LTP is a form of activity-dependent plasticity resulting in a lasting improvement of synaptic

transmission, and is input specific (changes can be brought about at one set of synapses without affecting other synapses). LTD is the opposite process to LTP and results in a long-lasting decrease in synaptic efficacy. Storage of information is enabled by these two mechanisms (Johansson 2004).

▪ Plasticity in the Spinal Cord

There is now a solid basis of knowledge from studies demonstrating plasticity at various levels and locations within the CNS following SCI (Onifer et al 2011). The plasticity of spinal neuronal circuits is also task specific and use dependent.

After an SCI, neuroplasticity depends on multiple factors: the level and extent of injury, postinjury medical and surgical care, and rehabilitative interventions (Lynskey et al 2008).

Adaptive changes within spared neuronal circuits may occur, both above and below a spinal lesion, at the cortical, brain stem, cerebellar, or spinal cord level (Darian-Smith 2009). Almost half of all SCIs are functionally incomplete, meaning that there is some sparing of function below the level of the lesion (Lam et al 2008). The potential for functional recovery is higher in incomplete SCIs than in the completely severed spinal cord (Lam et al 2008).

Following an incomplete SCI collaterals sprout from intact and injured axons in the neighborhood of the lesion (Rank et al 2015). These sprouts are assumed to make new synaptic contacts bypassing the lesion and contribute to improved functional recovery. These plastic changes are enhanced by exercise training (Rank et al 2015).

The short and long PSNs may also be important following spinal injury. It has been recently demonstrated that severed reticulospinal fibers spontaneously sprout and form contacts onto a plastic propriospinal relay, thereby bypassing the lesion (Rossignol & Frigon 2011).

Exercise and training have profound effects on cellular and molecular functions involved in plasticity (Cotman et al 2007). Treadmill training is the most studied training parameter to promote plasticity in SCI using body weight support (BWS) techniques to allow for gait training to promote plasticity in an activity-dependent manner. BWS gait training can start before the patient is able to fully bear weight and prior to developing adequate motor control.

Sensory inputs play a crucial role in the regulation of normal locomotion, which can be altered after SCI (Rossignol & Frigon 2011). The spinal cord circuitry is highly sensitive to proprioceptive and cutaneous inputs, and treadmill training might therefore be used to "reprogram" existing circuitry in the spinal cord (Onifer et al 2011). In addition, sensory information is important in shaping CPG function and in guiding postlesional plasticity mechanisms (Molinari 2009). An important parameter for training is to provide sensory stimuli that closely match normal conditions (i.e., appropriate sensory cues). Treadmill training may help to engage the spinal circuitry with sensory input associated with weight bearing and stepping, which is essential to activate the locomotor circuitry so that effective locomotion may be regained (Molinari 2009). Weight bearing and ground contact are essential for leg muscle activation; therefore, full BWS in complete paraplegic patients does not lead to significant muscle activation (Dietz 2002).

Human walking does not only involve the ability to move the legs; it also requires the coordination of neural commands to regulate upright balance and posture, as well as the ability to adapt gait to context. Therefore the recovery of postural control is a prerequisite for the recovery of locomotion after SCI. However, the effects of SCI on postural mechanisms have been much less investigated than the effects on stepping (Boulenguez & Vinay 2009).

Also, the essential sensory cues that may be provided from treadmill training through loading of the body and hip joint afferents require a focus on trunk muscle activation to keep an upright posture.

Plastic changes within the brain can be maladaptive, which is also the case in the spinal cord; for example, changes in pain pathways are involved in the post-injury development of neuropathic pain and allodynia (Onifer et al 2011). Other maladaptive changes due to plasticity following SCI include autonomic dysreflexia and spasticity (Onifer et al 2011).

Theories of Recovery after a CNS Lesion

Several mechanisms have been hypothesized to contribute to the process of functional recovery and can generally be categorized into two main stages: (1) spontaneous reorganization; and (2) training-induced recovery (Chen et al 2010). Recovery after brain damage in *the absence of interventions* is often referred to as a *spontaneous recovery*. Spontaneous recovery after stroke is generally said to plateau roughly at about 3 months postlesion (Kwakkel et al 2006), and after traumatic brain injury (TBI) approximately 6 months postinjury (Nakamura et al 2009). Three processes have been theorized to explain spontaneous recovery after injury (Dancause & Nudo 2011):

- Resolution of diaschisis.
- Compensation.
- Substitution.

Training-induced recovery is not time limited, has been observed years after injury, and is dependent on many factors, including individual experience and motivation. Depending on the stage of recovery, different neural mechanisms contribute to initiate recovery strategies, or they occur as a response to changes in experience (e.g., rehabilitation).

Resolution of Diaschisis

Brain regions remote to the damaged area show a reduction of function after an acute brain lesion due to a number of pathological changes in metabolism, blood flow, inflammation, edema, and neuronal excitability, which are particularly evident during the acute phase (Kleim 2011). These mechanisms are jointly referred to as *diaschisis* (Pekna et al 2012): activity in an area that is distant but anatomically connected to the lesioned region is depressed due to an interrupted functional input from the injured area. It is thought that at least some of the early functional recovery observed in both animal models and human stroke survivors may be due to the resolution of diaschisis (Dancause & Nudo 2011).

A role for the cerebellum in mediating functional recovery from stroke has been described (Makin et al 2013). Data suggest that patients with good recovery have clear changes in the activation of the cerebellar hemisphere opposite the injured CST, suggesting a possible link between cerebellar activation and behavioral recovery from hand paresis following a stroke. The underlying mechanism is not known, but it could be due to hemodynamic changes, such as diaschisis, or to the postulated role of the cerebellum in motor skill learning (Small et al 2002).

Compensation

After a CNS lesion the brain learns to use other sources of information for movement or different movement strategies to reach a movement goal

(Brodal 2010). *Motor compensation* refers to the use of new movements or movement sequences to perform a task in a different way from that used prior to injury (Kleim 2011). Compensatory use of muscles or movement patterns is commonly seen in humans after stroke. For example, excessive trunk movement, scapular elevation, shoulder abduction, and internal rotation of the glenohumeral joint may be used to compensate for upper limb impairment after a brain lesion. Compensatory movement of the lower limb may involve increased use of the least affected leg to stand up from sitting, excessive use of a walking aid instead of weight bearing on two legs, or hip hiking and circumduction to swing the leg forward during walking. To achieve early functional independence, a patient with a brain lesion may be encouraged to compensate for deficient motor control, where focus is on achievement of a task no matter how it is accomplished, and not on efficient and qualitative aspects of movement. It is possible that this focus on early independence achieved by compensatory movement strategies is limiting the individual's long-term potential for improvement in bodily function and structure and thereby activity. If a patient in the acute phase after stroke is not using the affected limb and relies solely on compensatory strategies, the patient may miss out on a time window of plasticity within which true recovery could be maximized (Levin et al 2009) (for greater detail see Maladaptive Plasticity and Motor Recovery after CNS Lesions).

■ Substitution

Various mechanisms of plasticity underlying functional recovery are included in the *theory of vicariation*, which refers to the ability of one part of the brain to substitute for the function of another (Brodal 2010). This mechanism may not be able to fully restore network function to prelesion level (Brodal 2010). The theory of vicariation of function involves recognition of several physiological processes, such as the unmasking of previously present but functionally inactive connections, collateral sprouting, synaptogenesis, and denervation hypersensitivity.

■ The Role of the Undamaged Hemisphere to Recovery

Normally, the two cerebral hemispheres are functionally coupled and balanced; however, recent studies have shown that a unilateral lesion, such as that caused by a stroke, may disrupt this balance, causing competitive interactions between the hemispheres that influence experience-dependent plasticity. In the subacute stage after a stroke, a reduction in motor cortex excitability and a decrease in the cortical representation area of paretic muscles have been found to occur in the affected hemisphere near the site of the injury (Bütefisch et al 2006). Furthermore, human fMRI and PET studies following a stroke have demonstrated increases activity in the contralesional (undamaged) hemisphere (Dancause & Nudo 2011). This interhemispheric imbalance is known as the hypothesis of *interhemispheric competition* (Allred & Jones 2008; Dancause & Nudo 2011; Takeuchi & Izumi 2012). In this hypothesis, the loss of neural tissue in the ipsilesional hemisphere results in a decrease of interhemispheric inhibition from the ipsilesional hemisphere. Excessive interhemispheric inhibition shifts activation of behavior over to the undamaged cortex (Allred & Jones 2008), which contributes negatively to diaschisis and may result in reduced motor activation and possibly decreased potential for recovery of the impaired body parts (Dancause & Nudo 2011; Jones et al 2009; Calautti et al 2010; Allred et al 2014). To counter this, blocking or reducing this maladaptive plasticity with noninvasive brain stimulation (NIBS) techniques like repetitive transcranial magnetic stimulation (rTMS) and transcranial direct current stimulation (tDCS) have been used (Raffin & Siebner 2014). The goal of treatment with noninvasive brain stimulation is to restore the excitability of the lesioned hemisphere and decrease the overactivity of the nonlesioned hemisphere (Mally 2014). Kheder and coworkers (Khedr et al 2009) showed that 5 days of noninvasive brain stimulation given to patients with acute stroke to inhibit the contralesional hemisphere increased the ipsilesional output to the paretic upper limb and enhanced recovery. The effects were still present 3 months after treatment. These findings suggest that the competitive interactions between the hemispheres influence experience-dependent plasticity. Excessive excitability of the unaffected hemisphere, activated by the use of the nonparetic limb, may inhibit the affected hemisphere through abnormal interhemispheric inhibition. To prevent this maladaptive plasticity, it is necessary to avoid excessive use of compensatory movement, which may limit genuine motor recovery after stroke; in other words, compensatory use of the intact body side can negatively influence the recovery of the most impaired side with unfortunate effects for any residual capacity in the impaired body side, including that which might eventually be realized with appropriate rehabilitative training (Allred & Jones 2008).

■ Functional Improvement after Brain Damage

Functional improvement in the damaged brain occurs due to two mechanisms: *recovery and compensation* (Kleim 2011). The terms *recovery* and *compensation* are not well defined, neither in the literature nor in the clinical field (Levin et al 2009). The term *recovery* has been used both to refer to restitution of damaged structures or functions within the CNS and to describe clinical improvement. Different understandings of terms used may confuse interdisciplinary communication; thus, in order to be meaningful for neurorehabilitation we are in need of clear definitions, by which neuroscientists and therapists can use a common language with clearly defined terms. Kleim (2011) suggests that, to differentiate *recovery* from *compensation* at neural and behavioral levels requires an understanding of the association between neural plasticity and rehabilitation-dependent changes in function. A clear definition will allow insight into the specific neural strategies that the individual patient employs or can be guided toward in the rehabilitation process. Considering motor function, Levin et al (2009) suggested definitions for both recovery and compensation using the framework of the World Health Organization (WHO); the International Classification of Functioning, Disability and Health (ICF) (**Table 1.1**). ICF differentiates between the underlying pathophysiology of the health condition, impairments in the body domain, and disability in the activity domain (see Chapter 3 for further discussion of ICF), thereby recovery and compensation can be understood at both behavioral and neural levels.

Levin and colleagues (2009) define recovery and compensation with regard to motor performance within the ICF framework (**Table1.1**):
1. Health condition (neural level).
2. Body functions and structure (performance).
3. Activity (functional).

Most researchers studying neuronal plasticity and brain reorganization after stroke agree on the definition of recovery and compensation at the neuronal level. However, this is not the case when it comes to the bodily and activity domains. Many studies use functional tests or assessments of patients' ability to perform activities of daily living (ADLs) as their outcome measures. These tests do not measure quality of movement, thus they cannot differentiate between recovery of impairment or recovery due to development of compensatory strategies (Kitago & Krakauer 2013). Consequently, this may result in confounding interpretations of the efficacy of different treatment interventions and misleading results (Levin et al 2009).

■ Maladaptive Plasticity and Motor Recovery after CNS Lesions

Injury and excessive training may drive neural plasticity in a maladaptive direction, referred to as "maladaptive plasticity," and contribute to the pathogenesis of phantom pain and dystonia, new-onset epilepsy, and autonomic dysreflexia after SCI as well as the gradual development of hyperreflexia and clonus (Cramer et al 2011; Ferguson et al 2012).

Maladaptive plasticity has been found to weaken motor function and limit motor recovery after stroke (Takeuchi & Izumi 2012; Takeuchi & Izumi 2013). Compensatory movement strategies, activated ipsilateral motor projections, and competitive hemispheric interaction after a lesion in the CNS can contribute to maladaptive plasticity (Allred et al 2010; Jones et al 2009; Takeuchi & Izumi 2013).

Learned Nonuse
Repeated failed attempts to use the affected limb have been hypothesized to underlie a worsening of the impairment by *learned nonuse*, which refers to conditions in which reduced motor control leads to further inactivity of the affected limb; for example, reduced control of the affected arm in hemiplegia may lead to compensatory strategies whereby a patient uses the least affected arm to compensate for loss of function in the most affected arm. The most affected arm is therefore not used, not stimulated, and increasingly inactivated, leading to shrinking of the motor map representation area in the lesioned hemisphere. This predisposes to secondary muscular and soft tissue changes (Ada & Canning 1990). At the same time, the least affected limb is used more than normal, and the motor map of this limb increases in size. Thus experience (or lack thereof) impacts on the cortical representations of MI during the stage of spontaneous recovery. Learned nonuse may also contrib-

Table 1.1 Text definitions of motor recovery and motor compensation at 3 different levels

Level	Recovery	Compensation
ICF: Health Condition (neuronal)	*Restoring function in neural tissue that was initially lost after injury* This may be seen as reactivation in brain areas previously inactivated by the circulatory event. Although this is not expected to occur in the area of the primary brain lesion, it may occur in areas surrounding the lesion (penumbra) and in the diaschisis	*Neural tissue acquires a function that it did not have prior to injury.* May be seen as activation in alternative brain areas not normally observed in nondisabled individuals
ICF: Body Functions/Structure (performance)	*Restoring the ability to perform a movement in the same manner as it was performed before injury.* This may occur through the reappearance of premorbid movement patterns during task accomplishment (voluntary joint range of motion, temporal and spatial inter joint coordination, etc.)	*Performing an old movement in a new manner.* May be seen as the appearance of alternative movement patterns (i.e., recruitment of additional or different degrees of freedom, changes in muscle activation patterns such as increased agonist/antagonist co-activation, delays in timing between movements of adjacent joints, etc.) during the accomplishment of a task
ICF: Activity (functional)	*Successful task accomplishment using limbs or end effectors typically used by nondisabled individuals[a]*	*Successful task accomplishment using alternate limbs or end effectors.* For example, opening a package of chips using one hand and the mouth instead of two hands

ute to interhemispheric imbalance (Takeuchi & Izumi 2012).

Sleep and Neural Plasticity

Sleep and synaptic plasticity seem to be strongly related. Sleeping seems to restore synaptic plasticity because different processes of synaptic remodeling seem to occur during sleep and may have a positive effect on recovery processes (Gorgoni et al 2013).

The promotion of sleep between therapy sessions may be important for consolidation of memory and therefore for learning.

> Motor training leads to reorganization of sensorimotor areas of the cortex.

Clinical Relevance

A CNS lesion works a sudden and dramatic change in a person's life situation. The physical and psycho-

logical consequences are serious for individuals and their family. Physically, even the simplest of tasks, such as sitting independently, or more complex activities, such as toileting and dressing, are difficult. The CNS is therefore driven to learn as quickly as possible to meet these functional needs.

Plasticity of the CNS leads to the potential for some degree of functional recovery as the learning ability of patients who have suffered an acute CNS lesion is heightened. Within the CNS, synapses need to be provided with the correct sensory information to guide the formation of useful connections. Work by Nudo and coworkers (1996a) and others has clearly demonstrated that the brain expansion in the monkey's hand representation area was counteracted by training-induced reorganization of areas adjacent to the lesion. Furthermore, several studies of use-dependent cortical reorganization have supported that training needs to be intense and behaviorally relevant to induce cortical reorganization (Demain et al 2006; Takeuchi & Izumi 2013).

The interaction between form and function influences plastic mechanisms; thus motor recovery and plasticity are dependent on the nature of motor rehabilitation. A major challenge is to match the right patients with the right training approach; interventions that aim to promote plasticity can be expected to have a maximum impact when coupled with optimal training and experience.

Knowledge of plasticity gives hope, along with considerable responsibility, to the health professionals caring for people with CNS dysfunction. Caregivers influence the patient through mutual interaction and play an important role in shaping the reorganization of the patient's CNS, and thereby the progress of the patient's abilities. Learning may lead to positive or negative developments in both physical function and behavior. How patients use their body, how they move or are moved by others, will influence the restructuring of the nervous and muscular systems. If a patient twists and turns on one leg as he transfers from a chair to the bathroom, while the arm flexes uncontrollably, this will be what the CNS learns. If an action is repeated time and time again, learning is established through functional and structural plastic changes in the CNS. Some authors suggest a time frame for the most acute plastic changes after a CNS lesion (Nudo & Milliken 1996a; Seil 1997). These studies were done mainly on animals (cat, rat, monkey), but some were functional imaging studies (PET, fMRI, among others) on humans after a lesion to the nervous system. The following discussion refers to these time frames, which are broad, with ample room for individual interpretation depending on the patient's premorbid status and general condition, as well as the type, location, and size of the lesion.

Acutely postlesion, the CNS is in shock, which may last for 2 to 3 days and may be caused by direct neuronal damage and increased inhibitory activity to protect the CNS from further damage. Changes in cortical and spinal function begin after a few hours as follows:

- The level of neurotrophic substances increases.
- Latent synapses and connections are activated.
- Synaptic strength increases (LTP).
- Denervation supersensitivity develops.

Initial restitution starts early, probably due to reabsorption of edema and degradation of necrotic tissue, and may last for days and possibly weeks depending on the size of the lesion. There is a gradual transition from the acute to the subacute and later stages.

The changes in activity and function observed in the patient after 3 to 4 weeks may be due to neuroplastic changes in the form of the following:

- Synaptic changes.
- Reorganization of cortical maps.
- Further unmasking.
  - Redundancy.
  - Collateral sprouting (starts after a few days).
- The formation of new connections also at the spinal level.

Clinical experience demonstrates that many patients suffering from stroke, head injury, MS, and so forth, may be hypersensitive to stimuli. Unexpected sounds, unrest, anxiety, fear of falling, and sudden or insensitive handling are examples of situations where the patient's tone may increase uncontrollably and may contribute toward the development of spasticity (Craik 1991; Stephenson 1993). Demands for activity that surpass the patient's balance and motor abilities and lead to malalignment during the performance of activities are a major feature in this regard. "Functional recovery after CNS injury may depend, in part, upon reorganization of undamaged neural pathways. Spinal cord circuits are capable of significant reorganization in the form of both activity-dependent and injury-induced plasticity" (Muir & Steeves 1997; Oudega & Perez 2012; Lynskey et al 2008). Neuronal circuits, stimulated by the specific activation of peripheral sensory afferents via training, can reorganize by strengthening existing and earlier inactive descending connections and local neural circuits (Bose et al 2012).

Clinically, therapists encounter changes in the viscosity of muscle, contractures, altered alignment and pattern of recruitment, edema, and reduced circulation and metabolism, which have a negative effect on muscular activity. As well as the physical limitations to the repertoire of movement, axonal transport may be reduced through inactivity. Improvement of the aforementioned factors should improve axonal transport and stimulate the production and transport of neurotrophic substances for the restitution and reorganization of the neuromuscular system, and thereby promote the patient's functional recovery. "To train and modify spinal circuits for a particular motor task, it is important that the movements performed during training are executed as normally as possible," and "In several studies, enhanced peripheral stimulation has been shown to improve limb action after spinal cord injury" (Muir & Steeves 1997; Hubli & Dietz 2013; Hubli 2011). The authors understand *normally* to imply that alignment and muscle activation patterns are appropriate for the activity to be performed.

> Improvement in motor control requires that the movements performed during training and exercising are executed as normally as possible, and that afferent information via skin, joints, and muscles is appropriate in temporal and spatial parameters.
> Neuroplasticity gives rise to possibilities throughout life.

Shortly after a CNS lesion many patients experience paresis or paralysis to varying degrees. The CNS very quickly compensates for the reduction of function by developing new strategies for achieving the goal; for example, an increased reliance on the least affected side for goal achievement or fixation of parts of the body to compensate for inadequate posture and balance. The use of compensatory strategies is unavoidable after a lesion in the CNS; however, through appropriate treatment the compensation can be minimized as necessary for functional achievement. The use of compensatory strategies can be reduced only if patients are given control over their own posture, balance, and selective movements.

Clinicians practicing the Bobath Concept differentiate between inappropriate compensatory strategies that will restrict improvement and the achievement of the patient's goal, and the use of strategies necessary for the performance of a specific task in a given environment at a certain time but that do not persist once the task has been accomplished (Graham et al 2009).

Inappropriate compensations have the following characteristics:
- They persist beyond the completion of a task.
- They limit other functions.
- They mask the potential for further recovery.

However, patients should not be stopped from moving in a certain way unless they have been provided with an alternate and more efficient strategy that achieves the same goal (Raine et al 2009). The therapeutic challenge is to adapt the task to encourage active participation without negatively influencing the potential for future task performance (Graham et al 2009).

The Bobath clinician aims to explore each individual's potential through the intrinsic plasticity within the system (Raine et al 2009). The brain lesion and the clinical presentations vary across the patient population. The impact of movement dysfunction is unique to each individual and is influenced by experiences prior to as well as postlesion. The factors underlying neurological impairment, recovery of activity, and participation are distinct to the individual. A key concept for effective rehabilitation interventions is recognition of the heterogeneity of mechanisms underlying stroke as well as the plastic processes that lead to recovery of function after a brain injury. A patient's health status, age, lifestyle, and time after injury, in addition to the nature and extent of the brain injury, will influence plastic properties of the brain.

Kleim and Jones (2008) proposed several principles that are important for effective treatment to maximize functional outcomes:

Use it or lose it. Several studies have shown that neural networks not actively engaged in task performance for an extended period of time will degrade. The reduction of sensory input, for example, lack of sensory information due to paralysis of a limb after a CNS lesion, will result in "invasion" of adjacent cortical representation areas in intact parts of the sensory cortex into the cortical representation area of the affected sensory part (Elbert & Rockstroh 2004). A permanent competition for cortical space enlarges those areas that are supplied by important information and leads to narrowing of others. If areas in the brain are not activated, transmitter production is lowered. This is important knowledge for neurorehabilitation; failing to engage a brain system due to lack of use may lead to further degradation of neural activity and function. If an object cannot be reached by a patient's most affected arm after a stroke, the patient quickly adapts to using the less affected arm. The most affected arm learns to be inactive, and the cortical areas representing this arm shrink and are taken over by intact areas. Behavioral experiences by the nonparetic body side may contribute to abnormal interhemispheric interactions after stroke. Learned nonuse is an additional factor in interhemispheric imbalance, coupled with the greatly increased use of the intact limb driving neuronal activity higher in the unaffected hemisphere (Takeuchi & Izumi 2012). Learned nonuse presents a major limitation to the patient's sensorimotor improvement. Positive changes in the brain after an intensive form of therapy called *constraint-induced movement therapy (CIMT)*, which is based on theories of *learned nonuse* (learned inactivity), have been described. A certain level of intensity seems important to optimize the potential for improved function (Feys et al 2004; Kwakkel et al 2004; Langhorne et al 2011).

Use it and improve it. In contrast to the foregoing, several experiments have shown that increased use results in an expansion of the respective cortical representation areas. Through intensive stimulation and requirement for use and activation, the brain is stimulated to produce more neurotransmitters in the activated areas. If not stimulated again within a certain time frame, the production may return to its original low level. This implies that patients who are in a restitution phase may need daily focused treatment to improve sensorimotor function. Exercise that drives a specific brain function can lead to an enhancement of both function and structure of the neural mechanisms involved in that behavior. This generally implies an intense training schedule of several hours a day for several successive days.

Specificity is needed. The nature of the training experience dictates the nature of the plasticity. Changes in neural functions may be limited to the specific function being trained. The clinical implication is that training in a specific modality, such as skill training or endurance training, will determine the plastic changes in specific areas.

Repetition is needed. Long-lasting neuronal changes require not only the acquisition of a skill but also the continued performance of that skill over time; that is, sufficient repetition for consolidation. Consistent with findings from randomized, controlled trials (RCTs) in stroke rehabilitation, there is strong evidence from recent animal studies that the number of repetitions also impact the extent of use-dependent cortical plasticity, which are similar in animals and humans. Studies on motor learning in neurorehabilitation have shown that, rather than blocked massed practice (repetition of one task) a varied repetition—"repetition without repetition"— is more effective for retaining motor learning over time. Varied practice has also been shown to increase generalization of learning to new tasks.

Intensity is needed. Induction of plasticity requires sufficient training intensity. There is, however, no consensus on how much treatment, and how intensive stroke rehabilitation started early may be linked to greater and faster improvement of activities after stroke. The importance of a multidisciplinary approach in the rehabilitation of neurological patients is well established. How patients are helped/trained/facilitated every time they get out of bed or dress themselves, contributes to enhanced experience-dependent plasticity. In the acute phase, patients need to learn to include their affected limb and not to rely on compensatory strategies to gain early independence. In the Bobath Concept, the 24-hour approach is considered an important means for creating opportunities for practice, thus maximizing the intensity of appropriate therapy throughout the whole day. This includes involving all members of the multidisciplinary team when appropriate.

Motor imagery is a cognitive technique by which physical skills can be rehearsed in a safe, repetitive manner. Motor imagery may serve as an adjunctive therapeutic tool for patients to continue their skills training when supervised therapy sessions have ended. Thus motor imagery can considerably increase the patient's intensity and time used for rehabilitation and has, in some studies, been shown to increase motor skill learning. Some of the same neural networks are activated when movement is mentally practiced compared to physical practice of the same skills (Calayan & Dizon 2009).

Time matters. The mechanisms of neural plasticity fundamental to motor learning occur as a process and not as a single event. Different forms of neural plasticity may occur at different time periods. Therapy that boosts neural plasticity should work any time, but there may be time windows in which it is particularly effective. Early and intense rehabilitation seems to be important to the patient's functional improvement to promote learning (Winstein & Stewart 2006). This is supported by studies on survival, psychosocial functioning, and the patient's home situation (Aboderin & Venables 1996; Karger 2008). How early and how intense this rehabilitation should be is not clear (Bernhardt et al 2009). Some authors claim that there is no use in continuing active rehabilitation after 6 months (Aboderin & Venables 1996). Ashburn (1997) stated that these studies had limitations because of their use of insensitive outcome measures, which do not detect qualitative changes in the patient's physical function. Even though neurorehabilitation may be predicted to have the most optimal effect early in life and as soon after injury as possible, there is no reason to assume that helpful training effects cannot be achieved late in life or several years after injury (Nielsen et al 2015).

Salience matters. Salience (meaningful to the individual), motivation, and attention can be critical modulators of plasticity (Woldag et al 2010; Kleim & Jones 2008; Takeuchi & Izumi 2013;

Nielsen et al 2015). This implicates that the intervention must be important and meaningful to that specific individual. Patients respond to meaningful interventions more successfully than interventions with less meaning (Feuerstein et al 2013). This has been described as the *salience* of the intervention. Meaningfulness can be directly related to creating awareness, that is, the patient becomes aware of his or her functioning, of its value, of the changes that are experienced, and the importance (value, salience, etc.) of these changes (Feuerstein et al 2013).

Several experiments on animals and humans have found that there is a neural system by which salience is mediated (Kleim & Jones 2008). The salience network has been observed in resting-state fMRI studies and includes the bilateral anterior insula, anterior temporoparietal junction, and dorsal anterior cingulated cortex (Luo et al 2014). This network associates with detection of relevance among several interoceptive and exteroceptive stimuli and guides behavior, while it updates our expectations about the internal and external environment (Luo et al 2014). Engaging this system is critical to stimulating experience-dependent plasticity. It is known that emotions modulate the strength of memory consolidation; thus neural plasticity may be enhanced when the movement/behavior that is trained feels purposeful for the individual. The engagement in the training process may therefore be enhanced. Motivation and attention are necessary for learning; thus movements must be "owned" by the patient. After a stroke, the brain must learn the new properties of the hemiparetic limb to predict the sensory consequences of motor commands accurately, which can be done by increasing the representation of the affected parts of the body in the body schema.

Age matters. The aging brain is responsive to experience; however, training-induced plasticity occurs more readily in the younger brain.

Summary

The goal of physiotherapy in neurological rehabilitation is to minimize functional disability and optimize functional motor recovery, achieved by modulation of plastic changes in the brain. See page 62.
Neuroplasticity has been defined as "the ability of the nervous system to respond to intrinsic and extrinsic stimuli by reorganizing its structure, function, and connections. See page 62.
Neurorehabilitation is based on the assumption that principles of motor learning can be applied to motor recovery after injury, and that training can lead to permanent improvements in motor function in patients with motor deficit. See page 63.
The result of motor learning is a (new) internal model of a particular task, which is used to predict the sensory consequences of self-generated action. See page 64.
Motor learning includes two distinct types of motor learning; motor adaptation and skill acquisition. See page 65.
Plastic changes within the CNS can be maladaptive. See page 73.
Activity and movement facilitate plastic changes in the CNS, both positively and negatively. See page 69.
Both appropriate and inappropriate movement may be learned. See page 70.
Muscular activity enhances the transport and production of neurotrophic substances. Stimulation may cause changes in the metabolism, structure, and function of muscle. See page 69.
Neuroplasticity has several ways of expressing itself in both the intact and the lesioned CNS, and occurs at many levels, from molecular to cortical reorganization. See page 67.
The sensory and motor cortices have a significant ability for reorganization throughout life, both in an intact CNS and after damage. See page 72.
Excessive interhemispheric inhibition shift activation of behavior over to the undamaged cortex, which contributes negatively to diaschisis and may result in reduced motor activation and possibly decreased potential for recovery of the impaired body parts. See page 74.
Improvement in motor control requires that the movements performed during training and exercising are executed as normally as possible, and that afferent information via skin, joints, and muscles is appropriate in temporal and spatial parameters. See page 78.
Neuroplasticity gives rise to possibilities throughout life. See page 78.
A certain intensity of treatment is necessary to improve the patient's sensorimotor function. See page 79.

1.4 Consequences of and Reorganization after CNS Lesions

The consequences of a lesion to the CNS depend on the interaction of many factors:
- Diagnosis: a vascular lesion, trauma, or disease process.
- Localization: one localized focus or many foci.
- Extent of the lesion(s).
- Speed of development: acute or gradual onset.

How the condition develops in an individual is related to the extent of plastic changes in the CNS, the individual characteristics of the lesion, and whether complications arise, as well as the patient's premorbid physical status, social situation, mental status (resources and coping strategies), and social network (family, friends, and colleagues).

The initial paralysis or paresis after a stroke is due to the acute onset of a lesion (shock), neuron destruction and death, edema, decreased circulation, and, possibly, increased inhibitory activity that protects the brain against further damage (**Fig. 1.30**). As a result of the biochemical sequence of events, changes in the circulatory output and blood pressure occur in ~75% of stroke patients. In most patients these levels return to normal in 7 days. Severe hyper- or hypotension is associated with a poor prognosis.

Too high or too low blood pressure, hypo- or hyperglycemia, and increased temperature are factors that may cause further destruction of the penumbra. The goal of acute stroke therapies is to normalize perfusion and intervene in the cascade of biochemical dysfunction to preserve the maximal amount of penumbral tissue (Maas & Safdieh 2009).

Turton and Pomeroy (2002) found that ~50% of stroke patients showed an increase of the infarcted area 2 weeks poststroke, and 50% experienced a reduction of the infarcted area. They advocate caution in stimuli or activity that may cause further cell death in the penumbra due to an increased blood supply in other, activated regions of the CNS. A gradual return of reflexes and motor activity is related to resolution of edema and necrotic tissue as well as initial reorganization of the CNS. Several authors also report pathological signs and symptoms on the least affected body half after acute stroke—weakness more proximally than distally, as well

as altered stretch reflexes (Mani et al 2013; Bohannon & Andrews 1995; Haaland & Delaney 1981; Rothwell & Lennon 1994).

▰ Upper Motor Neuron Lesions

Stroke, MS, and other causes of brain lesions from trauma or disease are classified together as upper motor neuron lesions. Upper motor neurons (UMNs), or Betz cells, are pyramidal neurons located in the MI that connect the brain to the spinal cord. Motor dysfunction after UMN lesions is classified into *positive and negative signs* (Canning et al 2004). The *negative signs* are the direct results of the lesion itself, and the *positive signs* relate to secondary changes. This classification does not encompass cognitive or perceptual dysfunction or psychological reactions, although these may be major reasons for a patient's limitations toward learning or regaining independence.

▰ The Negative Signs

- Weakness.
- Loss of dexterity.
- Fatigue.

The negative motor impairments following stroke contribute most to disability through functional limitations (Burke 1988; Bohannon 2007; Canning et al 2004).

Unilateral stroke causing hemiparesis is commonly thought of as affecting only the contralateral side; the effect of a stroke on the body ipsilateral to the lesioned hemisphere has been much less explored. Stroke patients may experience weakness not only on their affected side but also on their so-called good side, or, more correctly, their least affected side (Canning et al 2004; Kitsos et al 2013). Contrary to common belief, the trunk muscles can be impaired on both sides of the body in patients with stroke (Fujiwara et al 2001). Ipsilateral to a brain lesion, muscle strength tends to be more impaired proximally than distally (Bohannon & Andrews 1995). The weakness is first and foremost due to reduced or changed neural activation (i.e., weakness in systems and pathways in the CNS). Secondarily, inactivity and reduced muscular activation may cause atrophy and changes in the muscle fiber population (Patten et al 2004; Gray et al 2012). Reduced force production is also caused by fewer than normal functioning motor units and the inability to activate as many units as before (Toft 1995).

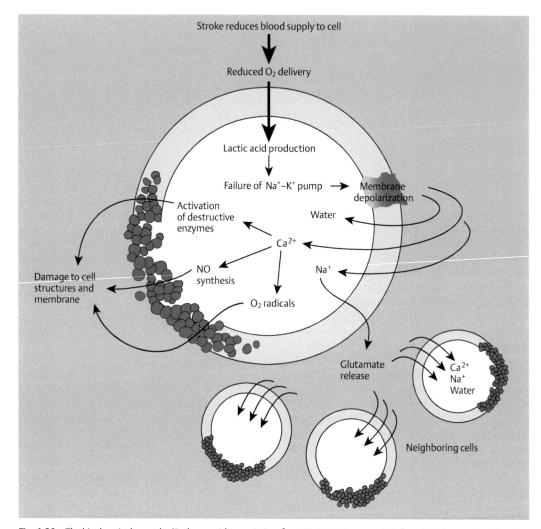

Fig. 1.30   The biochemical cascade. (Redrawn with permission, from Turton A, Pomeroy V. When should upper limb function be trained after stroke? Evidence for and against early intervention. NeuroRehabilitation 2002;17:215–224.)

Weakness

After a CNS lesion, the central executions of motor commands are disrupted, resulting in immediate weakness or paresis (Gracies 2005). Paresis may be defined as "the *quantitative lack of command* directed to agonist muscles when attempting to generate force or movement" (Yelnik et al 2010). This lack of command can occur through insufficient synchronous recruitment of the number of motor units and/or an insufficient discharge frequency (Yelnik et al 2010).

After a stroke, muscle mass decreases, muscle fibers may change in length (become shorter or longer

depending on use), and tendons become more (or less) compliant, all of which contribute to muscle weakness (Gray et al 2012).

Loss of Dexterity

Dexterity is the ability to adapt to the needs of the moment and depends on postural control for background stability. Canning and coworkers (2004) define dexterity as the ability to solve any motor task precisely, quickly, rationally, and deftly, where flexibility with respect to the changing environment and the ability to coordinate muscle activity to meet environmental demands are important features.

Fatigue

Fatigue has been described as an awareness of a lack of physical and mental energy (Lerdal et al 2009). Many patients report fatigue after a CNS lesion. In MS, fatigue is one of the major symptoms (Giovannoni 2006), and it may also be seen after other diseases or infections (Soderlund & Malterud 2005). Many patients suffer from fatigue after stroke (Canning et al 2004). A systematic review by Lerdal and colleagues (2009) reported frequencies ranging from 38 to 77%. Successful recovery takes place in patients who return to relatively normal patterns of brain activation, whereas patients who, on MRI, demonstrate continuing bilateral cortical activation commonly have a poorer recovery (Ward et al 2003). However, even in patients who recover well, noninvasive studies of brain function demonstrate considerable changes in activation (Ward & Cohen 2004; Cramer & Bastings 2000; Cramer et al 1997). The altered pattern of brain activation may constitute one reason for fatigue. Considerable energy and brain activation is recruited just to move an index finger—even after good restitution (Cramer & Bastings 2000). Reduced force production causes an increase in the effort required to move (Toft 1995). Therefore, weakness may be another source of fatigue. However, several studies have examined determinants related to poststroke fatigue, but there is inconclusive or insufficient evidence to pinpoint one source or cause (Lerdal et al 2009).

Current evidence suggests that, generally after stroke, the negative signs limit recovery of function, rather than the positive signs (Canning et al 2004) and should therefore be a primary target for neurorehabilitation.

■ The Positive Signs

The positive signs after an upper motor neuron lesion include the following (Pandyan et al 2005; Canning et al 2004; Thibaut et al 2013):

- Increased tendon reflexes with radiation.
- Mass reflex.
- Clonus.
- Dyssynergic patterns of co-contraction during movement.
- Spasticity.
- Associated reactions and dyssynergic stereotypical spastic dystonias.
- Flexor spasm.
- Extensor spasm.

These symptoms are mainly related to the reorganization of the CNS, which implies that learning may have a major role in the development and establishment of secondary changes (positive signs). In the clinical situation, the terms *spasticity* and *associated reactions* are often used. Spasticity is used in a variety of contexts with different meanings.

Spasticity

The term *spasticity* is widely interpreted, from Lance's definition (1980) (in Young 1994) of hyperreflexia and velocity-dependent resistance to passive stretch to a problem complex consisting of both neural and nonneural changes in tissues. Lance's definition has been criticized for being too restricted by describing spasticity only as a form of hypertonia. Spasticity has been described as a syndrome (Burke 1988; Brown 1994), a condition (Toft 1995), as a result of development (Carr et al 1995), and is related to functional plasticity in the CNS (Burke 1988; Brown 1994; Barnes & Johnson 2008). A literature review of the definitions used showed that 31% of the references with regard to spasticity were using Lance's definition, whereas 35% used increased muscle tone without further defining this. Furthermore, 3% were using other definitions, whereas 31% failed to apply any definition at all (Malhotra et al 2009). This lack of a precise definition makes it difficult to compare studies of spasticity and outcome after treatment interventions. The Support Network for the Assembly and Database for Spasticity Measurement (EU-SPASM) group was charged by the European commission with the task of reviewing and evaluating methods for the measurement of spasticity and building a framework of expertise in Europe. This group reviewed the literature and highlighted different aspects of the use of the term *spasticity*. The results were published in the journal *Disability and Rehabilitation* in 2005 (Pandyan et al 2005; Platz et al 2005; Wood et al 2005; Voerman et al 2005; Burridge et al 2005).

Spasticity is defined by Pandyan and coworkers (Pandyan et al 2005) as "Disordered sensorimotor control, resulting from an upper motor neuron (UMN) lesion, presenting as intermittent or sustained involuntary activation of muscles." This definition includes changes in the structure and function of the CNS and excludes both the negative signs of upper motor neuron lesions and the biomechanical changes in soft tissues and joints (nonneuronal changes).

Disordered motor control may involve the following:

- Loss of modulation from higher centers causes reduced inhibition of α-motor neurons, which react with an abnormal firing frequency and duration to an excitatory stimulus. The loss of descending fibers to the spinal cord causes reduced activity in many different types of inhibitory interneurons.
- Activity in other afferent pathways (e.g., cutaneous, proprioceptive). Cutaneous pathways seem to have a role in spasticity.
- Disordered feedforward modulation of reflex activity.
- Nonclassical behavior of motor neurons/interneurons described as *plateau potentials*; a stable membrane potential that is more depolarized than the normal resting potential causes a cell to fire action potentials in the absence of continuous synaptic excitation. The threshold for firing is maintained at a lower level, causing the neuron to depolarize, even without continuous synaptic excitation.

The mechanisms underlying spasticity are complex and multifactorial. The spastic syndrome in humans is considered to be a complex collection of clinical conditions, including excess muscle tone (hypertonus), changes in muscle properties, excess reflex activity (hyperreflexia), and muscle oscillations (clonus) (Dietz & Sinkjaer 2007). All the foregoing factors are clinical signs of spasticity, can exist independently of each other, and do not necessarily share a common pathophysiology. Changes in structure and function of the CNS can include the following:

- Increased gain (amplification) in the stretch reflex networks; that is, for a given afferent input [Ia and II] the response from the respective α-motor neuron is greater than normal, and may be due to several different mechanisms:
  - Increased excitability of motor neurons.
  - Changes in the characteristics of the α-motor neuron.
  - Reduced Ia presynaptic inhibition.
  - Changes in inhibition from the efferent pathway.
  - Altered reciprocal inhibition.
  - Reduced recurrent inhibition.
  - Increased excitability in the flexor reflex pathways (withdrawal).
  - Altered force feedback (feedback about the actual force production in muscle).

- Decreased threshold of the stretch receptors (i.e., the stretch reflex is more easily elicited in people with spasticity). This may be caused by increased receptor sensitivity and an increased drive to the muscle spindle efferents. Current evidence suggests that spindle afferent activity is not necessarily abnormal in stroke patients (Pandyan et al 2005).

Yelnik and colleagues (2010) state that "'Spasticity' is a term that is often used beyond its definition, to refer to various types of muscle over activity. The term 'muscle over activity' is more appropriate and should be used preferentially."

■ **The Complex Problem of the Upper Motor Neuron Syndrome**

The complex problems that health professionals experience in patients with UMN lesions may therefore be a combination of negative signs, spasticity, or muscle overactivity as already defined, as well as other factors. Pandyan and colleagues (2005) state that "There is insufficient evidence in the literature to support the hypothesis that the abnormal muscle activity in spasticity results exclusively from stretch reflex hyperexcitability. It would appear that activity in other afferent pathways (e.g., cutaneous), supraspinal control pathways (or systems) and even changes in the α-motor neuron may also contribute to signs and symptoms associated with spasticity and other features of the UMN syndrome." Other factors may be associated with the UMN syndrome:

- Components of inertia from extremity segments.
- Changes in viscoelastic properties of soft tissues and joints.
- Abnormal voluntary activation of muscle.
- Abnormal involuntary activation from phenomena other than the stretch reflex hyperexcitability.
- The patient's cognitive and/or perceptual abilities (the ability to understand instruction, etc.).

Clinically, altered sensory feedback and altered sensory perception also seem to have an important role. What therapists see in patients are the *consequences* of the lesion for the patient as a whole. Therefore, the patient's resources and problems must be analyzed and interventions planned on an individual basis.

Muscle overactivity is associated with lesions affecting the CRS pathways; lesions to the corticoreticular pathways at the level of the cortex or internal capsule, and the reticulospinal and vestibulospinal tracts at the level of the spinal cord (Pandyan et al 2005; Burke 1988; Burke et al 2013; Brown 1994; Brodal 2010). The reticulospinal system plays an important part in the stability of proximal body segments, and lesions that affect the CRS are often associated with dysfunction in postural control and balance and also with spasticity. Studies on the corticospinal system suggest that lesions to this system probably do not cause spasticity but produce a loss of distal dexterity (Brodal 2010). Indirectly, the functions of the cerebellum and the BG may be disturbed, causing clumsiness.

■ Clinical Reflections: Spasticity and Associated Reactions

The term *associated reactions* is both understood and used differently by different clinicians. This section presents clinically relevant reflections about spasticity and associated reactions and the formation of some hypotheses of possible causal relations, factors that initiate these responses, and consequences for the patient's motor control.

The term *associated movement* refers to natural activity that either requires considerable effort or is complex or new and is a normal feature of movement. Associated movements have many features in common with associated reactions, but some aspects are different. As a new skill is being learned, associated movements gradually disappear. This is not the case with associated reactions. Associated reactions are characterized by an activation of motor units or muscles not normally involved in the performed movement, and they get stronger through practice of the movement. They may also be called *dyssynergic patterns of movement*. Many patients with different CNS lesions experience similar symptoms irrespective of the exact diagnosis (e.g., cerebral infarctions, intracerebral hemorrhage, subdural hemorrhage, TBI, MS, and other upper motor neuron lesions, as well as incomplete SCI).

The following discussion is related to changes seen after stroke. A few hours or days after a stroke the patient starts to show some initial motor activity, some controlled and often some uncontrolled movement in the most affected parts of the body (the so-called hemiplegic side). Uncontrolled activity is usually first observed in situations that require motor control that the patient has not yet developed (e.g., balance), and usually observed first in the arm or leg, but is also often present in the trunk. It seems like a compensatory involuntary motor response

when the task is too difficult or associated with effort (too much effort for the needs of the actual situation), or in situations where the patient feels insecure, unstable, or unhappy — often connected to fear of falling or the feeling of having too little control to cope. As time goes on, this involuntary recruitment of muscle activity may increase; it presents itself in more situations, is more easily triggered, and may develop into—for the individual patient—a stereotypical involuntary pattern of activity. The patterns are characterized by little variety and may be activated progressively more easily in more situations to different degrees. In the literature they are often described as follows:

- Abnormal synergic muscle activity (Carr & Shepherd 1983).
- Abnormal movement or mobility (Shumway-Cook & Woollacott 2006).
- Abnormal movement synergies (Tyldesley & Grieve 1996).
- Spastic patterns of movement (Stokes 1998).
- Associated reactions (Bobath 1990; Dvir & Panturin 1993; Edwards 1996; Pandyan et al 2005; Burke et al 2013).

The author perceives these motor disorders to refer to the same aspect of motor activity, and in the following text the term *associated reaction* (AR) will be used. Previously, from a hierarchical model of the CNS, ARs were thought to be the release of primitive reflexes due to a CNS lesion (Bobath 1978). Research related to the structure and function of the CNS, plasticity, and different aspects of movement science has shown that the CNS is not governed by reflexes as such in context-based movement and is not hierarchically organized, but it is a multidirectional, integrated system that is developed through the interaction of the individual with the environment.

ARs are related to CNS reorganization postlesion, and viewed as an activity-dependent process of learning as the patient attempts to interact with the environment without the necessary prerequisites for motor control (i.e., as a result of altered behavior).

Walshe (1923) was the first to describe associated reactions as postural reactions in muscle deprived of voluntary control that is tonic in nature. If motor control is reduced generally or locally, balance is affected. Spasticity and associated reactions are associated with damage (indirectly or directly) of the CRS and vestibular systems, which have important roles in postural control. Clinical experience implies that associated reactions are more often present in balance-challenging activities than in lying or sitting. Walking is a challenge to human balance, and might result in increased drive to antigravity muscles through vestibulospinal pathways (the extensor muscles of the legs and flexor muscles of the arm and hand). Therefore, one explanation for the flexed arm posture often seen clinically in walking or in sit to stand could be due to an increase in the excitability of the vestibulospinal pathways (Kline et al 2007). If a stroke patient presents with positive features one might assume that a patient's postural control will be reduced to some degree. The patient therefore needs to compensate for both reduced postural control and motor function. The (re)organization of the CNS is activity dependent, that is, dependent on how the body is being used (form–function). Conversely, motor control is dependent on the structure and function of the CNS and the integrated systems control, as well as biomechanical factors (form–function). Probably there is no *one* cause of the development of ARs. It is multifactorial and the exact mechanism varies between individuals. ARs are what the clinician observe or perceive as involuntary, disorganized activity, an expression of the activity in the CNS and the interaction with external and internal demands. ARs may lead to secondary changes in the muscles, connective tissue, skin, and malalignment (i.e., *nonneuronal changes*).

■ Other Factors Contributing to Muscle Stiffness: Non-neuronal Changes

Recent studies indicate that, in addition to pathological changes in motor neuron activation (involuntary supraspinal descending inputs and inhibited spinal reflexes, etc.), changes in muscle properties also contribute to the clinical appearance of limb spasticity (Dietz & Sinkjaer 2007). After a stroke, muscle hypertonia seems to be associated with subclinical muscle contracture rather than reflex hyperexcitability; changes in collagen tissue and tendons, an enhancement of intrinsic stiffness of muscle fibers, and a loss of sarcomeres leading to subclinical contractures. In addition, changes in mechanical muscle fiber properties might also contribute to an increase in muscle tone (Dietz & Sinkjaer 2007).

Many authors describe secondary muscular and connective tissue changes as part of a patient's motor disorder (Goldspink & Williams 1991; Voerman et al 2005; Wood et al 2005). Some studies show that there may be a gradual transition of muscle fibers after a UMN lesion: Goldspink and Williams (1991) and Hufschmidt and Mauritz (1985) found type I fibers to atrophy quickly due to changes in the activation pattern leading to immobilization or altered use. They also demonstrated that muscles which were originally more phasic partially transformed to musculature with more tonic characteristics. Patients with stroke exhibiting spasticity demonstrate increased muscle atrophy, especially of type II fibers (Dietz & Sinkjaer 2007). The researchers found an increased population of type I fibers in the gastrocnemius, which normally contains more type IIa fibers. Different studies have shown different results, depending on the patients and muscles studied, but they all do demonstrate that changes in muscle fibers occur as a response to a UMN lesion.

When a paralyzed muscle is held in a shortened position it loses sarcomeres: the muscle "adjusts" so that it can produce optimal force at the shortened muscle length, and consequently a start to contracture formation.

Patients with TBI who were comatose for more than 3 weeks were found to exhibit a significant increase in contractures, probably due to the period of immobilization. Of the patients who suffered hemiplegia after TBI, 97% were found to develop contractures also in their least affected extremities (Yarkony & Sahgal 1987).

Increased resistance to passive movement after a lesion in the CNS is possibly also a result of another phenomenon in muscle called *thixotropy* (Vattanasilp et al 2000). The term *thixotropy* has been used with regard to substances that can be changed from gel to solution after being stirred. Both muscle and connective tissue demonstrate this phenomenon. Muscle behaves as a *thixotropic* substance in that its stiffness depends on the history of limb movement. For example, when the paralyzed limb has been kept in a shortened position over time it might show increased resistance to passive movements; however, after the paralyzed muscles have been stretched, moved, or activated, the resistance to movement decreases and the muscles become "looser" (Vattanasilp et al 2000).

The question of whether changes in properties of muscles or changes in neuronal activity are more important depends on the individual patient and the muscle studied. It is therefore of utmost importance that the treating team analyzes which factors trigger the individual's ARs, motor resources, and deviations. The combination of impaired balance and motor control together with demands for independent function may predispose the patient to develop associated reactions and secondary nonneural complications (Ashburn & Lynch-Ellerington 1988; Cornall 1991). Clinically, it is important to differentiate between neural and nonneural components of the motor disorder. Interventions used to treat the gradual development of contractures differ from the treatment of the motor disorder as such, and may involve splinting, surgery, more rigorous positioning, and a comprehensive management program.

Summary

Intense, specific stimulation should be performed with care the first week poststroke. Clinical decisions should be based on the patient's level of arousal, alertness, blood pressure, intracranial pressure, and temperature. Later, patients probably suffer more from too little activity. See page 81.

Stroke, MS, and other causes of brain lesions from trauma or disease are classified together as UMN lesions. See page 81.
Motor dysfunction after UMN lesions is classified into positive and negative signs. See page 81.
The negative impairments—weakness, loss of dexterity, and fatigue—seem to be the major factors that —limit recovery of function in stroke patients. See page 81.
The mechanisms underlying spasticity are complex and multifactorial. See page 84.
Spasticity is defined by Pandyan and coworkers (2005) as "Disordered sensorimotor control, resulting from an upper motor neuron (UMN) lesion, presenting as intermittent or sustained involuntary activation of muscles." See page 83.
Changes in muscle properties (nonneuronal changes) also contribute to the clinical appearance of limb spasticity. See page 86.
Associated reactions are postural reactions in muscle deprived of voluntary control that is tonic in nature. See page 85.

2 Human Movement

Introduction

Human movement is complex. Many books have been written on the subject, and more recently there has been a lot of research in different branches of movement science. Movement science is the study of movement from different perspectives, for instance, physiotherapy, psychology, pedagogy, physics, neurophysiology, biomechanics, and biology. It provides a basic knowledge of movement important for all therapists. Much research on movement is, however, still conducted in research laboratories with healthy, younger people, and thus is not always directly applicable to patients in a clinical setting.

This book presents physiotherapy based on the experience, knowledge, and point of view of the authors, qualified instructors within the International Bobath Instructors Training Association (IBITA). The word *concept* refers to "something understood, an idea" (Thomas 1997), or it is "an element used in the development of a theory." Here, *concept* is applied to the knowledge base that forms the foundation for clinical reasoning. A conceptual understanding is therefore not simply learning a method, but learning to *analyze* and *understand connections* in an individual's movement problems—*Why* does the person move in this way? This chapter enables readers to develop their own understanding of balance and movement, and it highlights some of the reasoning therapists use to make choices in their treatment of individuals with central nervous system (CNS) lesions.

We now know that the CNS undergoes changes depending on what input it receives and the re-

sponse to this input. There is a constant interaction between the individual and the environment that shapes the body and brain—plasticity is the bridge between brain and behavior. As a consequence, human movement is adaptable, and humans have a capacity for learning, both with a healthy CNS and after CNS lesions. Therapists form an important part of the patient's environment and training; treatment induces changes in cortical activation patterns over time (Nelles 2004). Our aim should be to help patients develop and optimize their own potential. But "we are currently being forced into interventions to 'get the patient out' that are supposedly cost effective. However, are we training compensatory strategies that will prevent true recovery, thus lengthening the time and increasing the level of care that the person will need in the long run?" (Held 1987). This statement seems as true today as when it was written nearly 30 years ago.

Health professionals face this dilemma; often we know what is possible but rarely have the resources to see it through. We may limit the patient's potential; perhaps we lack optimism and vision and do not believe that the patient can improve. The goals are set at a level we can reach based on our resources (time, economy, competence) and beliefs, not necessarily according to the patient's real potential for regaining function based on the localization and extent of the lesion and the patient's premorbid status, general condition, and plastic ability—the patient's capacity to learn.

First of all, we as therapists need to change our operating assumptions. We should expect recovery and work for that by preventing rather than encouraging compensation to occur. We should carefully analyze each person's problems, and we must intervene early (Held 1987).

In rehabilitation, goals are related to the International Classification of Functioning, Disability, and Health (ICF) domains:

Participation:
- Participate in life, fulfill roles.

Activity:
- Master activities.
  - Daily functions.
  - Function in the patient's own environment.

Body functions and structures:
- Control balance, movement, and function.
  - Improve postural control and selective movement.
  - Regain the ability to interact with the environment.
  - Control the recruitment of tone by learning through early and gradual interaction with gravity with good alignment to optimize muscle activation and with support or facilitation where and when it is needed.
  - Develop appropriate strategies and patterns of movement.
  - Develop appropriate strength to interact with gravity.
  - Maintain muscle length and range of movement.

Physiotherapy-related goals are set by the patient and therapist together. The patient's needs and goals and therapy goals must be in harmony. The therapist's challenge is to increase the patient's competency, insight, and understanding for a process leading to greater participation and independence, and this takes time. Treatment for many patients will first and foremost be aimed at improving selective postural control and balance in functional situations to strengthen carryover to daily activities in the patient's own environment. If patients regain their postural control to a level that enables them to more fully participate in their environment and become more oriented toward and integrated with the world around them, they will, in our understanding, have greater opportunities for participating in a variety of social settings.

People are unique in terms of their own interests, wishes, goals, needs, previous experiences, likes and dislikes. To be able to create a constructive patient–therapist relationship, the therapist has to adapt to many different individuals and meet each one with a positive attitude, empathy, professionalism, and respect for the person's integrity. It is important to create a positive learning environment to motivate and inspire the patient, and at the same time give realistic information without taking hope away. Evidence supports the theory that patients should be exposed to an enriched environment to develop their potential for learning (Virji-Babul 1991). Motivation and focused attention are important factors for learning (see Motor Learning and Plasticity). Assessment and treatment are built upon the following:
- Analysis of human movement.
- Analysis of deviations from human movement.
- Clinical reasoning.
- Appropriate treatment techniques to facilitate the patient's regaining of motor control.

The next sections describe and discuss aspects of the following:
- Balance and movement.
- Conceptual understanding for treatment rationale and choice of individually adapted treatment techniques.
- Other forms of treatment/interventions.

2.1   Balance and Movement

▮▮▮ Human Movement Control

When we study humans in movement we are able to recognize whether they are sitting, standing or walking, standing up or sitting down, or turning around normally, because we all perform these activities in a basically similar way. We recognize when people have good balance, and observing their movement strategies enable us to recognize common features in the average population, which define our genotype. There are many common aspects to how individuals problem-solve a movement task:
- Appropriate sequence of recruitment and tension development of muscles.
- Necessary range of movement in different single joints.
- Necessary ranges of movement between the extremities and the trunk.
- Appropriate development of torque.
- Appropriate alignment, which is essential for the sequencing and selective activation of muscles.
- Appropriate effort—no more than needed for efficiency and successful goal achievement.
- Rhythm, tempo, variation.

Basic components of movement that are coordinated in time and space have to be activated for us to interact with gravity and at the same time use our arms functionally. Our daily activities demand both postural and movement control. Which components are most important depends on the person, the goal, the environment, and the actual situation. Individual have their own, personal way of moving, the individual expression—the phenotype. We recognize a person by the way he moves. It may be enough to hear the steps in the hall: rhythm, step, tempo, firmness, light, hard or shuffling steps—all characteristics of the individual. The movement expressions may even reflect the person's state of mind: the extended, self-assured person or the flexed, modest, insecure or anxious person—just two possible extremes. A movement is referred to as voluntary (focal or goal directed) when its purpose is to perform a given task (i.e., as a means to complete a motor task) (Le Bozec & Bouisset 2004; Bouisset & Do 2008). According to the laws of mechanics, voluntary movement causes internal forces and torques, which are spread throughout the whole body to the base of support (BoS), where ground reaction forces (GRFs) are produced (read more about BoS and GRF in Postural Sets). These forces and torques induce perturbation to human balance. Therefore, voluntary movements are exposed to two antagonistic constraints: (1) to move the focal segment(s) toward a goal, and (2) to stabilize the "postural" segment(s) (i.e., the body segments not directly involved in the voluntary action) to maintain balance (Yiou et al 2012).

> Human movement is varied and without inappropriate effort. It is efficient, effective, precise, and successful, developed through the interaction between the person, the task, and the environment.

The expression *human movement* reflects both the common features of humankind and the individual expression. A person's build and posture inform the therapist of her movement experience and how she has used her body before. Through analysis of movement, the individual expression is evaluated, as well as how movement is performed in relation to the goal activity, the environment, and the ability to vary during different activities in different situations. Analysis of movement involves both observation and handling (hands-on) during activity, with attention directed specifically toward the following:

- Balance.
  - Postural control.
  - Postural activity, build, and posture—postural tone.
- The relationship to gravity and to the environment, the base of support.
- Coordination, reciprocal innervation.
- The relationship between body segments and their function (stability–movement).
- Coordination of the individual components in sequence, time, and space (i.e., the recruitment of movement patterns).
- The selective movement of single components.

Balance

Through movement we interact with the environment and learn to perceive ourselves in relation to the world around us, and balance is the foundation for our daily activities. Balance is the result of the interaction between motor, sensory, and cognitive processes, and it allows us to be stable and active in relation to gravity and the base of support while at the same time using our arms—which are free—for functional activities. Maintaining balance is, in the most basic sense, defined as *not falling*. Nevertheless, balance control is complex and includes maintaining postures, facilitating movement, and recovering equilibrium (Mancini & Horak 2010). Therefore, one can say that balance is movement as well as a prerequisite for movement. Balance is a holistic sensorimotor and perceptual interplay between our surroundings and us, and it requires graded and coordinated neuromuscular activity of the whole body at the same time. Normally, most people can adapt to the actual situation. Balance provides the body with harmony and safety in relation to the environment and is the foundation of our motor system. Patients with neurological conditions have lost some of their movement repertoire and are unable to adapt to the same degree as before. Therefore they have fewer choices open to them if balance is threatened. With reduced or no balance we have to use other strategies to prevent falls. Falling may occur in 50 to 70% of patients after a stroke due to balance impairments associated with impairments in the motor, sensory, cognitive, or integrative aspects of movement control (Kamphuis et al 2013). The ability to maintain balance is described as "the acts of maintaining, achieving or restoring the body center of mass (COM) relative to the base of support

(BoS), or more generally, within the limits of stability" (Pollock et al 2000).

To be able to maintain balance, the nervous system must meet the "degrees of freedom" problem first presented by Nikolai Bernstein (1967). The degrees of freedom, that is, the large number of elements that need to be controlled during human movement, give us numerous different possibilities, allowing the nervous system flexibility in performing a task. But how does the CNS make choices from an apparently unlimited number of possibilities? For example, how does it choose a combination of joint angles to produce the required movement? or the correct muscles, using the appropriate muscle force? The neural principles and mechanisms underlying the CNS's ability to control the degrees of freedom problem are still unknown. Bernstein proposed a neural strategy for simplifying the control of multiple degrees of freedom by grouping output variables. This hypothesis was based on Bernstein's experimental observations that, during motor tasks, joint angles appeared to be controlled together, rather than independently. This has been supported by several studies, and recent findings support Bernstein's hypothesis that the CNS simplifies motor control by limiting muscles to be activated in fixed groups, or synergies (Ting & McKay 2007; Safavynia & Ting 2012). A *synergy* can be defined as "a set of muscles recruited by a single neural command signal" (Torres-Oviedo et al 2006). Therefore, activating muscle synergies may be a mechanism by which the nervous system achieves repeatable and correlated multijoint coordination (Ting 2007).

The language used to describe balance is unclear (Tyson et al 2006). The terms *balance* and *postural control* are used interchangeably, and there are no commonly accepted definitions of these terms; however, in our understanding, *balance* is a holistic overall term encompassing the following:

- Postural control.
- Anticipatory postural adjustments (APAs) or feedforward postural control.
- Protective reactions/reactive strategies.

■ Postural Control

One of the most important functions of the CNS is to coordinate posture and movement to stabilize the body during self-initiated movements and externally triggered disturbances (Horak 2006). The nervous system automatically has to balance the body's center of mass over the feet during all motor activities performed in a bipedal posture: every movement necessarily begins and ends with a postural adjustment (Dietz 1992). Postural control has been extensively investigated in healthy subjects as well as in individuals with musculoskeletal and neurological disorders (Jacobs & Horak 2007; Sousa et al 2012; Gribble et al 2012). Postural control is no longer considered one system or a set of righting and equilibrium reflexes (Horak 2006). Postural control is organized in relation to the individual, the task, and the context in which the task is being performed (Shumway-Cook & Woollacott 2006). The postural control system includes all sensorimotor and musculoskeletal components involved in maintaining balance. In other words, postural control is the support system for motor action by ensuring that we are maintaining our balance during motor activities.

Postural control develops through the interaction of sensory, perceptual, cognitive, and motor systems as well as the musculoskeletal apparatus of the body. The desire to move combined with information received and modulated from all receptor organs and senses of the body form the basis for execution of movement. Movement is constantly adapting to variations in the environment, goals, and situations. Postural control is recognized as a key component in the acquisition of independence in activities of daily living (ADLs) and instrumental ADLs (IADLs), for instance the ability to go shopping (Hsieh et al 2002).

A vital function of the nervous system is to ensure efficient coordination between movement and posture: "Posture and movement are like Siamese twins: inseparable but, to a certain extent, independent" (Morasso et al 2010), or "posture is the foundation upon which movement rides" (Cram & Criswell 2011); hence the efficiency of our balance system will affect the efficiency of our voluntary movements. To optimize the control of balance, humans develop postural adjustments in anticipation of the forthcoming perturbation. Bouisset & Le Bozec (2002) called the body's ability to develop such a counterperturbation posturo-kinetic capacity (PKC). It involves the "ability of the stabilizing segments of the human body to assist the voluntary movement in terms of their speed and forcefulness." According to the PKC theory, the performance of a functional task depends highly on the role of the postural component to develop an efficient counterperturbation (Yiou et al 2007). This theory is supported by several authors claiming that the performance of a voluntary motor task, for example, pointing and reaching with an arm, is dependent on the exact coordination between proximal (e.g., trunk) and distal body segments (e.g., hand). Mononen et al (2007) gave evidence that shooting accuracy is dependent on the accurate trunk and lower-limb postural control. Some of this evidence arises from pathology. For example, Hsieh and colleagues (2002) have shown that trunk control early poststroke was one of the strongest predictors of upper-limb functional recovery; Stoykov and colleagues (2005) reported that speed and movement accuracy of the ataxic upper limb improved when a patient, who suffered a brain stem stroke, was specifically trained to improve sitting balance and trunk control.

The PKC theory highlights the fundamental need to develop postural adjustments in anticipation of the expected perturbation to optimize the control of balance (Yiou et al 2007). These postural adjustments correspond to the APAs (APAs are discussed in more detail later in this chapter). To ensure an efficient postural control, the PKC theory emphasizes the importance of postural joint mobility. Specifically, this theory predicts that any factor constraining postural joint mobility (e.g., through aging or pathology) would change the focal movement performance.

The control of posture can be divided into two different but interacting systems: the *anticipatory or feedforward* system, where postural corrections are made prior to movement; and the *feedback or reactive system*, where corrections are made in response to perturbations. Muscles are the effectors of the postural control system and contribute to both feedforward and feedback postural stability. The postural activity is therefore a result of changes of tone—a functional adaptation (i.e., altered distribution of activity in different motor units for the maintenance of stability).

■ Anticipatory Postural Adjustments

APAs or feedforward control is the pretuning of sensory and motor systems in expectation of postural demands based on experience and learning (Shumway-Cook & Woollacott 2006). APAs are active before movement starts and involve activity in muscles not directly involved in generating the movement (the goal-directed movement), but in maintaining postural control. Anticipatory control is used when the need for balance and stability is predictable and the CNS can preprogram a postural alignment before the planned movement starts. Belenkiy and colleagues (1967) (Massion et al 2004) were the first to describe the APAs for an arm-raising task, and they

have since been studied in a wide variety of voluntary movements. The CNS learns through experience to precisely estimate the effect of a *predicted perturbation* and use synergistic anticipatory activation of selected muscles to provide the best body stabilization (Santos & Aruin 2008).

APAs represent two different phenomena: one is the early postural adjustments preceding the movement; these are sometimes referred to as preparatory APAs (pAPAs) (Schepens & Drew 2004; Leonard et al 2009), or early postural adjustments (EPAs) (Klous et al 2011; Krishnan et al 2012). The second phenomenon is the postural responses occurring *during* the movement, by which the body or body segments are stabilized during the execution of the movement itself. These are often referred to as accompanying APAs (aAPAs) (Schepens & Drew 2004). Both the pAPAs and the aAPAs are considered to be feedforward in nature because they are produced before feedback from the ongoing movement can influence them (Massion 1992). pAPAs and aAPAs are not a single phenomenon with variable timing, but two distinct aspects of postural preparation to perturbation (Krishnan et al 2012). The main goal of the pAPAs is to ensure efficient mechanical conditions for the planned action (Klous et al 2011), whereas the aAPAs are the postural response accompanying the movement to generate net forces and movements of force acting against those associated with the expected perturbation.

Anticipation requires prediction of the upcoming perturbation, which implies that internal models are developed through movement experience and stored in the CNS to be used during the performance of a task; the key factor of being able to anticipate is based on learning (Massion et al 2004).

Research has showed that APAs are tailored to specific characteristics of focal movements, such as the direction and speed of the expected perturbation (Berg & Strang 2012). Furthermore, when a perturbation is unpredictable, APAs are diminished, leading to bigger feedback strategies, for example, when we step to avoid falling. If the displacement is very sudden and the feet are free to move, APAs may not always be present (Santos & Aruin 2009; Santos & Aruin 2008). Also, in conditions of postural instability in healthy subjects, the CNS may be reluctant to activate strong APAs because the APAs themselves may cause perturbations to balance. Therefore, the CNS will try to avoid exposing a vulnerable unstable condition to another source of perturbations (Yiou et al 2012).

■ Protective Reactions/Strategies

The second type of adjustments deals with the actual perturbations of balance and is termed protective reactions or compensatory reactions (or compensatory postural adjustments [CPAs]) (Santos & Aruin 2009). These reactions are the coordinated activation of muscles that stabilize the body *following a perturbation* (Ting et al 2009), and are not simple reflexes, but the synergistic activation of muscles, and therefore strategies (Kandel et al 2013). CPAs in general cannot be predicted and are initiated by sensory feedback (Alexandrov et al 2005). Each protective strategy activates different muscular patterns and provides postural stability in the appropriate direction.

In standing, humans mainly use three main types of protective strategies to return the body to equilibrium: two strategies keep the feet in place (referred to as feet in place strategies) and the third changes the base of support through stepping or reaching (Horak 1987; Horak 2006). The latter is also referred to as a change-in-support strategies.

Feet in place strategies:
- The ankle strategy opposes body sway in standing and is based on a distal-to-proximal activation (Horak & Nashner 1986; Rothwell & Lennon 1994; Shumway-Cook & Woollacott 2006).
- The hip strategy activates the lower trunk-, pelvic-, and hip-related musculature first (i.e., a more cranial–caudal [proximal–distal] sequence of recruitment). In many conditions stepping occurs even if the line of gravity is within the base of support, when balance is not threatened (Maki & McIlroy 1997; Shumway-Cook & Woollacott 2006)

change-in-support strategies:
- Taking a rapid step and reaching movements are important to restore equilibrium. These protective reactions are much faster than volitional limb movements and can be very effective in decelerating the center-of-mass (CoM) motion induced by sudden unpredictable balance perturbations (Maki & McIlroy 2006). Stepping is, in this situation, reactive, but elements of planning and strategy are present at most times: we place the foot in the direction in which we are likely to regain balance. However, when we step to initiate locomotion, we plan ahead and initiate feedforward strategies. Stronger cognitive elements are now present, and this is therefore not a protective reaction.

- Protective reactions to restore balance disturbances are not restricted to the lower limbs during standing or walking. Rather, whole-body responses are frequently observed (Marigold & Misiaszek 2009). These responses show themselves as coordinated lower limb and arm reactions as well as stabilizing muscular activity of the trunk (Marigold & Misiaszek 2009). The arms are recruited in a protective reaction if stepping is not possible or is inadequate. Often some elements of planning will be present: we place the arms where they may most appropriately save us or lessen or grade the fall, for example, using the handrails for grasping to maintain balance when one slips while walking down a flight of stairs or when standing on a bus (Marigold & Misiaszek 2009).

Early theories of postural control viewed compensatory strategies as developing from fixed support, that is, ankle strategy to hip reactions with increasing perturbation amplitude, only engaging change-in-support reactions for extremely large perturbations that forced the CoM outside the BoS. However, it is now known that changes in support strategies are often selected, even at smaller perturbation magnitudes (McIlroy & Maki 1996).

Humans are normally able to use different strategies when displacement occurs. The ability to choose the appropriate postural control reactive strategy reflects complex and integrative sensorimotor processes. Efficient human postural control depends on having accurate knowledge of the entire body configuration in space (body schema) as well as the location of the body CoM relative to the line of gravity and the base of support (Bouisset & Zattara 1981). Therefore, the strategies that are used will depend on the situation; the sequence of muscle activation varies in relation to needs and possibilities, and the choice of strategy will depend on prior experience, habituation, expectation, and fear (Ting 2007). The response also varies depending on the feet; if they are free to move or kept stationary when displacement occurs, whether the base of support is smaller or larger than the feet, how displacement is given, and if the study participants are instructed to stay still or are allowed to move. Research with regard to change of support strategies in patients with stroke have reported that stepping responses are "least affected" limb dominant, even when obstacles block this limb (Lakhani et al 2011; Mansfield et al 2012). Furthermore, when using the most affected limb to step, patients with stroke demonstrate a time lag in the foot-lift, poorer clearance of the floor, the need for several steps, or even an inability to initiate a step (Lakhani et al 2011; Martinez et al. 2013). Improved use of the paretic limb is associated with better balance recovery (Mansfield et al 2013; Mansfield et al 2012). Balance research in patients with Parkinson's disease (PD) has showed freezing of step or decreased velocity and step length of the stepping response (Jacobs & Horak 2007; Smith et al 2012).

A relationship between APAs and CPAs has been demonstrated. Santos and colleagues (2010) studied the role of APAs in compensatory postural adjustments and demonstrated the existence of an interplay between anticipatory and compensatory mechanisms of balance control. The results of this study also suggest the importance of optimizing the use of APAs in rehabilitation of individuals with balance impairments.

▬ The Neural Mechanisms Contributing to the Origin of Postural Control Mechanisms

How the coordination of balance and movement is accomplished is far from being understood. However, it is known that several neuronal networks in the CNS contribute to this coordination; areas in the spinal cord, cerebellum, basal ganglia, cortex, and brain stem are vital for balance (Jacobs & Horak 2007; Deliagina et al 2008).

The cerebral cortex probably influences postural responses both directly via corticospinal loops and indirectly via communicating with the brain stem, and as a result influences the postural responses by providing both speed and flexibility for preselecting task specificity and appropriate postural responses to a balance threat (Jacobs & Horak 2007). Behavioral experiments have shown that healthy subjects receiving information about the magnitude of a postural disturbance about to happen can scale and modify their postural responses in relation to this information, evidencing that feedforward adaptations need the involvement of the cerebral cortex (Papegaaij et al 2014). The supplementary motor area (SMA) is thought to play a part in the generation of APAs (Jacobs et al 2009). Also, reduction in executive functions, such as attention, mental calculation, orientation, and memory, interfere with balance, further indicating the involvement of cortical circuits in postural control (Jacobs & Horak

2007). The basal ganglia likely act as the "middle man" between the cerebral cortex and brain stem for automating the selection and implementation of context-specific postural responses (Takakusaki et al 2004). This gives us the possibility to change the balance strategy according to the actual needs of the task. Furthermore, the BG are probably associated with the cognitive features of postural control, including the handling of unpredictability and the ability to give priority to the most vital elements of a complex postural task (Visser & Bloem 2005).

The cerebellum plays an essential part in the control of upright posture and is involved in adjusting postural control to ongoing movements (Massion et al 1999). It contributes to feedforward the adjustments in trunk and extremity movements during complex motor programs, or in coupling postural control to limb movements (Thach & Bastian 2004; Gramsbergen 2005).

Several studies in both cats and humans have looked into the neural mechanisms contributing to the origination of the postural control mechanisms (Massion 1992; Schepens & Drew 2004; Schepens & Drew 2003); two different modes of central organization have been put forward (Robert et al 2007):

1. A single-process control, where the APAs and the voluntary movements would share a common command (Aruin & Latash 1996).
2. A parallel process control (dual-process control) where the APAs and the voluntary movements would be independently controlled through parallel commands (Massion et al 1999; Schepens et al 2006; Schepens & Drew 2004; Tagliabue et al 2009).

The parallel relationship between postural control and movement hypothesis can be justified by the connection between the cortex and the reticular formation. Several studies have shown that neural commands for feedforward postural adjustments can be identified in the pontomedullary reticular formation (PMRF) of the brain stem (Schepens & Drew 2004; Schepens et al 2006; Schepens et al 2008). Schepens and Drew (2004) and Schepens et al (2006) demonstrated that neurons in this area discharged either during the pAPAs, the aAPAs, or both, during reaching movements in the standing cat. They found independent channels within the PMRF for initiating the postural responses and for producing the reaching movement. This research is thus in support of the dual-process control.

▨ The Function of Postural Control

The two main functional goals of postural control are *postural orientation* and *postural equilibrium* (Horak 2006).

▩ Postural Orientation

Postural orientation is the ability to orient the body to environmental variables and align various body parts. Human posture can actively be oriented to a variety of reference frames depending on the task and movement goal. Postural orientation is based on the interpretation of sensory information. The frame of reference can be visual, somatosensory, or vestibular (Horak 2006), or the internal representation of body orientation to the environment, such as an estimated reference position from memory (Popovic & Sinkjær 2008).

Postural orientation involves the following:
- The ability to maintain an appropriate alignment between body segments.
- The ability to maintain an appropriate relationship to the environment.
- The need to establish a vertical orientation to oppose gravity.
- Creating a reference frame for perception and action.

Information needed to maintain postural control is important for conscious awareness of our own bodies, spatial orientation, and internal models (Brodal 2004). *Internal models* are the stored information needed for specific activities, such as walking down stairs or reaching for something in space (see Chapter 1 Cerebellum,). Neural networks in the cortex coordinate the different sensory modalities and give them meaning. Postural control therefore creates a reference frame for perception and action in relation to the world around us (Brodal 2004).

The postural orientation of the individual relative to the base of support and gravity determines the movement strategies that will be accessible and effective (van der Fits et al 1998). The orientation of the trunk is probably one of the most vitally controlled variables of the body because the orientation of the trunk will influence the positioning of the limbs (Popovic & Sinkjær 2008).

The *midline* is a term that is frequently used clinically. It is a broad term that is difficult to define precisely. *Midline* refers to the interplay of body segments and alignment, and involves both phys-

ical and perceptual factors, such as body schema. We explore and adapt to our environment, and action requires perception, balance, and movement. We have to perceive our body in space to adapt to the environment. The term *midline control* refers to both ability to and an experience of being balanced. The perception of midline (i.e., verticality) is critical for balance control and for interaction with the environment. In an upright human, the perception of the vertical, also referred to as the subjective vertical (SV), is perfectly aligned with the earth vertical. This requires an updated internal model (Barbieri et al 2008). This internal representation of verticality is constructed from multisensory components, including visual, auditory, somatosensory, and vestibular inputs (Mittelstaedt 1996; Mittelstaedt 1992). There are different modalities to evaluate the subjective vertical: the visual vertical (VV), the haptic vertical (HV), and the postural vertical (PV), with the latter being the most relevant in explaining balance disorders (Pérennou et al 2008). As stated by Mittelstaedt (1992), the subjective PV is first determined by information from the visceral graviceptors in the trunk and secondarily by somatosensory information.

▩ Postural Stability

Equilibrium may be defined as stability—the resistance to both linear and angular acceleration—and will therefore be referred to as *postural stability*. Postural stability involves the coordination of sensorimotor strategies to stabilize the body's CoM relative to the BoS during both self-initiated and externally triggered disturbances in postural stability (Horak 2006).

Some activities may push stability to the limit and beyond, and necessitate a change of base of support (e.g., taking a step). Some tasks will focus on attaining the goal rather than maintaining stability limits (e.g., the football keeper who throws himself to catch the ball, while the fall itself is as controlled as possible). Stability is a result of forces being balanced in relation to each other or equal to each other. In human movement, stability is always dynamic (i.e., movement also occurs in stabilizing segments). Dynamic stability ensures dynamic equilibrium at every instant (i.e., dynamic stability allows a task to be performed efficiently, from the onset to the end) (Bouisset & Do 2008). Even as we stand still, there is a segmental adjustment through the body (i.e., stability in standing is dynamic); the ability to hold a position demands continuous adjustment of neuromuscular activity.

Stability allows movement between body parts; to reach out for an object, the body must stabilize and stay, then gradually move with the arm to reach further if necessary. As we reach, the hand initiates the actual movement of the arm while feedforward mechanisms (APAs) stabilize the body. Stability during walking (dynamic stability) can be defined as the ability to maintain functional locomotion despite the presence of external disturbances or internal control errors (Hilfiker et al 2013).

Controlling postural stability during walking is more complex than maintaining upright stance (Winter 1995). During forward locomotion, the neuromuscular activation of the hip and pelvis has to maintain the stability of these segments at the same time as we are moving forward in space, and the hip joint rotates and changes from flexion to extension. As we reach the swing phase, the activity changes; tone is reduced to allow a free swing (**Fig. 2.1**).

Stability areas vary continuously, depending not only on the function but also on all phase changes of movement. Therefore, mobility is essential for stability, as is stability for movement. The trunk may stabilize for movements of the extremities, the extremities may stabilize for trunk movement, the upper trunk may stabilize for pelvic mobility, the pelvic area may stabilize for trunk movements, the right side may stabilize for movements of the left half of the body, and so on. Even distally, the lower arm must stabilize for movements of the hand, and the wrist for movements of the fingers. The same is true for the lower leg and foot. Stable areas of reference adapt and change as movement evolves.

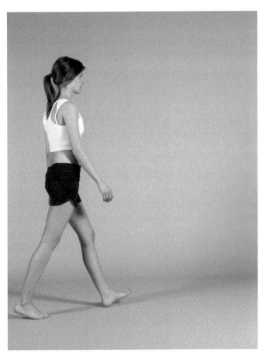

Fig. 2.1 The stability areas vary during locomotion.

■ Multisensory Integration for Postural Control

To produce a context-dependent postural activation, the CNS must first establish the current status of the body relative to its environment. To accomplish this, humans use multiple sensory references: gravity (the vestibular system), contact with the environment (somatosensory systems), proprioceptive signals of body position (Mergner et al 2003), and the relationship between the body and objects in the environment (vision) (Horak et al 1997). The integration of all three systems enables us to maintain balance (Marigold et al 2004). The sensory information is translated into appropriate motor responses to ensure both anticipatory and reactive aspects of balance control. Human postural control has to be adaptable and stable under many different conditions, which require a process of *reweighting* of multisensory stimuli. Sensory reweighting is the ability of the CNS to suppress incorrect or weak sensory information while becoming more sensitive to other available sensory information (Pasma et al 2012). Visual, vestibular, and somatosensory inputs are dynamically reweighted to maintain upright posture as environmental or nervous system conditions change (Logan et al 2014). To give an example of this, studies have shown that in a well-lit environment with a firm base of support, healthy individuals rely on a combination of somatosensory (70%), vision (10%), and vestibular (20%) information to maintain an upright standing posture (Peterka 2002). However, upon a change from a stationary to a tilting surface, humans shift sensory weighting from somatosensory to vestibular cues (Peterka 2002). Therefore, when sensory integration is intact, the weight of one type of sensory input is enhanced to compensate for a decrease in or absence of information from another sensory channel. Thus a neurologically healthy human does not lose balance during visual deprivation (e.g., when moving from a light to a dark environment) because the information provided from vestibular and somatosensory input will be upgraded to guide the postural demands needed in a dark environment. Ongoing reweighting of the different types of sensory information is required for efficient, flexible, context-dependent postural control (Bonan et al 2013). The CNS selects the type of sensory information estimated to be the most significant in a given situation and to ignore information assumed to be less reliable. Sources with variable input tend to be ignored (Brodal 2004). Sensory deficit is a well-known consequence of many neurological disorders, and most stroke patients have been found to be excessively reliant on visual information to control their posture (Bonan et al 2006; Yelnik et al 2006), this has also been demonstrated in patients with PD (Brady et al 2012). This behavior makes the patient rely on visual information, even when inappropriate, and regardless of normal vestibular or somatosensory function (Yelnik et al 2006). Decreased multisensory integration with excessive reliance on visual information and consequently poor balance control, has been demonstrated during the chronic stages (> 1 year) after a stroke (Bonan et al 2004) and in the later stages of PD (Keijsers et al 2005). The ability to sensory reweight is critical with regard to recovery of balance control in pathological conditions (Bonan et al 2013). Research has shown that sensory integration can improve after specific multisensory training programs and can have positive effects on postural stability in neurologically intact elderly people (Alfieri et al 2010) as well as in stroke subjects more than 6 months poststroke (Bayouk et al 2006).

To choose the appropriate postural response, the nervous system must be able to judge the positions of the body parts to one another and to a representation of the external world. This is achieved by an internal model of the arrangement of the body and its orientation in space—the body schema (see Chapter 1). *Body schema* includes all information relevant for action and is continuously updated through movement. Body schema is a representation of the body in the brain that informs us of the position of the body segments in relation to each other, and also takes into account the length of the limb segments and muscle length (Gandevia et al 2002). The body schema therefore provides a foundation for the exploration of space—the environment—for perceptual analysis and motor action. Hence the appropriate response is developed based on the body schema, and the postural muscle synergies are activated to perform the appropriate head, eye, trunk, and limb movements to maintain posture (Horak 1997; Horak 1987; Kandel et al 2013). We need detailed

information from all sensory modalities to create and continuously update a body schema to balance and move; thus reduction of one or more modalities drastically impairs the body schema (Blouin et al 1993).

Several modalities of sensory information are available for the CNS for postural control. Visual information contributes to establishing the orientation of objects in space and to detecting movements; there is a close relationship between vision and postural control. The simplest connection between vision and posture has been demonstrated by asking people to close their eyes, as a result of which postural sway increases. Visual cues exert their effect on posture both through feedforward information on postural demands and feedback information of one's own body movement as well as that of the surroundings. For example, in standing, vision provides information about self-motion to detect movement and monitor the displacement of the head and body in relation to the environment. This allows for corrective adjustments to deviations from the vertical. The functional role of central and peripheral vision in the control of posture indicates a greater contribution of peripheral vision than central vision to the control of quiet standing (Berencsi et al 2005). During locomotion, vision is important for setting the level of neuromuscular activity through feedforward planning (Wade & Jones 1997). Also, it has an important predictive role in navigation and obstacle avoidance (Logan et al 2010), in picking up information about our surroundings resulting in alteration of direction or speed if appropriate. Vision does not direct the placement of the foot in detail under normal circumstances. If the terrain is uneven or difficult, vision becomes more involved but has no role in the actual adaptation and adjustment of the foot to the ground; the feet respond immediately to unevenness and changes. When one is standing on a mobile base, as in a bus, on a train, or in a boat, or on an unsteady rock, there is a flood of information from the feet to the CNS about the properties of the surface and the line of gravity in relation to the feet. Postural tone is automatically adjusted to the situation and the goal. This adaptation is in response to information received through the somatosensory systems, that is, feedback. Activity—the interaction with gravity—demands continuous interplay between feedforward and feedback.

Somatosensory information provided by muscle, joint, and cutaneous receptors informs the CNS about head, trunk, and limb position in space. The vestibular contribution includes the detection of head movements in space, specifically rotation and translation. They are active even at rest to sense the pull of gravity and thus determine the earth vertical. Vestibular information plays a part in head stabilization during dynamic tasks by which successful gaze control is achieved (Pozzo et al 1990), and provides a stable reference frame for the head from which postural responses can be generated (Pozzo et al 1995).

The last sensory system important for postural control is the graviceptor systems in the internal organs (Mittelstaedt 1996; Vaitl et al 2002; Trousselard et al 2004; Clément et al 2014) *Graviceptors* are specialized sensory receptors detecting displacement of weight in relation to gravity, for instance the weight of shifting fluid in the intestines and kidneys. The graviceptors may monitor the force vector exerted at each joint to oppose gravity, and this information contributes to an internal representation of the vertical axis (Mittelstaedt 1996). Research has argued for graviceptors as a separate pathway in humans for sensing body orientation in relation to gravity (Karnath & Dieterich 2006).

■ Light Touch Cue

The term "haptic" sense was introduced by Jeka and Lackner in 1995. Haptic sense relates to the cutaneous and kinesthetic sensory information from mechanoreceptors in the skin, muscles, and joints of the hand and fingers while touching or manipulating an object. In their pioneering work, Jeka and Lackner (1994, 1995) showed the important role of added haptic information provided by a light touch of the index fingertip on a stable support surface in the control of upright posture. *Light touch cue* is somatosensory information from the fingertip that is obtained by lightly touching an object with a contact force of < 100 g (Boonsinsukh et al 2011). Since this original work, several studies have demonstrated that, when one is touching a rigid immobile object, sensory cues are provided to the CNS about the direction of body sway, which improves the postural stability in standing even when the applied forces provided are inadequate to give a significant biomechanical support (Jeka 1997; Franzén et al 2011; Lackner & DiZio 2005; Boonsinsukh et al 2009). Because light touch does not provide a significant biomechanical support, changes in postural sway have been attributed to central neural integration of somatosensory information provid-

ing an additional spatial reference frame for postural control (Jeka 1997; Jeka & Lackner 1994; Jeka & Lackner 1995). Franzén and colleagues (2011) showed in their study that light touch cue from the hands resulted in significant changes in axial tone (hips and trunk). The authors suggest that this is due to the provision of an additional reference system by which axial muscle tone is increased leading to a reduction of postural sway. This is supported by Creath and colleagues (2008), who suggest that the benefit from light touch is primarily in increasing trunk control. Light touch cue has been shown to reduce postural sway in both healthy individuals and those with postural control dysfunctions due to diabetic neuropathy, cerebellar disease, PD, multiple sclerosis, stroke, and vestibular impairments (Lackner & DiZio 2005; Boonsinsukh et al 2009; Kanekar et al 2013; Baldan et al 2014).

■ Postural Control and Biomechanical Conditions

According to Horak (2006), the size and quality of the base of support are the most important biomechanical constraints on balance. In standing the foot provides the only direct source of contact with the ground, and therefore plays an important role in all weight-bearing tasks. Changes to foot structure and any impairment in strength, range of movement, pain, or control of the feet will therefore affect the control of balance (Horak 2006) (**Fig. 2.2**). The foot is an active and flexible structure under balance control and is sensitive to minute perturbations (Wright et al 2012). With more than 100 muscles, tendons, and ligaments, 26 bones, and 33 joints, the foot, specifically the arches of the foot, is evolved for the vital role of balance control (Wright et al 2012), among other functions. A study of balance control in older people suggests that ankle flexibility, toe plantar flexor strength, and plantar sensation are significant and independent predictors of standing balance control (Menz et al 2005), and it is hypothesized that manual handling applied to the foot and ankle may be beneficial to augment other therapeutic modalities when working with patients with balance problems (Wassinger et al 2014).

Postural control in humans is dependent, to a large extent, on the efficient function of trunk and neck muscles, as well as on antigravity muscles in the legs (Gramsbergen 2005). Reduction of muscle strength may affect the available postural control

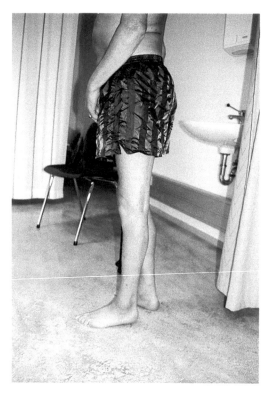

Fig. 2.2 Reduced adaptability in the foot in standing. The left knee is hyperextended and the left hip flexed. In walking there is a reduction of forward motion of the body over the left foot causing a posterior displacement of the center of gravity leading to displacement feedback and consequently associated reactions of the left arm.

mechanisms and shift the postural responses away from the area of weakness. For example, muscle weakness around the ankle joint may result in large compensatory hip and trunk motions to correct disequilibrium in standing (Horak 1987), reduced muscle strength, especially of the lower limbs, has been indicated as one of the most important risk factors for falls (Orr 2010; Horlings et al 2009). Alignment of the different body segments over the base of support influences the effort required to support the body against gravity and determines the type of movement strategies that will be effective in controlling posture (Woollacott & Crenna 2008). This may be due to altered length–tension relationships between muscles working together, which might disrupt the normal functioning of the muscle synergies necessary for postural control. For example, two muscles important for optimal postural strategies

in the hip and ankle, the gluteus maximus and the tibialis anterior, have been found weak or "underactive" in several common postural disorders (Daubney & Culham 1999). If these muscles are too weak to adequately respond to external perturbations and make necessary corrective movements, balance may be reduced.

■ Trunk Control

Trunk control is the ability of the muscles in the trunk to keep the body upright against gravity, to adjust weight shift for various functional movements, and to perform selective movements of the trunk compartment by which the center of mass is kept within the base of support during postural adjustments.

The various body segments are linked together in a functional kinematic chain connecting the eyes to the feet (Massion 1992) in which the trunk serves as the center (Borghuis et al 2008). Trunk control is thus an essential component of postural control (Borghuis et al 2008; Dickstein et al 2004; Karatas et al 2004; Kibler et al 2006) and is a complex, ever changing, and dynamic neuromuscular function.

The trunk constitutes over half of the body mass and greatly influences the rest of the body (Kang & Dingwell 2009). The core of the body consists of the musculoskeletal areas of the trunk, pelvis, hips, and proximal lower limbs (Kibler et al 2006). The abdominal muscles, especially the m. transversus abdominis, together with the diaphragm above, the pelvic floor below, and the back muscles, contribute to postural stability (Ebenbichler et al 2001). The muscles of the trunk and pelvis are responsible for dynamic stability of the trunk in functional activities (Kibler et al 2006; Borghuis et al 2008). The segments of the trunk and the pelvis are interconnected and interdependent in human functional movement because most of the deep and superficial muscles of the back and abdomen attach the trunk to the pelvis and spine. Trunk control is important and complex; therefore, careful clinical assessment is required for accurate diagnosis of dysfunction in this area.

Limiting the definition of core stability to "the ability to control the position and motion of the trunk over the pelvis" (Kibler et al 2006) seems to leave out the base of support as an important prerequisite for trunk stability and movement. Trunk control is therefore understood as the selective control of the trunk over the pelvis as well as the pelvis/

hips in relation to the base of support, encompassing the simultaneous control of stability and mobility. In the following discussion, the term *trunk control* will be used to cover both trunk control and core stability.

The human trunk receives bilateral supraspinal input (Carr et al 1994), and a postural role for muscles on both sides of the trunk during limb movement has been indicated (Dickstein et al 2004). APAs precede and accompany limb movement and provide proximal stability for distal mobility (Borghuis et al 2008; Dickstein et al 2004; Ebenbichler et al 2001; Kibler et al 2006; Massion 1992) to minimize postural destabilization and orient the trunk to allow the limbs to carry out the desired movement (Borghuis et al 2008).

Lower trunk postural muscles (axial, erector spinae, and rectus abdominis) are involved more in maintaining trunk postural control, whereas upper trunk muscles are involved more in counteracting the destabilization brought on by a moving limb (Dickstein et al 2004). The recruitment and timing of appropriate muscles are extremely important for trunk control, more so than endurance and muscle strength alone (Borghuis et al 2008). Modest levels of trunk muscle coactivation are required to give sufficient stability for the optimal and complex balance between stability and mobility for task performance (Borghuis et al 2008). To control the three-dimensional forces applied to the trunk, the CNS probably differentially activates individual regions of musculature in the spine. Recent research findings by Park and colleagues (2014) demonstrated that muscle activation in the trunk appears to be based on the mechanical advantage of the muscle (how the muscle can create torque for stability), rather than motor unit size (Henneman's size principle). The recovery of trunk control thus seems to be a prerequisite for more complex functional abilities.

Postural Control and Cognition

Postural control represents the most automatic activity in human movement (Massion 1994; Massion 1992; Mulder et al 1996), although it is probably less automatic than previously thought. There is growing evidence from research in both psychology and neurophysiology that human motor control and emotion are largely interconnected and reciprocally interrelated; thus there seem to be strong interactions between cognitive processes and balance con-trol (Teasdale & Simoneau 2001; Niedenthal 2007; Yogev-Seligmann et al 2012). Postural control in ADLs occurs while at least one other simultaneous task is being performed, for example, standing while talking. This is referred to as dual-tasking postural control. Dual tasking involves dividing cognitive resources between a cognitive-type task and a postural challenge. Recent research has shown that the ability to maintain postural stability in every situation demands a certain level of attention, and that attentional demands increase with increasing balance demands (Hunter & Hoffman 2001). Simultaneous demands for cognition and balance increase the tendency to fall in elderly people (Brown et al 1999); dual tasks demonstrate the same relationship (Mulder et al 1996). Furthermore the combination of a cognitive task and a balance task results in a poorer solution of the cognitive task if it contains spatial elements (Brodal 2004). Recent studies have shown that psychological factors, such as fear of falling and low balance confidence, may induce adaptive changes in postural control (Yiou et al 2012).

Additional evidence for the involvement of cortical networks in balance control is that impairments in executive functions, such as attention, mental calculation, orientation, and memory, interfere with balance control (Jacobs & Horak 2007).

Postural Tone

In the following section the term *postural tone* or *tone* is used instead of *muscle tone* to emphasize that the CNS activates many muscle groups for the maintenance of postural activity. Shumway-Cook and Woollacott (2011) describe postural tone as an increased level of activity in antigravity muscles (i.e., the background tonic muscle activation that supports the body against gravity), and Ivanenko and colleagues (2013) define postural tone as "an unconscious, low-amplitude, long-lasting muscle tension distributed in a specific pattern along the entire body axis." The function of postural tone is to supply adequate joint torques to maintain equilibrium against gravity (Ting et al 2009).There is a continuous adjustment of postural tone before, during, and after every movement. The most important factor in altering the level of tone is muscular contraction (Brodal 2010). Let us consider postural tone in the axial muscles and the functional relevance for this. These muscles have an extensive anatomical origin, with insertions linked to several structures, such as the pelvis, rib cage, spinal column, shoulder girdles, and head. Several axial muscles run long distances and have multiple attachments. The descending control of axial muscles originates from cortical and subcortical structures. The bilateral and ipsilateral descending pathways from the brain stem provide an important source of control to these muscles as they innervate the spinal interneurons and motor neurons both uni and bilaterally (Gurfinkel et al 2006). Postural stability and controlled mobility require constant activity of axial muscles because the axis (trunk) links all parts of the body together; hence axial tonic activity from various descending structures must take the actions of all parts of the body into account. For coordination of movement, tonic regulation of axial muscles is a necessity (Hasan 2005).

Postural tone gives an automatic background for activity and may vary from moment to moment. It needs to be high enough to withstand the effect of gravity and at the same time low enough to allow dynamic adaptation through small movements; therefore the control of the appropriate level of postural tone is related to the effect of gravity on the human body and to the base of support (Raine et al 2009). The BoS is the contact area between the body and the environment: the feet in standing; the thighs, buttocks, or back (if there is a backrest on the chair) in sitting; and the contact area between the hand and an object. The quality of the base, its size, material, texture, softness, and temperature, and the distance between the base of support and the center of gravity, are all important factors in setting the level of postural tone and the motor response: we lie down to rest, and sit, stand, or walk when we want to be active. Postural tone has a wide spectrum in normal movement: it is normally at its lowest in a relaxed supine position, when the base of support is large and the center of gravity is low. It may change in a millisecond, as when we jump out of bed to answer the phone. In normal daily activity postural tone is at its highest in toe-off in the stance phase, just before weight transference to the opposite heel. Humans may grade activity in the postural system as needed and through experience and exercise. The ballet dancer who dances on tiptoes and the tightrope walker are examples of postural activity on a much higher level than needed for ADLs. Tone is highest in those areas of the body where the need for maintaining and sustaining activity against gravity is highest, and varies in relation to the base of support and the effect of gravity. There are individ-ual differences in postural tone; some people have a naturally higher level of tone, and others have a lower tone. There are several possible explanations for why the distribution of muscle tone differs in healthy individuals. Psychological factors may play a role; people who are anxious often have a higher tone than those who are relaxed. In addition, the body is not structurally designed to optimize stability because the masses of the different axial segments of the body are not vertically aligned (Wright & Horak 2007). The CoM of the head is in front of the neck, thus the neck muscles must be active to prevent the head from falling forward. The same applies for the trunk, which has a center of mass that is anterior to the spinal column and the hip joint. With the trunk and head stooped forward in a flexed posture, the center of mass of the upper body requires back and hip extensors to oppose a larger torque than optimal (Wright & Horak 2007).

Gravity acts on the body at all times, whether at rest or during activity. The level of activity in different muscles depends on the orientation of the body and the extremities to gravity and the base of support, the relative relationship between body segments, the activity to be performed, the environment, and experience.

All ADLs demand that we relate to and oppose gravity, from turning over in bed, shifting our position, turning over pages in a book, and reaching out to turn off the light in bed, to initiating head movement for sitting up, getting dressed, and managing the bathroom, lifting a fork to eat, writing a letter, running after the bus, or walking in the mountains. The musculoskeletal system is constantly adapting to modify activity during changing relationships. Outdoors, even weather and wind conditions act on our bodies and demand postural adjustments.

Descriptions that may seem artificial in relation to healthy people may seem logical in clinical situations: *against gravity* is a term used in the treatment of neurologically damaged persons. The inability to adopt a natural, upright posture might be thought of as an interruption of the habitual distribution of postural tone (Ivanenko et al 2013). Acutely after stroke, a spinal cord injury, or relapse of multiple sclerosis (MS), many patients suffer from severely low postural tone (**Fig. 2.3a, b**) and are unable to activate or sustain activity against gravity and therefore also have problems moving.

These factors are not all-important, however; postural tone is not always low in supine. Most people will recognize the situation in the dentist's chair:

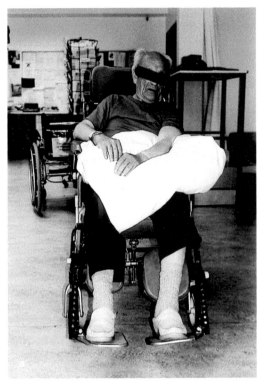
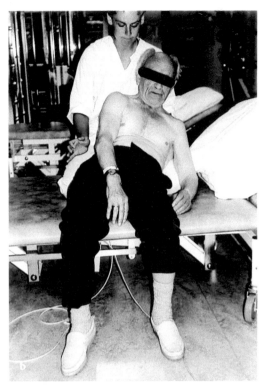

Fig. 2.3 The patient has had an acute stroke. **(a)** It seems as if he is either falling or pushing himself up with his right arm. He has very low postural tone and balance. He is unable to stay upright and interact with gravity. **(b)** He compensates by increasing his flexor activity in the right side of the head, neck, and trunk in an attempt to pull himself up. Notice his right foot in both **(a)** and **(b)**, which seems to push against the floor and footrest. There is very little activity in his left side.

if you are uneasy or nervous, your postural tone is higher. In this situation, adaptation to the contact area is not appropriate, and you may have a feeling of being suspended in the air above the chair through muscular tension instead of resting *in* the chair. If a person sits uncomfortably, too still, unable to adjust or change position, postural tone may increase.

The interaction with the environment demands a constant adjustment of tone, alignment, balance, and movement. This interaction depends largely on the ability to receive and perceive information from peripheral receptors and to adapt and adjust in response to this information. Our initial evaluation of conditions of the base of support is based on tactile information from the BoS: feet (soles), bottom, and hands. We evaluate the support conditions by tactile contact. Our next calculation is of inertia; a smaller support means that inertia is more easily overcome and more quickly evaluated and assessed. The larger the estimation of the tactile area, the more difficult

it is to overcome inertia. The relationship between the body and the base of support is the foundation for adjustment of tone to varying environments and activities. Tone needs to be optimal for the actual activity, whether it is to relax, initiate movement, balance, or perform functional activities.

> In a functional context, the sensorimotor and perceptual interaction between the body and the base of support is more important for the level of postural tone than the size of the support base.

The human foot is a very complex structure, which allows it to carry out many different functions. It is a flexible and adaptive body segment with precise active control (Wright et al 2012; Zelik et al 2014). The control specificity of the foot muscles in different functions is described as reminiscent of the fine motor control of the hand (Zelik et al 2014). During standing, it provides our base of support, whereas during walking, it must be stable at the initial heel contact and pushoff phase. On midstance, the foot must be mobile to adapt to the ground. The feet transmit information directly between the body and the environment and must *adapt* and *respond to* the BoS and not *react to* the base with inappropriate tension—pushing or clawing—for balance and movements to be optimal.

The feet are our base of support, our foundation. They are sense organs that communicate the information they pick up about the BoS—unevenness, texture, hardness, direction, incline, and the distribution of body weight—to the CNS. The structure of the foot determines which rotatory components are available in the foot and leg during walking and running (Nawoczenski et al 1998) (i.e., patterns of movement). The foot has springlike characteristics by which elastic energy is stored and released (McKeon et al 2014). This is possible due to the architecture of the foot, and especially due to the development of the arch of the foot, which is distorted during walking and running. The deformations result from the stretching of passive tissues (i.e., plantar fascia and ligaments) (McKenzie 1955) as well as from contractions of the intrinsic and extrinsic foot muscles. Sensory information from these passive and active structures is used to control movement and posture (McKeon et al 2014). McKeon and colleagues (2014) propose that the concept of *core stability* may also be extended to the arch of the foot. They claim that the *foot core system* includes interacting subsystems that deliver relevant sensory input and functional stability for accommodating to changing demands during both static and dynamic activities (McKeon et al 2014). Comparable to the lumbopelvic core, the arch of the foot is controlled by both local and global muscles. The local stabilizers are the intrinsic muscles of the foot, and the global muscles are the muscles originating in the lower leg and insert onto the foot. During walking the intrinsic muscles are controlling the degree and speed of arch deformation. Without this control the foot becomes unstable and malaligned, resulting in abnormal movement of the foot (McKeon et al 2014).

Alignment and neuromuscular activity in the feet have a significant influence on the alignment and neuromuscular activity in the rest of the body (Neely 1998; Cote et al 2005) (**Fig. 2.2**). Thornquist (1985) states that the load and tension condition of the feet influence our way of moving and determine to a great extent the movements available to us. She uses the words *interplay*, *balance*, and *interdependence* to describe the relationship between our foundations, physical and psychological factors, and the environment (Thornquist 1985). However, changes in alignment and neuromuscular activity proximally will also influence the ability of the feet to function as balance organs.

Reciprocal innervation is the coordination of muscle activity for efficient, harmonious, rhythmic, and smooth movement without involving more effort than is appropriate for the actual activity (Bobath 1990; Edwards 1996). All complex movements are a result of finely graded interaction between external forces (gravity, inertia, and passive, biomechanical characteristics in involved structures) and variations in the tension-length relationships in the different motor units in agonist, antagonist, and synergic muscle groups. Reciprocal innervation tunes and balances muscle action, and we understand this to be the same as that which Sahrmann (1992, 2002) calls muscle balance (see Chapter 1, Neuromuscular System). Reciprocal innervation is described as the harmonious interplay in and between muscles (i.e., coordination between eccentric and concentric muscle activity leading to selective control of movement). Reciprocal innervation involves the following:

- Differential activation of motor units in a muscle.
- Coordination of different muscles surrounding a joint: agonists, antagonists, and synergists (i.e., eccentric and concentric interplay).
- Coordination of different body parts: right and left, proximal and distal, through neuromuscular activity.

Neurophysiologically, the recruitment principle is an important element of reciprocal innervation; the motor units involved in an activity are sequentially recruited and modified through presynaptic inhibition (see Chapter 1, Presynaptic Inhibition). Reciprocal innervation is the foundation for stability, selectivity, and coordination in normal movement.

> Mobility is essential for stability, as is stability for movement.

Selective Movement

Selective movement is understood as the controlled, specific, and coordinated movement of one joint or body part in relation to other segments. Selective movement is the result of precisely graded neuromuscular activity based on reciprocal innervation.

Stability and selectivity are both dependent on adequate ranges of motion, muscle length, alignment, and the coordination of agonists, antagonists, and synergists in concentric and eccentric work. Eccentric muscle activity is the result of active, neurophysiological processes. Reciprocal innervation leads to the ability to do the following:

- Automatically adapt muscle activity for postural adjustments.
- Stabilize for selective movement.
- Grade the activation and interaction of agonists, synergists, and antagonists for precision in timing and direction.

Patterns of movement are sequences of selective movements that vary from person to person, the task at hand, and the situation (see **Fig. 2.4a, b**). Movements are the output of a dynamic interaction between muscular forces and peripheral field effects (e.g., gravity, friction, joint reactive forces) and can be described in terms of their pattern, displacement, or topology (Mulder et al 1995). The motor system has to contract the agonist with the right force at the right time as well as time and organize the contraction patterns of the antagonists, synergists, and postural muscles necessary for the agonist in the actual function. The number of muscle fibers and motor units recruited in a muscle varies depending on the function and other muscles that are recruited in relation to the task. The anatomical construction of the skeleton enhances coordination and rotation between the different body parts. The muscles cause rotation to varying degrees depending on the anatomical form and arrangement of the muscle fibers, their function, and the organization of different

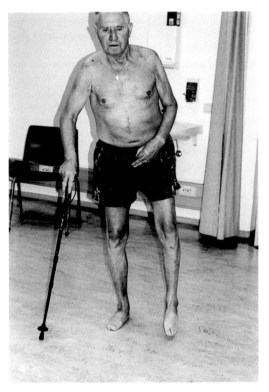 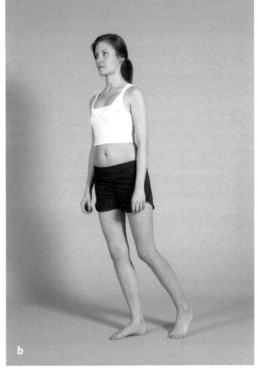

Fig. 2.4 Compare the patterns of movement in the two pictures. **(a)** The patient's center of gravity is to the right of his right leg, and he presses actively down on his walking stick. Therefore, the flexor activity in his right side is increased at the same time as he seems to lift his left side forward with his right. There is decreased mobility and interplay between body segments generally, but especially proximally. The patterns of movement in his arms and legs are stereotypical. Rotation in his left leg does not change to swing the leg forward. There is reduced dorsiflexion in the foot. This could be caused either by stiffness of his calf muscles or weak dorsiflexors, or malalignment of the whole leg negating the activation of dorsiflexion. **(b)** A healthy young woman is taking a step forward with her left leg. Notice the extension over the standing leg and the interplay between body segments. On the swinging side the pattern of movement changes from stance phase activity (more extensor/abductor/external rotation activity) to let go of the same activity through rotation to swing the leg forward. The left dorsiflexion ensures clearance of the floor.

parts of the muscle to each other (alignment) and their attachments. Examples are the tendo-Achilles, which is rotated 90° before its attachment to the calcaneus, and the pectoralis major, which is rotated 180° before its attachment to the humerus.

Rotation is an essential component of normal movement, and it gives enhanced proprioceptive feedback to the CNS compared with, for instance muscle palpation or tendon tapping. Humans move along three planes: sagittal, frontal, and transversal (or horizontal), and this is combined through rotation. All weight transference and movement demand rotational components. We vary between symmetry and asymmetry caused by interplay between body segments through rotation. Rotation is based on the ability to grade and combine flexor and extensor components in infinite variations of movement patterns, and gives flexibility and resilience. Rotation, for instance, between the upper and lower arm and between the thigh and lower leg, in relation to their proximal segments, and through trunk rotation, causes a functional diversity that allows anything from fine motor activity and distal dexterity to coarse grasping and locomotion.

Basic patterns of movement are *reach* and *grasp* and *stance* and *swing*. These patterns vary infinitely depending on the task and the environment. *Reach* and *stance* are both patterns that are mainly dominated by components of extension, outward rotation, and abduction. *Grasp* and *swing* have more flexor components to their patterns, often with components of outward rotation and adduction. When the arm is by the side, the hand is brought to the mouth through flexion/adduction/external rotation initially, and changing to graded internal rotation of the shoulder, flexion of the elbow, and supination of the forearm. The patterns interchange and vary in all our activities: we position ourselves in more extension if we need to reach out for something above shoulder height; when performing activities that demand fine eye–hand coordination we often choose to sit in a more flexed position based on eccentric trunk extensor activity. Normal postural tone and normal reciprocal innervation allow individuals to choose their own background neuromuscular activity most appropriate for the situation.

■ Deviations from Normal Human Movement and Balance Control

Neurological patients are heterogeneous in terms of their disease, lesions, degrees of impairment, and disabilities. They show individual characteristics; lesions in a similar location and of a similar size in two patients will manifest differently. Patients have different personalities, talents, and experiences that have shaped their body and mind. Some patients may present with other medical diagnoses as well, such as diabetes and cardiac problems. Some patients may be in poor general condition for different reasons. The aim of treatment is to enhance the patient's potential as much as possible, keeping this heterogeneity in mind. Many patients will not reach the same level of function as before the lesion and will have to compensate to be functional within their environment. Clinically, reduced postural control seems to be one of the main problems for many patients with CNS lesions. Biomechanical components, sensory inputs, integration and reweighting, as well as motor strategies, cognitive processing, and perception of verticality, all contribute to balance control to different extents in different patients. A loss of a stable reference frame as a basis for voluntary movement causes balance problems, reduced coordination and interaction between muscle groups, as well as a reduced tempo and ability to react. Postural control counterstabilizes movements of the extremities; if the body is not kept stable as a person reaches out in space, the body moves with the arm and the person is destabilized. As a consequence, the person's choice of how to solve different motor tasks becomes limited, which again may reduce the person's ability to be independent and master daily activities. Postural control and precise, goal-oriented movement are not separate phenomena in the CNS; they are coordinated to allow successful achievement of motor tasks in a context-based environment. Postural control requires segmental displacement and interaction with gravity. Therefore, the therapist should ensure that the patient has segmental mobility, for instance of the spinal column.

Many patients with stroke tend to demonstrate insufficient trunk control, affecting their functional ability in many activities, such as turning in bed, sitting up/lying down, rising from sitting to standing, and standing and walking (**Fig. 2.5**). Impaired anticipatory activity of the superficial lateral trunk muscles (latissimus dorsi, rectus abdominis, and external oblique) on the paretic side has been found to influence the ability to perform daily activities (Dickstein et al 2004). Impaired APAs have also been documented in a variety of conditions, such as aging, atypical development, and neurological disorders (Aruin & Almeida 1997; Inglin & Woollacott 1988; Latash et al 1995; Slijper et al 2002).

Patients have demonstrated an altered trunk position sense after stroke (Ryerson et al 2008) and mislocalization of tactile stimuli to the trunk in the presence of neglect (Rousseaux et al 2013). Several studies

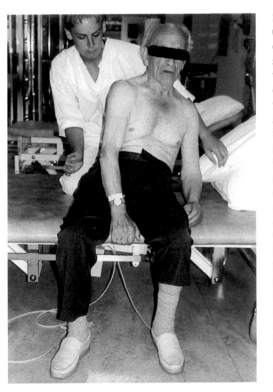

Fig. 2.5 This patient shows reduced balance as a result of an acute stroke. He has reduced tone in his trunk and lacks the interplay of movement between body segments in all three planes.

ments were found for patients compared with controls (Genthon et al 2007; Perlmutter et al 2010). A greater dependence on vision to maintain stability on an unstable base of support was found in patients compared with controls (Van Nes et al 2008). These studies indicate that patients suffer impaired trunk control at all times after stroke. Because trunk control is essential for sitting balance, impairments of the trunk might also affect functional activities involving the use of the arms and hands (e.g., in dressing and reaching) possibly due to altered alignment, stability, and movement of the shoulder girdles affecting distal precision. Robertson et al (2012) found reduced protraction of both shoulder girdles in left hemispheric stroke of patients with a dominant right hand. In right hemispheric stroke this was found only for the left shoulder girdle, suggesting a different role of the two hemispheres. They also found reduced dexterity of the nonparetic hand after stroke. This is supported by increasing evidence about involvement of the ipsilesional side (Sousa et al 2013). In fact, after a unilateral lesion of the subcortical medial cerebral artery territory, damage can occur not only in the crossed fibers responsible for movement execution in the contralesional limbs but also in the corticoreticular networks, which may have consequences for the function of the reticulospinal pathways, thus interfering with the muscle activity of the ipsilesional postural muscles. Especially trunk control is essentially modulated by the descending ventromedial system, which projects mostly ipsilaterally (Stapley et al 2008; Schepens & Drew 2004).

In addition to impairments, compensatory strategies seem to affect the postural role of the trunk in functional activities. With impaired skills in movements such as reaching, the trunk may exhibit compensatory strategies with increased flexion and/or rotation, as described by several authors (Robertson & Roby-Brami 2011; Reisman & Scholz 2006; Roby-Brami et al 2003; Michaelsen et al 2006; Thielman 2013; van Kordelaar et al 2012; Woodbury et al 2009). Empirically, some patients seem to compensate for deficits in selectivity of leg movement during walking by using their trunk to lift and rotate the pelvis to swing the most affected leg forward during walking (hip hiking, circumduction) (see **Fig. 2.4a**). The use of compensatory trunk activity to move a limb implies a secondary source of trunk instability, potentially increasing the patient's functional disability.

The foregoing studies show that dysfunction in trunk control is a substantial problem after stroke. However, dysfunction in trunk control is also seen in other neurological disorders, such as MS, incomplete spinal cord injuries, traumatic brain injury, and PD.

have demonstrated decreased trunk muscle strength (Dickstein et al 2004; Karatas et al 2004; Pereira et al 2014; Pereira et al 2010; Winzeler-Merçay & Mudie 2002), and muscle strength has been found to be positively correlated with balance as measured with Berg's Balance Scale (Karatas et al 2004). Increased activation of the erector spinae muscle on the paretic side has also been described (Dickstein et al 2004; Winzeler-Merçay & Mudie 2002).

Altered recruitment patterns for head and trunk rotation in sitting, whereby patients with stroke move the head and trunk simultaneously instead of in a cranial–caudal pattern, has been reported (Verheyden et al 2011). Deficit in segmental rotation between the thorax and pelvis was found to be associated with poorer postural control and walking ability (Hacmon et al 2012).

Upright sitting has been examined by posturography in both the early (Genthon et al 2007; Van Nes et al 2008) and the chronic stage after stroke (Perlmutter et al 2010). A larger sway area and larger displace-

■ Compensation

Shumway-Cook and Woollacott (2006) define compensation as behavioral substitution, that is, alternative behavioral strategies that are adopted to complete a task. The two terms *compensation* and *compensatory strategies* are perceived to mean the same.

In the acute phase there is often seemingly severe paresis or paralysis after an upper motor neuron lesion. The CNS is vulnerable in this phase (see Consequences of and Reorganization after CNS Lesions); the concentration of neurotrophic substances increases and facilitates the formation of new connections. We learn by doing, and the patient's CNS quickly learns new strategies that may seem appropriate for the moment. What the patient is stimulated to do, or required to manage more or less independently by carers, himself, or the environment, drives the formation of new connections in the CNS. Many patients are required to master independence in activities of daily living without having the postural or movement control needed to do so. The patients who sit alone on the side of the bed in the first few days are driven to compensate if they lack the postural control to do so safely.

If compensation leads to goal achievement, the drive for improvement may stop. The brain is oriented toward immediate success and rewards, not to the process involved in reaching the goal. The compensatory strategies will be learned as relevant and appropriate for this stage. Held (1987) describes it as follows: "In other words, if compensation is allowed to occur, there is apparently no stimulus to the partially damaged system to recover and behavioral substitution will occur." This may be explained by reactive synaptogenesis (the formation of new synapses and collateral sprouting) forming abnormal connections that compete with more appropriate connections. Compensation may therefore limit the neural functions that are spared after lesions.

Clinical experience supports the theory that therapy may influence the restructuring processes in the lesioned CNS (see Chapter 1.3 Motor Learning and Plasticity). The CNS recovers very quickly after the initial shock, and some functions may be spared: as edema and the penumbral zone shrinks and circulation improves, neurons start working again and some functions return; this is called spontaneous recovery. If the patient learned to use compensatory strategies during the acute phase, these may not be necessary any longer. But if the CNS experiences these strategies as appropriate in the acute phase, they may be established and difficult to change. The strategies will often have developed based on the need to balance because balance and movement control is inadequate with regard to prevent falls or the feeling of insecurity. Thus the compensatory strategies often involve fixing with the arms, grasping and holding on, weight transference to the least affected side in stroke, fixing through flexion of the trunk or flexion/adduction of hips, or pushing off the floor.

This development may be illustrated as follows (Edwards 1996); reduced postural tone and loss of reciprocal innervation as the basis for coordination as well as weakness influence the patient's balance and quality of movement negatively. Postural stability and orientation are reduced and therefore also the control of movement. The main aim of the CNS is to ensure the person's safety; thus available alternative strategies are recruited and enhanced. The sequence of recruitment (Henneman's recruitment principle) and the sensorimotor organization of activity are altered as a response to balance impairment. The feedback to the CNS of the execution of movement through peripheral receptors will be different due to the movement being different and to the altered integration and modulation of sensorimotor activity: previous responses, feedback from a healthy system, and normal movement repertoire. The basis for the execution (i.e., APAs), of the next movement and movements in the future will therefore be altered. After a CNS lesion patients alter their strategies to compensate for loss of or reduced balance control. Many patients develop cognitive and visual strategies that seem to override the integration of information from somatosensory receptors—they do not listen to their bodies any more. Movement becomes slow, and patients poke their head forward and look down to enhance visual information (this change in alignment of the head and neck will influence the vestibular system). With this increased dependence on cognitive strategies and vision, patients are increasingly prone to falls if they are distracted or people catch their attention. Mulder et al (1996) propose three measures for the improvement of balance: reduced cognitive regulation, decreased dependency on vision, and increased sensorimotor adaptation. When we have the ability to balance, we rarely think of it; if we do not have it, we think of it all the time. CNS lesions result in a move away from automatically regulated background control of balance and postural control to increased awareness and cognitive regulation of balance. Which balance strategy the patient adopts depends on build, experience, personality, and the consequences of the lesion.

> Inappropriate compensatory strategies—alternative behavioral strategies—may delay or hinder the development of balance and selective motor control in patients with CNS lesions.

Clinical Examples

Balance develops through interaction with gravity. We have to be exposed to gravity to develop postural control in standing, sitting, step standing, and walking. Asberg (1989) found that patients with stroke had improved orthostatic blood pressure, improved ADLs, and fewer severe functional impairments and limitations after being placed in the standing position early and on a regular basis (every day for 12 days after admission) compared with patients in the control group. The differences between the groups were significant, and no other interventions could explain these differences. At the same time, it is not proven that early standing alone caused this, but Asberg recommends early standing as a treatment intervention. Jakobs et al (1985) found that a group of trial participants significantly improved their perception of trunk orientation (trunk positional sense) in relaxed standing compared with lying. These studies support the importance of early standing both for functional improvement and for the patients' perception of their body.

Standing seems to improve both trunk positional sense and overall function.

Normally the hip and pelvis are stabilized in stance phase for the swing of the opposite leg. This stability is dynamic: the pelvis and hip move in relation to each other, the trunk, and the base of support to allow the translation of the center of gravity in the direction of movement. Stability is maintained over the standing leg throughout this movement. Neuromuscular stability is a prerequisite for selective movement control.

In clinical practice the therapist will meet patients who have reduced or altered recruitment of appropriate stability and movement. Many patients have reduced trunk control (core stability) and instability of the pelvis and hips. Reduced stability or increased trunk flexion seems to prevent activation of hip extension, necessary for stability. At the same time, reduced stability over the pelvis and hip may influence trunk stability negatively. Weight transference in standing may increase compression of the ankle and thereby deform the foot. As a result, alignment is changed distally, further compromising the recruitment of neuromuscular activity proximally.

Patients compensate in different ways: shifting their weight onto the least affected side or body parts (**Fig. 2.6a**), using the environment for support, enhancing the support and protective reaction of the arms, fixing within their own body, recruiting activity more proximally—a shift from ankle to hip strategy, and patients with neurological dysfunctions will often over-rely on the hip strategy (Maki

et al 2000; Raine et al 2009) (**Fig. 2.6b,c**). There is an infinite variety of possibilities. Many patients are not able to step due to reduced stability of the standing leg. They move their strategies more proximally to their arms (see **Fig. 2.6**). Patients use arm support in different ways: fixing through adduction, inward rotation of the shoulder, and increasing their flexion activity in the trunk, fixing through increasing flexion/adduction, compression of the hip, among others. The muscular interplay and muscle balance for selective stability necessary for maintaining a freestanding position, weight transference, and walking are disturbed, and stepping strategies are often used prematurely due to a lack of appropriate antigrav-

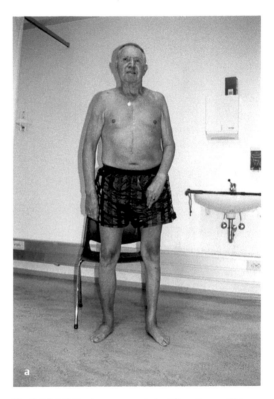

Fig. 2.6 (a) Patients compensate in different ways. This patient's right shoulder is medially rotated, the right trunk is laterally flexed, and the left shoulder girdle and pelvis are retracted, the left leg is pulled back with the pelvis and therefore seemingly outward rotated and adducted. The left arm is pulled back with the shoulder girdle but is observably inwardly rotated and adducted with flexion/pronation of the elbow and lower arm. The right hip and knee are flexing. The stability and movement control are reduced on both sides (see also **Fig. 2.4a**) but more on the left, most affected side. His body weight shifts toward the right in both standing and walking. (*Continued*)

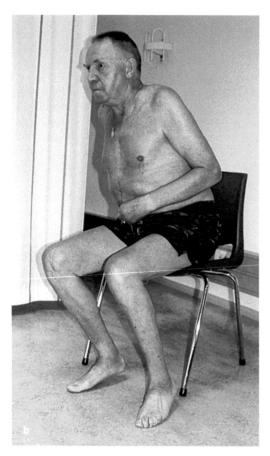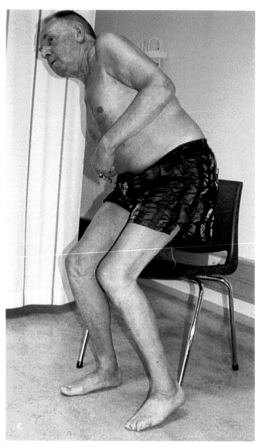

Fig. 2.6 (*continued*) **(b, c)** When this patient stands up from sitting he uses a lot of effort. Note the facial expression and the associated reactions in the arm. Compare with **Fig. 2.6a**, where the associated reactions are less when the patient has been standing for a short time. The transfer to standing demands interplay between body segments and the base of support. The patient has very little mobility generally, and his left foot is not adapting to the base of support; therefore weight transference to the left is not possible. The propulsion torque into standing should be initiated from distally to proximally; however, one cannot fire triceps surae if the forefoot is inverted. He has to compensate by pushing up through his right side. This patient had two strokes ~30 years ago. He manages most activities and is active in participation. But it is costing him a lot of effort, and he becomes tired, more so as he is getting older.

ity activity and feedforward controls (Raine et al 2009).

Clinically, it may be necessary for two or three therapists to work together to facilitate trunk, pelvis, and hip activity for the stance phase to allow for the swing phase. If appropriate and available, a treadmill with bodyweight support may be of some help to ease the facilitation and rhythmic interplay between stance and swing as well as finding the right speed to facilitate central pattern generation in the individual (see Chapter 1.2, The Spinal Cord: Central Pattern Generators and Locomotion; Clinical Relevance). Speed is very individual. Rehabilitation of individuals with neuro-

logical impairment may benefit from using training principles aimed at eliciting whole-body coordination.

Sometimes an orthosis or splint may be appropriate to stabilize the ankle. Heel-strike and heel-off seem to be important to signal phase changes to the patient's CNS; therefore the heel should, if possible, be free to receive and transmit somatosensory and weight information. An orthosis that stabilizes the ankle medially and laterally or taping may therefore be of use in a period of transition (**Fig. 2.7a–f**).

In patients with PD, one of the early symptoms is a flexed posture and lack of rotation (Vaugoyeau et al 2006). One of the early motor symptoms is reduced muscle function in the trunk, which causes reduced postural control (Bridgewater & Sharpe 1998; Wright et al. 2007; Hubble et al 2014). Flexion causes a forward lean of the trunk and displacement of the CoG, and the patient develops a tendency to fall forward. In fact, a study done by Wright and colleagues (2007) demonstrated that the ratio of hip-to-trunk torque increases in PD subjects, and this finding suggests that increased tone in the hips is a compensation to the stooped posture in PD. Patients have a shuffling and tripping gait with short steps and seem to be running after their own CoG. Some patients develop compensatory strategies in an attempt to bring the CoG back by pressing their feet into the floor through plantar flexion. Bridgewater and Sharpe (1998) refer to other studies in which dorsiflexion was found to be reduced. Trunk flexion and rigidity combined with pushing back from the feet cause the patients to lose mobility, and plantar flexion contractures may develop. Patients with PD seem stiffened in their total expression of movement. Improving mobility of the spinal column, shoulder girdles, and neck, together with facilitating selective extension, often spontaneously regain rotation. The feet and muscles of the lower leg should be maintained at an appropriate length for mobility. Through improved distal mobility patients will be able to receive and perceive somatosensory information and orientation of their body in relation to space and the support surface. These interventions may improve their ability to adjust their posture and thereby balance.

An internal model of verticality is necessary for the postural control system to function properly (Massion 1992; Massion 1994). Some stroke patients seem to develop a tendency to push away from the midline through their least affected extremities (ipsilesional to the brain damage). Many names have been given to this syndrome; postural hemineglect (Schädler & Kool 2001), the Pusher syndrome (Davies 2003), contraversive pushing (Karnath et al 2000), among others. This is a complex combination of symptoms, and several studies have shown that Pusher syndrome can occur in patients with lesions in both hemispheres, although more often after a right brain lesion (Abe et al 2012), and that it is distinct from neglect (although several patients have both Pusher syndrome and neglect) (Karnath et al 2000; Pérennou et al 2000). The high prevalence among patients showing Pusher syndrome and other neurophysiological deficits is suggested to be due to an increased vulnerability of certain brain regions to stroke-induced injury rather than any direct involvement with the occurrence of Pusher syndrome (Santos-Pontelli 2011). Pusher syndrome has been reported mainly in stroke patients;

however, it has also been described in nonstroke conditions (Santos-Pontelli 2011). Imaging studies have suggested the posterolateral thalamus as the brain structure that is typically affected in patients showing this behavior. However, other cortical and subcortical areas, such as the insular cortex and postcentral gyrus, have also been emphasized as structures that are potentially involved in the pathophysiology of Pusher syndrome (Ticini et al 2009). Karnath and Dieterich (2006) argue that the superior temporal area, insula, and temporoparietal junction form a multisensory area where vestibular information is also processed in relation to spatial orientation. These areas are integrative for vestibular, auditory, and visual information coming from the surrounding space to form multimodal spatial representation and may thus be involved in the pathophysiology of this syndrome.

The mechanisms underlying Pusher syndrome have been associated with a dysfunction of the patient's perception of body posture related to gravity that leads to postural reactive behavior (i.e., pushing/fixating). Nevertheless, in contrast to the disturbed perception of upright body posture, stroke patients with Pusher syndrome demonstrate almost undisturbed processing of visual and vestibular inputs; therefore abnormal labyrinthine function does not seem to be a central impairment in pusher patients (i.e., the origin of pushing does not seem to be vestibular in patients with a hemispheric stroke) (Pérennou et al 2000; Pontelli et al 2005; Barra & Pérennou 2013). This supports the assumption of a separate neural pathway in humans for perception of orientation of gravity and controlling upright body posture (i.e., the existence of a separate system from the interoceptive receptors/trunk graviceptive system) (Mittelstaedt 1996; Barra et al 2010).

As was discussed earlier, normal postural function depends partly on the ability of the postural control system to integrate visual, proprioceptive, and vestibular sensory information. Verticality can be perceived through different modalities (see also under Postural Orientation):

- Subjective postural vertical (SPV) is a sensitive direction-specific orientation for vestibular function, which receives input from sense organs in the trunk—a trunk gravitation–dependent system.
- Subjective visual vertical (SVV) is a visually perceived sense of being vertical that depends on visual, proprioceptive, and vestibular inputs.
- Haptic/tactile vertical.

Normal postural perception of the vertical, being a prerequisite for normal body orientation with respect to gravity, requires the integrity of neural cir-

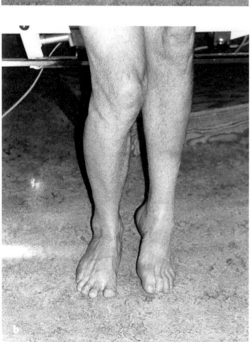

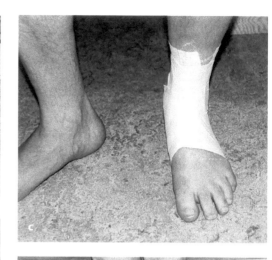

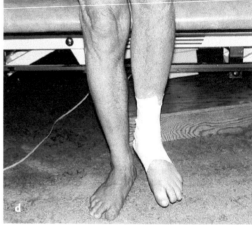

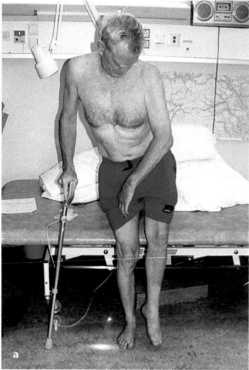

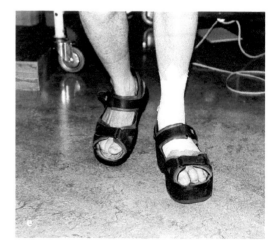

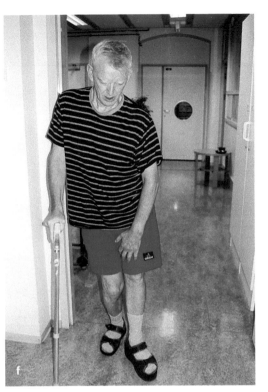

Pérennou and colleagues (2008) suggest that pushing is a postural behavior that leads patients to align their erect posture with an incorrect reference of verticality; hence the patients with Pusher syndrome make a postural response to control their balance and so actively align their erect posture with a verticality reference tilted to the side opposite the stroke.

Clinically, patients with Pusher syndrome are often totally paralyzed on their affected side for a relatively short time initially. The severity of the pushing disorder varies across patients. In the most serious conditions patients are unable even to sit without assistance, whereas patients who are less severely affected may lose balance only when circumstances are particularly challenging. They fall to the left side (usually) and their eyes perceive the world on a slant to the right. There is increased flexor activity throughout the right side of the trunk and neck while pushing away from the right using the right arm and leg, and little or no activity throughout the left side (**Fig. 2.8a, b**).

Certain perceptual problems are frequently observed in patients with Pusher syndrome:

- Visual neglect: Some patients do not seem to perceive visual information from the most affected side.
- Auditive neglect: Some patients do not seem to perceive what they hear from the most affected side.
- Neglect of the most affected side of the body: the patient has reduced perception of the most affected side and does not integrate information from this side. But, as previously stated, this syndrome often involves flaccid paralysis initially; thus there is very little somatosensory information to receive or integrate.
- Spatial problems, both in relation to one's own body and to the relationship between the body and the environment.
- Reduced sensory perception: But the patient may have normal sensation if the two body halves are tested separately. Often the therapist finds that the patient has severely affected bilateral simultaneous perception of sensation.
- Altered perception of the midline: The patient is afraid of falling to the least affected side.
- Other perceptual and cognitive problems. Physical problems that may occur include the following:
- Reduced postural control: Particularly reduced ipsilateral trunk control.
- Hemianopia: The patient may have a reduced visual field to the paretic side.

Fig. 2.7 (a–f) This stroke patient has congenital hip dysplasia and 7 cm difference in leg length, the shorter leg being his left. He has always walked on his toes on his left side, and perceived no balance or movement problems and no restrictions in function or participation. Among other things, he and his wife used to dance a great deal. He then suffered a stroke, resulting in left side affection and motor apraxia. He had a lot of instability on his left side, no hip, knee, or ankle stability or voluntary movement. To help increase the stability of the ankle, the ankle was taped to recruit more proximal stability. Notice the difference in alignment and therefore the ability to recruit more appropriate neuromuscular stability in (**a–f**). Note: Taping is not a long-term solution; it may cause skin problems and is difficult for the patient and his carers to put on. After some time this patient received a sport bandage, which gave adequate stability distally.

cuits centered around the superior parietal cortex (i.e., the primary somatosensory cortex and the thalamus) (Pérennou et al 2008). The posterior thalamus is a relay structure of vestibular pathways (Pérennou et al 2008; Lopez & Blanke 2011). and it is also assumed to be essentially involved in the control of upright body posture.

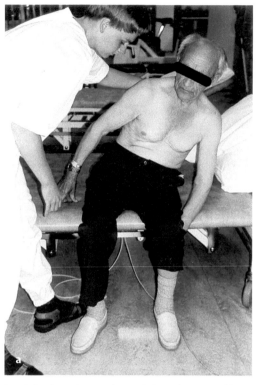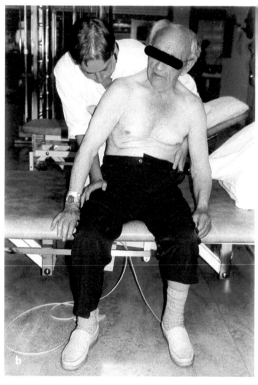

Fig. 2.8 The patient pushes with his right arm and leg. **(a)** There is severe side flexion throughout the right side, and the pelvis is elevated on the right side. His interaction with the base of support and between body segments is disturbed. He is malaligned and out of midline. **(b)** The therapist handles the patient to improve the alignment of his pelvis to the base of support. The patient pushes less, but there is still observable malalignment of his upper trunk and head.

- Initial paralysis, which seems to recover quickly in many patients. They may have relatively good selective movement in the most affected side but cannot use it because of severe midline disorientation.
- Reduced weight transference, reduced interplay between left and right.
- Use of the least affected extremities to push and or fixate with. In patients who have a right hemispheric stroke, the head, neck, and trunk are side flexed to the right, and the head is often rotated to the right. An increased use of protective reactions and strategies (the push from the right to avoid the perceived falling to the right) seems to inhibit the interaction of right and left in all three planes.

If this syndrome is not treated successfully, patients may develop severe flexor/retractor activity throughout their most affected side and are totally dependent on carers for all functions. They demonstrate inappropriate use of their least affected side, and their ability to vary patterns of movement is reduced. Often, carers and therapists experience severe resistance when attempting to correct the patient's alignment and relationship to the base of support. There may be bilateral problems, and problems arise in all practical situations that require balance and transfers as well as positioning in a chair and in bed.

Treatment is goal oriented toward regaining midline control. The following factors are important to evaluate:

- The patient's trunk stability, in particular the ipsilesional side.
- The patient's awareness of and activity in the paretic side.
- The compensatory activity of the pushing side. Aims of treatment include the following:
- To regain interaction of movement between body segments in all three planes, especially trunk, shoulder girdles, and pelvis.

- To improve integration between the two sides of the body, to increase midline orientation and postural control.
- To improve and facilitate distal sensorimotor integration, to increase orientation through contractual hand orientating response (CHOR).

The 24-hour management of stroke patients is always of great importance and no more so than in the case of patients displaying pusher behavior. Positioning of the patient is of crucial importance. Patients with Pusher syndrome do not appear to push when appropriately supported (Karnath et al 2000), therefore appropriate seating and positioning in bed are important from the early stages. The challenges in the physical management may prevent patients with Pusher syndrome from receiving accurate information about their postural and visual upright. Hence it is important to provide the patient with accurate, reliable, and consistent information served by reliable, valid cues, such as postural symmetry and visual and somatosensory information of the gravitational vertical. In a treatment situation perceptions need to be matched. Vertical orientation requires alignment of the pelvis and intra-abdominal pressure for stimulation of the trunk graviceptive system because postural verticality comes from within. Therefore, vision may be removed (the patient blinded or vision blocked to the right) combined with using a broad bandage or belt to assemble the trunk and abdominal contents in the midline to increase abdominal pressure and thereby stimulate the graviceptor system in the trunk. Lying on the right side or with the right side supported in sitting and standing may make the left side more available for increasing the somatosensory information through the affected (most often left) side.

Some patients develop a hypersensitive foot that pushes off the floor through plantar flexion and inversion. They may experience a primary hypersensitivity toward stretch, touch, or weight bearing to the forefoot, or this reaction may develop as a response to gravity to stiffen the leg to be able to stand on it to walk when the proximal areas are too weak or unstable to carry weight selectively. The severity of the reaction will vary in different patients and in different situations. Pressure, touch, or stretch to the foot in weight bearing causes plantar flexion with a backward translation of the tibia in relation to the foot. The pattern causes plantar flexion with varying degrees of inversion—a mechanical hyperextension of the knee—and is usually combined with flexor components at the hip (i.e., varying degrees of flexion/adduction/inward rotation). The mechanical hyperextension of the knee is a result of the knee being caught in the middle between a plantar flexed foot and a flexed hip during weight bearing. The quadriceps is rarely active in this reaction. The incoordination of the foot, ankle, knee, and hip negatively affect balance and reduce interplay and variation of movement.

Flexor withdrawal may be caused either by a hypersensitive foot or sensitive (short) hip flexors (flexor reflex afferents) and therefore either from a distal or a proximal initiation:

- Weight transference through the foot causes stretch of the soft tissues within the foot. In some cases initial stretch in attempted weight bearing produces withdrawal of the foot from the floor. The pattern varies in severity and rotational components but usually causes inversion of the foot and flexion of the hip and knee.
- A withdrawal reaction may also be caused by stretch to the hip flexors, often initiated as a reaction when the patient starts to raise himself to standing from sitting. The stretch of the hip flexors causes hip and knee flexion combined with dorsiflexion of the foot with varying degrees of inversion or eversion, depending on the neuromuscular rotational components of the hip.
- Both these reactions may retract the pelvis and therefore seemingly abduct and outwardly rotate the flexed hip. The apparent abduction is a result of the backward pull of the pelvis in retraction taking the hip with it, without the hip in reality being truly abducted or externally rotated.

All of the aforementioned deviations prevent normal weight transference, balance, and transfers. Treatment is targeted toward the impairments: the hypersensitivity, the immobility of the foot, and improving muscle length and flexibility to improve the patient's postural control. Improving postural control, especially the stability component in different situations, involves bringing all the following into activity through graded weight bearing and varied active movement over the foot in different weight-bearing activities: sitting to standing over one or two feet, controlled standing to sitting, standing and step standing, stepping in different directions, single-leg standing, stepping down from a height, sitting on one or two legs, stairs, and so forth. The restoration of dynamic interplay between the foot, knee, and hip is essential to the patient's ability to balance and move.

2.2 Intervention—Considerations and Choices

On the basis of continuous assessment and clinical reasoning the therapist chooses interventions that seem appropriate to the individual patient. The Bobath Concept does not give a solution or method for treatment of patients.

> **Definition**
> The Bobath Concept is a problem-solving approach to the assessment and treatment of individuals with disturbances of function, movement, and postural control due to a lesion of the central nervous system (IBITA, Theoretical Assumptions 2007; www.ibita.org).

Treatment is tailored to the individual patient and is response-based. Therefore interventions depend on patients as individuals, their sensorimotor dysfunctions, their perceptual and cognitive resources and problems, the adaptive compensatory strategies they have developed, the environment, and the goal or task. All interventions, even if impairment oriented, need to integrate activities to make treatment as functional as possible and the carry-over effect as strong as possible. Motivation is a crucial factor to learning. Treatment incorporates the following:

- Regaining movement control.
- Motor learning.
- An interdisciplinary approach to enhance learning and carryover.
- The use of compensatory strategies when further motor learning does not seem possible (may incorporate the use of aids and orthoses).
- Management strategies to prevent or minimize complications.

Postural Sets

Posture can be defined as the geometric relation between two or more body segments (e.g., trunk and leg, and the upper and lower trunk). A complete geometry defining the posture of the whole body should take into account the relationship between the body and the environment (e.g., body relative to support surface) (Nashner 1982). Berta Bobath described postural sets as "adaptations of posture" that "change with the intended movement—in fact, they may precede it" (Bobath 1990). Body segments have a biomechanical and a neuromuscular relationship, which are the basis for and a consequence of the build of the individual, movement, and the actual relationship with the environment. This relationship continuously changes during activity. Neuromuscular activity and biomechanical factors influence and are affected by each other. Changes in the relationship with the environment and alterations in the biomechanical relationships through changes in rotational components or direction of joint movement require adaptation of the neuromuscular activity, even if the goal of movement or task stays the same. Neuromuscular activity depends on where the person started the movement from (e.g., standing up from sitting on a low, soft cushion, or stepping down from a high seat). When a person flexes the elbow when sitting or standing, the biceps is the prime mover. The same movement performed in supine, with the arm stretched up in the air or the arm being held over shoulder level in sitting or standing, requires more eccentric control from the triceps as the prime mover and agonist.

The neuromuscular activity required to perform pelvic tilt varies in different positions because the biomechanical relations alter with the changing relationship of gravity to the BoS. Therefore, the activity is different in sitting, in the transition from sitting to standing, in standing, through sitting to supine, and in supine. Analysis of movement is the detailed analysis of movement during every phase of an activity to form hypotheses with regard to the patient's recruitment of neuromuscular activity in function. This analysis is the foundation for clinical reasoning, together with an analysis of the patient's performance that includes an assessment and evaluation of perceptual and cognitive function.

> Postural sets describe the interrelationship between body segments at a given moment.
> Movement may be described as a continuous change of postural sets.

If serial photographs of a movement or activity are taken, each photograph represents a postural set. Analysis of postural sets gives information about the following:

- The effect of gravity.
- The relationship to the BoS.
- Alignment.
- Patterns of movement.
- Neuromuscular activity.

There is a tendency to analyze basic postures, but humans move within and between postures. *Basic postures* are sitting, standing, step standing, supine, or prone, with symmetry or asymmetry if including step standing and even weight distribution. Postural sets are all different variations within a basic posture and the transitions between postures.

There is an interrelationship between postural control and postural sets. The analysis of postural sets in a functional activity allows the clinician to observe actual and gradual changes in alignment and to form hypotheses regarding the neuromuscular activation creating the movement. The chosen interventions may or may not support the hypotheses. If the patient's motor control is not improving, either the interventions or the hypotheses may be wrong and must be reconsidered. The clinician must continuously adapt the interventions to the patient's response and required movement.

Postural sets are also used in treatment to adapt and adjust requirements to suit the patient's ability. Individual components of the whole task can be trained in several postural sets before putting them together into the performance of functional activities (Raine et al 2009). The choice of postural sets depends on the patient's balance control and relationship to the BoS, and therefore the choice of goal activity or task. Patients who have low postural control or who are flexed with asymmetry, malalignment, and deviant tone distribution will not be able to recruit a more appropriate activity to interact or respond to the environment. Shumway-Cook and Woollacott (2006) describe *ideal alignment* in the standing position as follows: "muscles throughout the body, not just those of the trunk, are tonically active to maintain the body in a narrowly confined vertical position during quiet stance. Once the center of gravity moves outside the narrow range defined by the ideal alignment, more muscular effort is required to recover a stable position." Optimal or ideal alignments in any postural set allow us to use no more effort than necessary to maintain stability. Inappropriate alignment or malalignment may maintain an inappropriate neuromuscular recruitment pattern and thereby prevent patients adapting their response to the environment. Sahrmann (1992) states that a normal neuromuscular interplay, muscle balance, or adaptive muscular activity facilitates good alignment, and that good alignment facilitates normal, adaptive neuromuscular activity.

> A selective movement in one postural set requires a different neuromuscular activity in a different postural set. As the biomechanical alignment changes, so does the neuromuscular activity.

■ Analysis of Basic Postures and Postural Sets

During treatment, the therapist needs to be specific, critical, and selective, and use postural sets that are appropriate in relation to the patient's problem. The following are essential factors in the choice of postural sets:

- How easy or difficult it is to vary the patient's posture for the appropriate recruitment of neuromuscular activity.
- How easy or difficult it is to vary postural sets in the gradual transition from one position to another.
- How much effort is required.
- What motor strategies are facilitated.
- Whether the patient loses or strengthens the control he regained in one position as he moves into another.

We move from one postural set to another continuously in our daily activities; we rarely stay in one position to do anything. Therapy has to reflect this by facilitating the patient to regain control of movement, not static activity. The functional importance of the treatment is essential for learning.

The postural sets chosen as intervention have to be adapted to the patient's specific problems to enhance or facilitate success and motivation. Advantages and disadvantages, possibilities for variation, how easy or difficult it will be for the patient to move into and out of and between the postural sets must be considered in the light of the patient's movement control at the time. Balance and movement result from the interaction of many muscle groups and their eccentric/concentric work as agonists, antagonists, and synergists. It is not possible to analyze the activity in all muscles in all phases of different activities, and not possible to describe this variation in words. The following sections analyze the main features or qualities of standing, sitting, supine, and side lying. Any other position may be analyzed in the same way.

■ Standing

The control of human standing posture can appear to be a relatively uncomplicated task; however, maintaining an upright stance is rather complex due to the small base of support and the high vertical position of the CoM. Human standing requires the action of muscles distributed over the whole body to maintain the CoM over the BoS. Due to the postural function these muscles exhibit (i.e., their contribution to maintaining the upright posture against gravity) they are often referred to as *antigravity muscles* (Shumway-Cook & Woollacott 2006). Because the feet do not move during quiet standing, information from cutaneous plantar mechanoreceptors and muscle activity around the ankle has a critical role in maintaining the CoM in the ideal location within the BoS (Fitzpatrick et al 1994). In the standing position the calf muscles are continuously active (Loram et al 2011). For the control of the CoM in the anteroposterior direction, the ankle plantar flexors (the soleus and medial gastrocnemius) and the ankle dorsiflexors (e.g., the tibialis anterior), contribute (Winter 1995); in the mediolateral direction, activity of the ankle invertors, ankle evertors, and hip abductors is important (Winter 1995). Humans exist in a world subjected to the laws of gravity; hence, even when standing still we must work to remain upright to prevent us from collapsing due to the pull of gravity (Shumway-Cook & Woollacott 2006). The vertical projection of the CoM toward the ground is called the center of gravity (CoG) (Winter 1995). With regard to biomechanics, the forces between the human body and the ground are GRFs (Winter 1995). The vector sum of all of the GRFs under the feet is used to calculate the center of pressure (CoP) (Winter 1995). Winter (1995) define the CoP as "the point location of the vertical ground reaction force vector and it illustrates a weighted average of all the pressures over the surface of the area in contact with the ground." Because the ankle muscles are primary controllers of the CoP in standing, the location of the CoP is the effect of collective efforts of the individual ankle muscles (Winter 1995); therefore, increasing the activity of the plantar flexors will move the CoP anteriorly, and increasing the activity in the ankle invertors will move the CoP laterally. When humans are asked to stand normally, they are never completely still. Rather, small amounts of body movement, referred to as *postural sway*, can be observed. These movements are both forward and backward (anterior–posterior) and sideways (medial–lateral). Postural sway is primarily controlled by the immediate torque generated from the ankle plantar– and dorsiflexors in the sagittal plane and the hip loading/unloading mechanism in the frontal plane (King et al 2012).

Postural sway can be studied by recording the movement of CoP measured with a force plate under the feet. Sway area has been related to the effectiveness of the postural control system. Postural sway therefore indicates the reciprocity between the destabilizing forces acting on the body and actions by the postural control system to prevent loss of balance (Murnaghan 2013; Maurer & Peterka 2005). Hence balance impairments caused by altered sensory, motor, or CNS function with regard to such factors as older age and pathology (e.g., stroke, PD, peripheral neuropathy) will be reflected in altered characteristics of postural sway (i.e., increased postural sway = reduced balance) (Pavol 2005).

The GRF is a three-component vector representing the forces in the vertical, anterior–posterior, and medial–lateral planes. Each component measures a different characteristic of movement (e.g., the vertical component is primarily generated by the vertical acceleration of the body). The GRFs are the result of a pressure distribution under the foot (feet) reflecting the load coming through the body onto the ground. GRF measurements can be used to diagnose neuromuscular impairments and provide a quantified measure of asymmetries between a patient's legs. In healthy humans, the GRF magnitudes are the same for both legs; that is, healthy subjects maintain a symmetric position of weight distribution between the lower limbs, and the muscles are able to perform similar activity for both feet. Many neurological patients have a poor GRF activity on the hemiplegic side and an excessive GRF activity on the least affected side (see **Fig. 2.6a**). Studies have shown that greater load applied to the body during standing increases the magnitude of extensor muscle postural reactions in healthy individuals (Dietz 1992). Hence the GRF influences the whole extensor pattern in the lower limbs, which allows for selective movement of the pelvis. Without selectivity of pelvic movement, it is not possible to have optimal core stability, and this might again affect scapular setting and neck stability.

Many patients with hemiparesis secondary to a variety of neurological disorders demonstrate less weight bearing (i.e., loading) through their most affected lower limb than through their less affected lower limb (see **Fig. 2.6a**), which the literature refers to as *weight-bearing asymmetry (WBA)*. WBA is associated with a change in loading of the legs as well as a change in body geometry. Kamphuis and colleagues (2013) concluded in their review article that "WBA after stroke is associated with increased postural sway as well as with poorer between-limb synchronization of CoP trajectories." In addition, Aruin (2006) demonstrated the effect of body asymmetry on APAs; the subjects were standing with one leg externally rotated, inducing body asymmetry, which lead to an increase of APAs on the side opposite of leg rotation. Aruin therefore suggested that, in the presence of body asymmetry, the CNS might choose a strategy of activating muscles on the contralateral side of the body to compensate for the effects of an additional mechanical constraint. The ability to initiate and control weight transfer toward either leg is essential for several tasks, such as walking, turning when walking, and reaching. The ability to load the paretic lower extremity has been shown to relate to performance of functional tasks. Lee et al (1997) showed that patients with stroke who put less weight through their paretic leg during sit to stand had poorer mobility scores on the Functional Independence Measure; Cheng et al (1998) reported that asymmetric weight bearing during a sit-to-stand task is thought to contribute to falls in individuals with stroke (see **Fig. 2.6b, c**). In the contemporary Bobath Concept a goal of treatment is to get "two same legs" and thus to be able to initiate gait with either leg, depending on the task and the environmental constraints. An active and efficient standing leg will produce kinetic energy for swing (i.e., the longer and better you are able to stand on one leg will produce a more efficient swing on the same leg). Bobath practitioners believe that optimal standing alignment promotes better loading of the leg and therefore a better ability to store kinetic energy, which allows for active weight bearing and thereby optimal sensory feedback to update the body schema. Also, optimal alignment contributes to the ability to efficiently activate muscles needed for the task in demand.

Humans rarely stand for the sake of standing. Rather, we stand to accomplish a goal-directed task; we stand to initiate walking, to reach for something with our arms, or to sit down. Changing from stationary stance to walking involves a sequences of muscle activations (APAs) and thereby changes in the GRFs. This sequence of activity produces the forces and moments necessary to propel the body forward and toward the single-stance limb.

Limits of Stability During Standing

Limits of stability can be described as the maximum distance a person can intentionally displace her center of gravity and lean her body in a given direction without losing balance, stepping, or grasping (Melzer et al 2009). The planning and executions of movements like reaching in standing or bending over from the standing position depend on the limits of stability for that individual. Shumway-Cook and Woollacott (2006) define the *perceived limits of stability* as the distance a person is willing and able to move without losing balance or taking a step.

The basic standing posture is characterized by extension: trunk, head and neck, and legs. This selective extension is based on the interplay of trunk musculature, core stability, and the balanced muscular activity of the legs. The postural tone is relatively high if the person stands actively and the base of support is relatively small. The shoulders are slightly protracted but relatively relaxed and the arms hang by the side (**Fig. 2.9**). The rotation of the arms depends on the biomechanical alignment and neuromuscular activation of the individual, especially of the trunk and shoulder girdles. Increase of thoracic extension and of the shoulder girdles may give more outward rotation of the arm, whereas active protraction and flexion enhance inward rotation. Standing is generally facilitatory to the development of extension. The patient is exposed to gravity, which enhances postural tone and postural control if the alignment is good.

Advantages

There is a wide variety of standing postural sets; using different foot positions, or mobile or stabile supports behind, at the side or at the front to allow the patient to explore his motor control safely. All changes cause neuromuscular adaptations. The placing of the arms influences tonus distribution of the body: if the arms are placed above 90°, trunk extension is facilitated to a larger degree. The arms may be placed in different positions and at different heights (**Fig. 2.10, Fig. 2.11, Fig. 2.12, Fig. 2.13**).

An active arm facilitates postural activity, whereas the use of arm support may alter or negate postural control depending on how it is used (Jeka 1997; Jeka & Lackner 1994; Slijper et al 2002). Standing postural sets may vary from parallel to step standing and thereby enhance weight transference and access alterations of stance to swing in different directions. Changes in hip rotation require altered neuromuscular activity; physiological outward rotation in the standing leg may facilitate abduction and extension

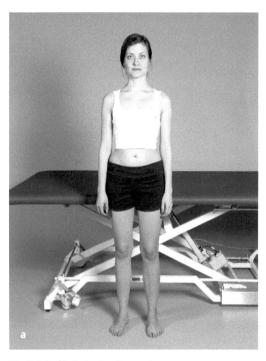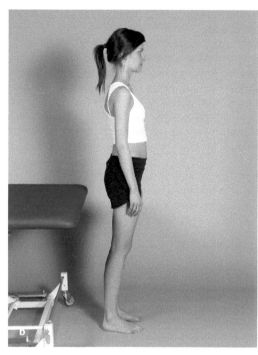

Fig. 2.9 (a, b) Basic standing postures.

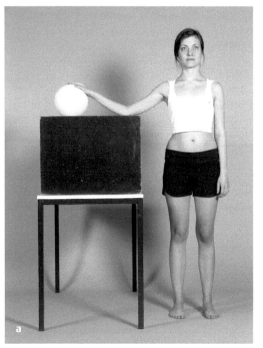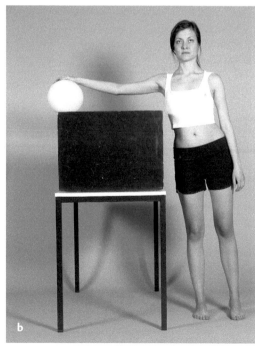

Fig. 2.10 (a, b) Lateral weight transference with the arm abducted at shoulder level as the model rolls a ball. The demands for extension and stability increase on the weight-bearing side if the model does not press down on the ball.

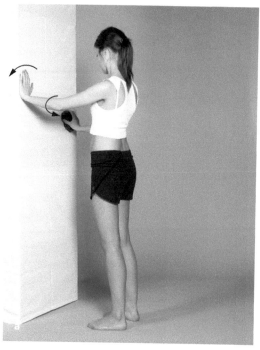
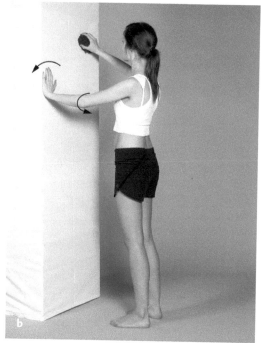

Fig. 2.11 The use of the wall may facilitate placing of the arms to create a contractual hand orientation response (CHOR). The CHOR is a frictional contact of the hand to a surface that allows for the hand to begin its functional roles (Porter & Lemon 1995; Raine et al 2009). Use of a CHOR can facilitate "light touch contact" for increasing axial tone (Franzén et al 2011), midline orientation, limb support, and limb loading (Raine et al 2009). The model has to stabilize both body and arms to maintain the postural set and move at the same time. **(a)** More outward rotation of the arm and hand combined with extension at the elbow and protraction of the shoulder facilitates abdominal activation as part of postural control. Improved postural control facilitates stability through the shoulder and arm. **(b)** Improved postural control and stability of the left arm facilitates freedom of movement for functions in the right arm.

and thereby stability. The "let go" or eccentric activation of hip extension/abduction/outward rotation facilitates initiation of the swing phase. There are good opportunities for therapeutic handling and correction of alignment, both distally and proximally, if the patient has a certain level of postural control, feels safe in this situation, and is willing to explore the possibilities. It is important to give adequate and appropriate support to knees, for instance, to allow the patient to experience and develop trunk control or pelvic movement with or without facilitation. The use of a plinth placed at different heights, at different positions in relation to the patient (at the side, at the back, diagonally, at the front) allows variation and active exploration between sitting and standing. In addition, it allows for an adapted standing position, reducing degrees of freedom (**Fig. 2.14a–d**).

The patient is facilitated to experience and explore variations in eccentric control and grade movement in different directions. Eccentric muscle activity seems to improve strength and generalization (carryover) to more varied muscle work and functional activities (Patten et al 2004). Strength training facilitates significant synaptogenesis on the motor neurons in the spinal cord and does not seem to have a negative impact on spasticity (spasticity as defined by Pandyan et al 2005). (See Chapter 1.4 Consequences of and Reorganization after CNS Lesions.) Patten et al (2004) state that skill training combined with task-specific training improves activity-dependent cortical reorganization. Therefore, treatment needs to be targeted, involves specific aspects of strength training, and is context-based because this combination seems to improve the patient's function.

Use of the standing postural set often motivates the patient. The patient is oriented to the relationship between body and space, which improves per-

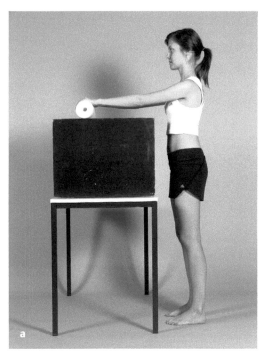

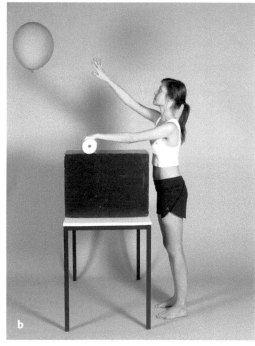

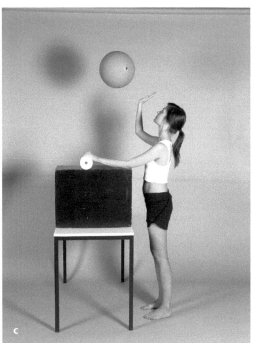

Fig. 2.12 (a) The practice of a dynamic task in standing is a functional challenge to postural stability and allows the exploration of stability limits. The ability to keep the trunk extended and back against expected perturbation when the limbs are moving forward demands both posterior and anterior muscle activity in the trunk. The demands for postural stability and orientation increase even more when the arms are active. When combining reaching for something in standing, an important factor contributing to performance of the task is anticipatory postural adjustments to stabilize posture. Anticipatory postural control and voluntary arm movement are thought to be controlled by different, but parallel, descending pathways, which need to be integrated for successful task accomplishment. Reach training should, if possible, be performed in the context of the demands of the chosen task. **(b, c)** The demands for postural control increase even more when arms are active.

ception. Standing is functional (**Fig. 2.15a–d**), as well as improves orthostatic control of blood pressure, circulation, lung function, and bowel and urinary functions.

Disadvantages

Some patients have very low postural tone and are unable to interact with gravity and to activate an upright posture. If the patient supports herself, leans

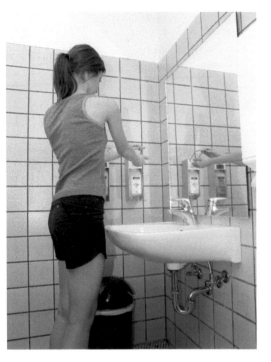

Fig. 2.13 Motor control research has demonstrated that there are inherent neural interaction patterns in the two hemispheres when both arms move simultaneously in homologous actions. This coupling may facilitate the functional recovery of the paretic arm. Cooperative action of both hands during training has always been an important factor in the Bobath Concept. However, attention is often on the fact that the two arms cooperate to complete a task but with each arm having a separate function that requires quite different activities, such as stabilizing one hand under the soap dispenser and manipulating it with the other.

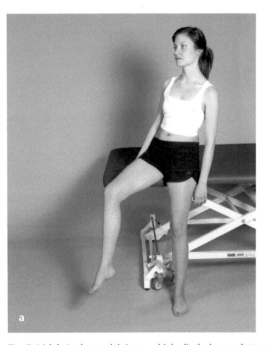
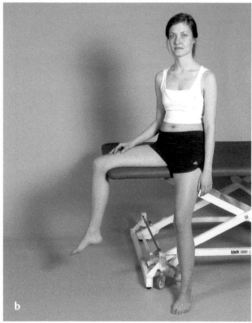

Fig. 2.14 (a) As the model sits on a high plinth she needs to stabilize and move over the standing leg. In this situation there are specific needs for abduction and outward rotation of the weight-bearing hip to lift the pelvis onto the plinth, as well as for aligning body segments to each other. **(b)** Components of rotation may be varied to alter the demands for postural control, balance, and movement both in standing to sitting and sitting to standing. (*Continued*)

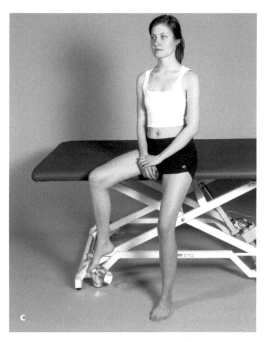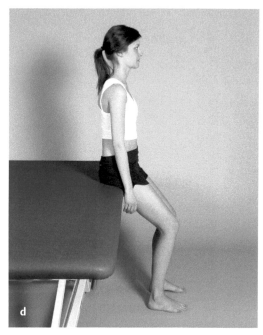

Fig. 2.14 (*continued*) **(c)** A postural set of high sitting. This posture demands good pelvic mobility (i.e., movement of the pelvis in relation to the hips and the lumbar spine) and facilitates the transition from standing to sitting and sitting to standing—stand-down. **(d)** Stand-down is an intervention to strengthen the extensor chain, fundamental for stance, propulsion, and reaching. The aim is to stimulate a balanced activity between vestibulospinal and corticoreticulospinal systems in the task of standing down onto the leg from a high plinth. Stand-down is used to facilitate single-leg stance, for enhancing an efficient extensor pattern in the lower limb for locomotion, and it may provide improved postural base for reaching in standing.

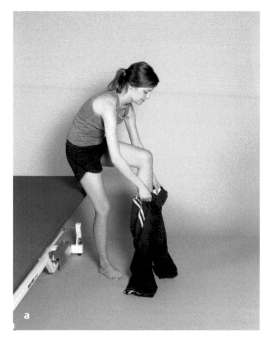

Fig. 2.15 Appropriate postural control allows for functional arm movement in standing. **(a)** Dressing in a standing position is normal. The model balances over her right leg demanding the ability to be postural stable over one leg, at the same time as putting her left leg into the trousers. This is a complex perceptual, cognitive, and sensorimotor activity demanding problem solving and a continuous adaptation to displacement over a small base of support. (*Continued*)

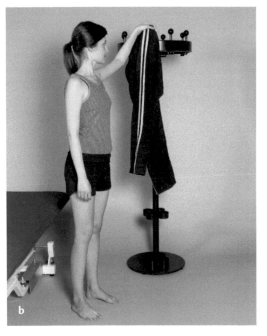

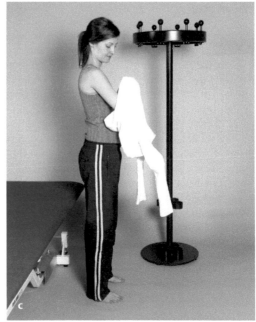

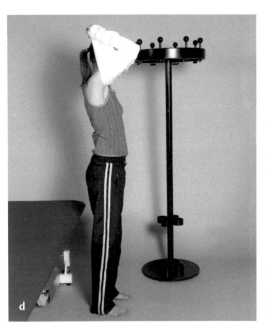

Fig. 2.15 (*continued*) **(b)** The model hangs her jumper on a hook above shoulder level. She has to locate the hook and problem solves the activity, weight transfer, and at the same time sustains her postural stability to free the arm to lift the jumper onto the hook. Dynamic changes will occur in the trunk and lower extremities prior to the initiation of the arm movement, serving to stabilize the body. Because the hook is placed at an arm's length, the trunk does not move with the arm. The trunk moves only if the target is placed in such a way that arm movements alone do not reach it. **(c)** When the model puts on her jumper, the hand and arm actively lead the movement through extension into the sleeve. Scapular stability is a stable reference for reaching and a prerequisite for optimal arm function. **(d)** As the jumper goes over the head, vision is obscured, and the integration of somatosensory inputs is weighted more for postural control. The need for sensorimotor adaptation to maintain postural control increases. Body segments align themselves in relation to each other.

onto, or presses down on an external support, she may recruit inappropriate active flexion components, which further negates interaction with gravity and the acquisition of postural control. Flexor strategies may increase if she feels insecure. Standing postural sets may require two therapists or the help of an assistant to make the situation facilitatory for the patient's postural activation. The use of a standing frame or similar device may be appropriate in some cases. Note that the patient needs to be placed completely upright in a vertical alignment at 90° to facilitate postural tone and activity over her BoS, her feet.

◼ Sitting

Unsupported sitting is different compared with standing at both the sensory and the biomechanical level. At the sensory level, somatosensory information from the feet contributes less to the position of the legs because somatosensory information from the buttocks and thighs is integrated instead. Compared with standing, at a biomechanical level there is a reduction in the biomechanical constraints; that is, there is a reduction in the number of joints to be controlled, there is an increase in the BoS, and the CoM is lower. The sitting position is mainly controlled by the trunk muscles (Genthon et al 2007), and unsupported sitting requires trunk postural stability, which is also necessary for almost all ADLs (Perlmutter et al 2010). Due to the importance of trunk control in transferring between sitting and standing, walking, and so forth, restoration of sitting posture appears determinant for recovering independent function (Hsieh et al 2002; Geurts et al 2005).

The basic unsupported upright sitting position is characterized by trunk extension balanced with abdominal activity, and head and neck alignment in extension. The hips are in a position of flexion biomechanically, but stability in sitting depends on the interplay of neuromuscular activation of extension/abduction/outward rotation balanced with flexion. The thighs rest on the plinth and serve as a reference for the trunk. Components of hip rotation may vary, but the optimal neuromuscular activity as a foundation for stability favors outward rather than inward rotation (**Fig. 2.16a, b**).

The arms rest in adduction when they are not active; rotational components depend on the neuromuscular and biomechanical relationship of the thorax, head, neck, and shoulder girdles. Sitting is a functional position for many activities and allows the therapist good handling opportunities and variations (**Fig. 2.17**).

Stability in sitting requires coactivation of trunk muscles, and how we sit influences trunk muscle activity (O'Sullivan et al 2006; O'Sullivan et al 2002). O'Sullivan and colleagues (2006) identified and measured the differences in kinematics and muscle activity between two sitting postures, upright versus slump sitting, in a pain-free population. They concluded that the upright sitting posture, specifically the "lumbopelvic" upright sitting with anterior pelvic rotation, neutral lumbar lordosis, and relaxation of the thoracic spine, is critical to ensure activation of superficial lumbar multifidus and concurrent re-

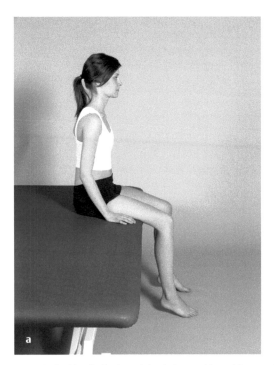
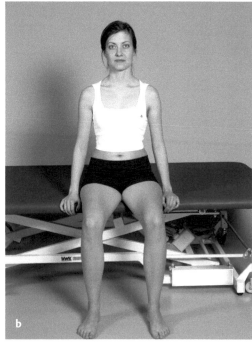

Fig. 2.16 (a, b) The basic upright sitting position with neutral lumbar lordosis and an upright thoracic spine.

laxation of thoracic erector spinae. Activation of the deep trunk-stabilizing muscles was reduced in slump sitting. Caneiro and colleagues (2010) studied healthy subjects being placed in three different sitting postures—lumbopelvic, thoracic upright, and slump—to investigate their influence on cervicothoracic muscle activity and head/neck posture. Slump sitting was found to be associated with increased thoracic flexion and head/neck flexion with a greater anterior translation of the head, as well as a significant increase in cervicothoracic muscle activity. The authors concluded that there is a clear link between different sitting postures on head/neck posture and motor activity in the neck muscles. These results support the role of the pelvicolumbar and thoracolumbar spine in postural activation of the head and neck region. This is supported by Griffin (2014), who states the following: "when addressing the hemiplegic shoulder complex, the first area to be assessed is the alignment of the trunk. The optimal alignment of anterior pelvic tilt, followed by lumbar extension and thoracic extension, provides a biomechanical foundation of all head, neck, and limb movement" (Griffin 2014). Therefore the sitting posture, and thus the activity in the trunk musculature, is important to address when training the upper limb; segmental movement and posture of the thoracic spine are important for scapular movements and scapular position on the thorax, and a normal scapular and thoracic spine motion allows optimal mechanics for the glenohumeral joint (Crosbie et al 2008) (**Fig. 2.18a, b**).

The control of the scapula during arm motion is an important component of normal shoulder function (Ludewig & Reynolds 2009). The shoulder complex must be considered a part of a larger kinetic chain made up of several joints. Stability of the scapulothoracic joint depends on coordinated activity of the surrounding musculature. The scapular muscles must dynamically position the glenoid so that efficient glenohumeral movement can occur. When weakness or dysfunction of the scapular musculature is present, normal scapular positioning and mechanics may become altered. Furthermore, limitation of thoracic motion is associated with functional restriction of arm movement due to the effects on the position and movements of the scapula (Crosbie et al 2008) because the thoracic spine forms a key link in the kinematic sequence of arm elevation. It is of great importance to consider whether the actual sitting posture is enhancing or inhibiting optimal trunk activity that further interventions may be

based on (e.g., when moving from sitting to standing or facilitating arm activity). Falla and colleagues (2007) compared activation of the deep neck flexors and lumbar multifidus during verbal and facilitated correction of sitting from a slumped posture to a neutral lumbopelvic posture. They demonstrated that activity of the deep neck flexors and lumbar multifidus were significantly greater when postural correction was facilitated by a therapist (hands on) than through verbal instruction. This has clinical implications with regard to the use of facilitation to correct a poor posture in sitting.

Sitting is a frequently used postural set for reaching activities in the neurological patient. In healthy subjects, upper limb reaching leads to APAs being generated in the trunk prior to arm movement, by which the flexor moment and orientation of the trunk is controlled (Cirstea & Levin 2000; Lee et al 2009). However, poststroke subjects demonstrate an increased trunk displacement and a delay in the APAs bilaterally while performing a reaching movement in sitting (Pereira et al 2014). Compensatory reaching strategies that involve the trunk have been shown to be inflexible and difficult to generalize to other tasks, as compared with reaching training based on trunk control (Thielman 2013). Limiting forward trunk flexion using a trunk restraint while practicing reaching has demonstrated improvement toward a more normal movement pattern of the arm trajectory. including increased scapular protraction and increased range of motion at the elbow and less trunk movement (Thielman 2013; Michaelsen et al 2001; Michaelsen et al 2006).

It is important to note that perfect alignment of body segments and postural control are not essential requirements for starting task practice in sitting. The use of task-directed activity in treatment does not require independent postural control. However, if the patient has reduced postural control it is important to adapt the environment to provide the appropriate external support. In this way, the patient may be able to perform task practice that in turn may improve postural control and selective movement (Graham et al 2009). However, attending to alignment of body segments and postural control may improve the patient's ability and efficiency of complex motor tasks (Raine et al 2009).

Advantages
Sitting postural sets (**Fig. 2.19**) may be varied infinitely, depending on the neuromuscular activity the therapist wants to facilitate: sitting straight, diagonally, more or

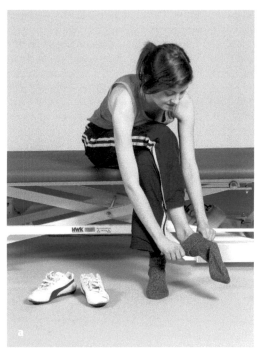

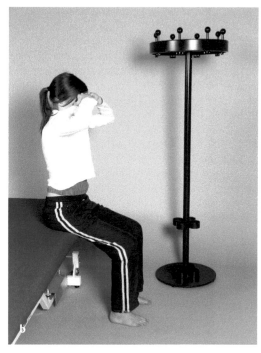

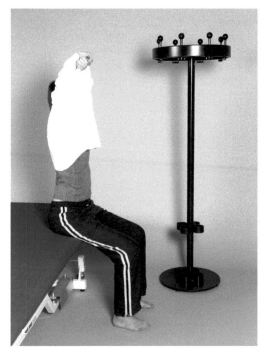

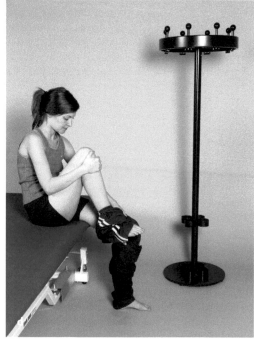

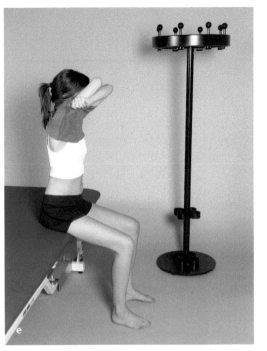

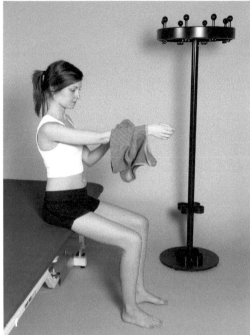

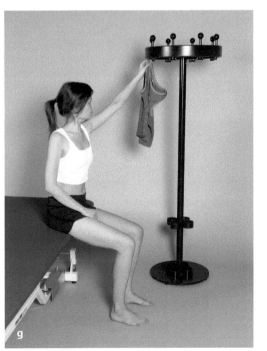

Fig. 2.17 (a–g) Undressing in a sitting position. Balance, movement, weight transfer, rotation, alignment between body segments, are all necessary elements for dressing or undressing in a sitting position. The trunk muscles are the primary muscles to keep the body upright, adjust weight shifts, and control movements against the constant pull of gravity. The lack of proximal stabilization in this task influences the limbs profoundly in that the arms cannot reach the toes to get the sock on or off, or be free to move easily in and out of the garments. Note the extension of the arms as the jumper and T-shirt are taken off **(c, e, f)**. The arms are free due to the stable trunk and may therefore move easily in and out of the garments. Proximal stability of the trunk is a prerequisite for distal limb mobility.

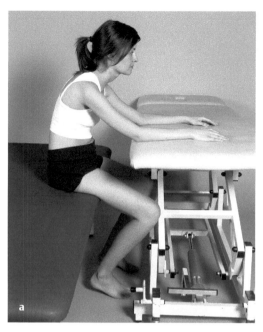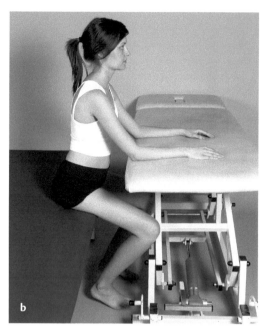

Fig. 2.18 (a, b) There is a clear effect of different sitting postures on head/neck posture and motor activity in the neck, trunk, and scapulae. The sitting posture and thus the activity in the trunk musculature is important to consider when using the sitting postural set to train the upper limb function, when facilitating a good sitting posture for eating, or when strength training the lower limb.

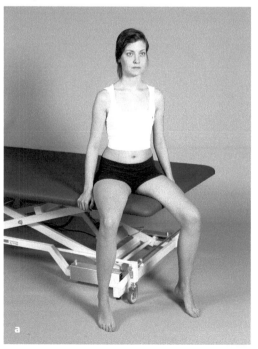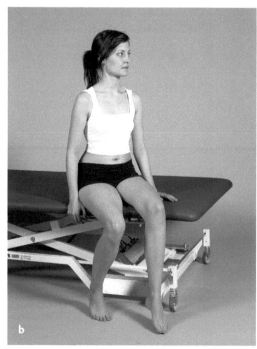

Fig. 2.19 (a) Increased adduction of the hips is a frequent problem in recruitment of stability and movement of the hips and pelvis. Enhanced abduction/outward rotation of the hips facilitate a more upright posture and postural control, and thereby interplay between body segments. A bigger and more open base allows for more movement of proximal segments. **(b)** Variation with rotation alters the weight-bearing areas and therefore stability requirements.

less rotated, leaning backward or forward, sitting high or low, far into the seat or toward the edge, different bases (bed, plinth, a variety of chairs, stools), different textures and hardness, or sitting on the floor.

Sitting postural sets are varied in relation to the task; where and in which direction the patient's next movement is going (i.e., the direction of the evolving activity), and therefore which neuromuscular activity is needed (**Fig. 2.20a, b**).

The position, posture, and activity of the arms influence the neuromuscular activity in the trunk. Normally, the activity of one upper limb will demand increased APAs bilaterally in the trunk (Lee et al 2009); first contralaterally as pAPA then ipsilaterally as aAPA. For example, activation of the left shoulder facilitates enhanced right trunk antigravity activity.

The use of arm support may reduce the patient's postural control by reorienting the reference for equilibrium responses to the support and the supporting arm instead of the feet in standing or the buttocks and thighs in sitting — depending on how the arm support is being used (Jeka & Lackner 1994; Jeka 1997). Arms above 90° with the glenohumeral joints toward outward rotation facilitate trunk extension and postural activation. If the patient can start to take over and carry the weight of the arms, postural stability and strength are enhanced throughout the body and arms. This is needed, for example, when placing dinner plates in a high cupboard or hanging a coat on a hook (**Fig. 2.21**). Movement of the body in relation to stable arms or moving the arms in relation to a stable trunk facilitates the interplay between stability and movement, which are facilitatory for postural control.

Sitting postural sets are easy to vary through different phases of treatment: from a more mobilizing hands-on intervention to facilitation of activity to the patient moving himself in the same treatment. Sitting postural sets are adapted to optimize the neuromuscular activity for the actual function the patient will perform; for instance, using high sitting, a more extensor-dominated postural set and more facilitatory to postural control to stand up from, or activate/stimulate/facilitate early arm and hand function. Sitting postural sets are used for the following:

- Mobilizing and activating the pelvis in relation to the trunk and the BoS.
- Facilitating segmental lumbar extension to facilitate components of hip stability and abdominal activity, which helps to achieve postural control and free arms.

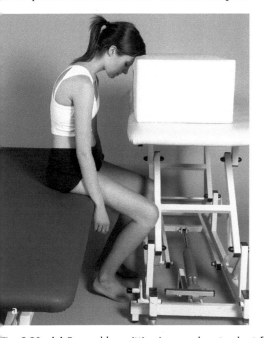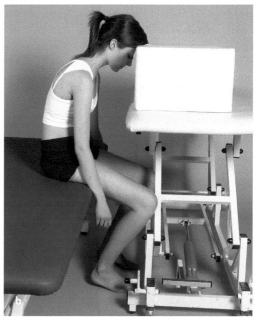

Fig. 2.20 (a) Forward-lean sitting is a good postural set for stabilizing the head and neck and facilitating interplay between body segments postural activation. This is a good postural set to assess the scapulae, activate scapular setting, and facilitate selective movement in the thorax. (b) In a clinical situation it is important to facilitate active sitting in the patient and not allow the patient to lower his tone and lean on the support because this might negate the aim of using this postural set.

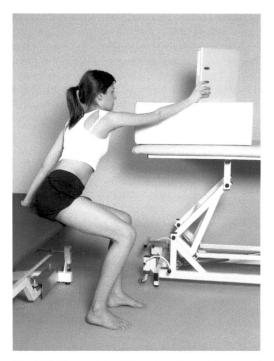

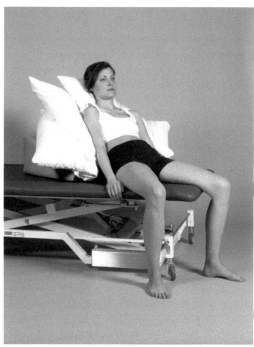

Fig. 2.21 The model stabilizes through her left arm and hand as she transfers weight and rotates to fetch a book on her left side with her right hand. The left arm becomes part of her base of support and allows her to move farther to the left, out of her original stability limits. She stabilizes over her left side and has to move in relation to her left arm. Note that she is not pushing into her arm but is extending the whole arm. Thus the arm gives her dynamic support; she has to move to and from the arm and needs to have good mobility, stability, and coordination in the shoulder girdle and between the body segments.

- Facilitating thoracic segmental extension on which scapula setting is based.
- Facilitating and activating scapular-selective movement and scapular setting.
- Facilitating head stability and orientation to midline.
- Facilitating gaze stability.
- Variation and movement from sitting to supine or sitting to standing.
- Stimulating and facilitating fine motor activity of the hand if postural activation is maintained, or using the arm and hand to facilitate postural control.
- Backward-lean sitting to access a stiff or hypersensitive foot or shortened hip flexors and adductors as preparation for improved stability in transfers and standing (**Fig. 2.22**)

Fig. 2.22 Backward-lean sitting. Note the importance of obtaining good alignment to the base of support. Depending on the adaptability of the patient's hip flexors, the position will have to be adapted with more or less support at the back to allow eccentric lengthening of the lumbar extensors. Good contact between the lumbar area and the support facilitates activation of abdominals for core control, to adjust the position, or to sit up.

Disadvantages

Because of the bigger base in sitting, patients with low postural tone easily sink into flexion and may start to fix in flexion because this may be the only strategy available to them. Patients who are already fixing in flexion may be stimulated to do so even more: short muscles enhance short muscles.

Use of supports influences the patient's postural tone, depending on how the support is used by the patient and the therapist. A support such as a table, plinth, stick, pillow, or wall increases the supporting base. If the patient leans on the support, the requirement for postural control is reduced. If the patient presses into the support, supports herself heavily, or fixes to the base of support, flexor activity is increased. However, the patient and therapist may use the support as a reference for movement or to reduce the weight of heavy arms and thereby facilitate postural control.

The material that the support base is made from is important for the neuromuscular activity that is promoted. A soft seat may stimulate more flexor/adductor/inward rotator activity, especially over the hips, pelvis, and lower trunk, than a firm support. A high support—a wall, high stick, high table, high cupboard—facilitates extensor activity more than a low support, depending on how it is being used.

Supine

How you stand dictates how you are able to "stop to stand" (i.e., sit down); this will further dictate the way you sit, by which the ability to selectively activate posture and movement in sitting is dictated. Therefore, creating the supine postural set should preferably start with the facilitation of *stop standing*. Stop standing is a therapeutic facilitation of the patient from standing to sitting in one continuous movement by which the patient actively controls various aspects of the movement to increase core stability and facilitate selective movement.

The aim of facilitation of *stop standing* is to create efficient postural control in the posture of sitting through the transition of postural sets, allowing the therapist and patient to move more directly to activities in sitting or in changing the postural set into, for example, supine.

In supine the therapist must assess the alignment of the head, neck, and shoulder girdles as well as the trunk, pelvis, and lower limbs in relation to each other because impairment or fixation in any of these segments can block selective activity in the supine position.

Supine postural sets are characterized by extension if the person is able to eccentrically lengthen his hips, lumbar spine, neck, and shoulder girdles. The base of support is large and the center of gravity low, and if the person is able to relate to the support and let go of muscular tension, the postural tone will be low. There is a tendency toward anterior tilt of the pelvis because of the weight of the lower limbs or sustained tone in the hip flexors, but if the person is able to eccentrically lengthen both hip flexors and lumbar extensors, he will have a better contact to the base of support and a more appropriate alignment, both for rest and for activity. With this alignment, the extremities will tend to be slightly abducted, outwardly rotated, and extended. The forearms are often pronated, and the elbows slightly flexed, which is normal. We tend to relate to the environment through the palms of our hands for orientation (**Fig. 2.23**).

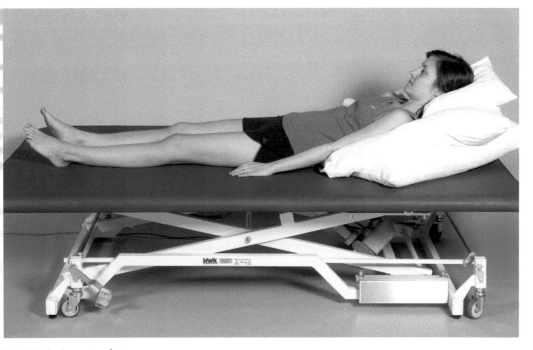

Fig. 2.23 Supine postural set.

Advantages

Supine postural sets may be varied in different ways: both legs may be flexed and the feet placed in different distances from the hips. The degree of hip and knee flexion will determine how difficult or easy it is to move the pelvis. If the feet are placed closely to the hips, weight transference onto the feet through pelvic tilt is facilitated due to biomechanical relationships (**Fig. 2.24a**). Hip extension and postural activation are enhanced if the knees move distally to be in line with the feet during bridging activity (**Fig. 2.24b**).

If the feet are placed further down and away from the hips, the biomechanical alignment changes, and the recruitment of pelvic and postural activity is made more difficult. The upper body may be supported with pillows to enhance eccentric lengthening of trunk extensors and thereby facilitate abdominal activity. The interplay between abdominal and extensor neuromuscular activation is essential for selective pelvic activity (in relation to hips and lumbar spine), mobility, and stability.

A common muscle imbalance is short and tonically active hip flexors with weakness of the gluteals, proximal hamstrings, and abdominals, resulting in anterior pelvic tilt with increased lumbar lordosis; the hip flexor component has to be treated to allow the patient to eccentrically lengthen the back extensors and flatten the lumbar spine because this is an important factor for the patient's ability to achieve selectivity of movement in the supine position (Raine et al 2009). Supine postural sets may be suitable for specific mobilization of muscles that are short or inactive if the patient is able to adjust to the position.

Different phases of the transfer from sitting to supine or supine to sitting are used clinically to facilitate a graded coordination and interplay between flexor, extensor, abductor, adductor, and rotatory components within and between body segments for the control of stability and movement.

Disadvantages

Postural tone is basically low in supine. Therefore the initiation of activity to oppose gravity may be difficult. The large contact area means that there are many frictional and inertial components to overcome. Therefore, to be active in supine and to

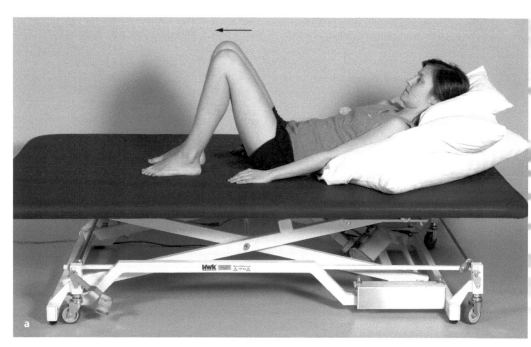

Fig. 2.24 Supine postural set. Crook lying. Important in achieving stability in this postural set is that the legs are actively "placed" in crook posture. Thus the postural stability within the hips can be achieved relative to the feet in efficient contact with the plinth and therefore context based to stance phase. This postural set can be used as a facilitator of postural stability within hips and lower limbs. Note the position of the knees in relation to the feet in the two pictures, and consequently hip extension and abdominal activation. **(a)** Facilitation of forward weight transfer over the foot in crook lying as a basis for selective pelvic tilt in bridging. (*Continued*)

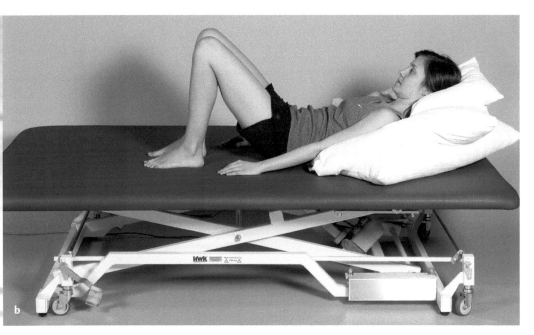

Fig. 2.24 (*continued*) **(b)** Selective pelvic tilt involves stability of ankles and knees together with activation of proximal hamstrings, gluteal muscles, and abdominal muscles.

transfer from supine to sitting requires a reasonable postural activation, or this activity to be facilitated. The transfer from supine to sitting is complex and requires a certain level of postural control combined with graded alterations of flexor, extensor, abductor, adductor, and rotatory components to be performed independently. At the same time, the patient is often required to perform this with no or little help or positional adaptations, even in the early stages after a CNS lesion, and this may drive the choice of compensatory strategies for other functions also. Supine may therefore not be the first position of choice in the treatment of the very low toned patient, but may be used more appropriately for the training of specific components of stability, movement, and strength with a patient who has more background activity.

Some patients have increased tone in supine. They may have a reduced ability to adapt to the base of support and feel uncomfortable, insecure, or vulnerable. Others may have reduced segmental mobility and interaction between body segments, and therefore reduced ability to actively move and transfer weight to change position. Weight and friction make movement less accessible, also for therapeutic handling.

◼ Side Lying

Side lying is characterized by extension through the weight-bearing side and a more flexor bias on the upper side (**Fig. 2.25a–c**). The stability requirements are greatest on the weight-bearing side because of the interaction with the base of support.

Side lying may be used in therapy to retrain components of gait (Raine et al 2009), such as the following (**Fig. 2.26**):
- Create stability in the leg and trunk of the weight-bearing side.
- Contextualize the sensory information in side lying to create a stable alignment on the weight-bearing side through plantar pressure information to the foot.
- Selectively activate the hip, knee, and foot of the uppermost leg to promote perception of the relationship between a stance leg (weight bearing, undermost side) and a moving leg (uppermost), which is context based to locomotion.

Advantages
Side-lying postural sets may be varied by changing rotatory components within the trunk or extremities or by using more or fewer pillows to influence stability (**Fig. 2.25**). Side-lying postural sets allow for great mo-

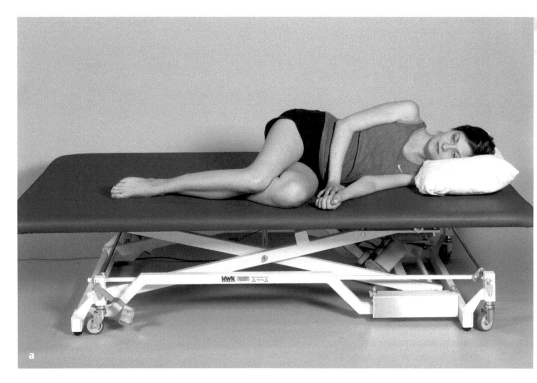

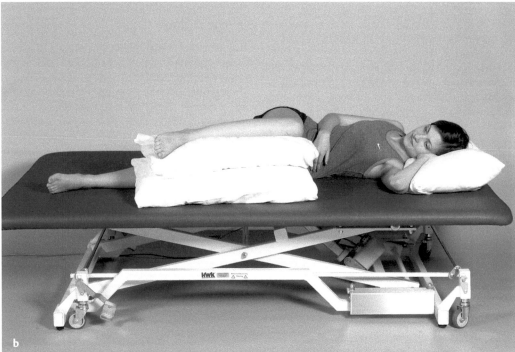

Fig. 2.25 (a–c) Side lying with different supports. (*Continued*)

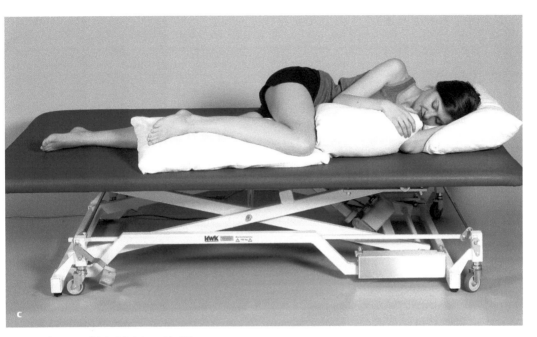

Fig. 2.25 (*continued*) **(c)** Side lying with different supports.

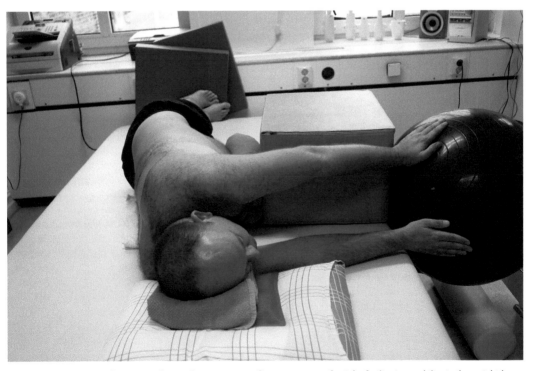

Fig. 2.26 Side lying may for instance be used to retrain specific components of gait by facilitating stability in the weight bearing leg and trunk; contextualizing the sensory information to facilitate a stable alignment of the leg (weight bearing side) with plantar pressure information; and using bilateral contractual hand-orientating response to enhance trunk stability.

bility between proximal body segments and facilitate placing of the upper arm or leg to enhance postural stability and strength. Side lying on the most affected side in stroke may stimulate this through weight bearing and tactile input, and facilitate postural activity in both central and proximal segments. Side lying on the least affected side in stroke may improve the stability of this side as a background for movement of the more affected limbs in space.

Disadvantages

Side lying may be very unstable because the base is long and narrow with a slightly higher center of gravity than supine. Therefore, it may be a difficult postural set to use in treatment. If the adaptation to the base of support is inadequate, for instance, if the patient has reduced ability to eccentrically lengthen the supporting side, then the uppermost shoulder girdle will be very unstable. The stable position of the scapula depends on the activation of intercostal muscles and the muscles of the trunk. If these are stretched or inactive, the scapula will glide upward on the trunk, with inappropriate alignment for selective placing of the arm. The stability of side lying may be enhanced by placing tightly rolled towels closely into and very slightly under the patient's trunk posteriorly and anteriorly as well as by using pillows to stabilize the upper leg in neutral.

▰   Key Areas

Movement causes continuous displacement of body segments in relation to each other, as well as for intrasegmental alignment and distribution of tone through neuromuscular activity. This may be analyzed through observation and handling (Taylor et al 1995). Several authors call some of the body segments *key points (of control)* (Bobath 1990; Bader-Johansson 1991; Kidd et al 1992; Edwards 1996). This term is easy to misunderstand because it refers to segments, regions, or areas, and not to points. *Key areas* or *functional units* are more accurate names, also because these areas have their own activity at the same time as they interact with the rest of the body. The key areas are central, proximal, and distal.

▪   The Central Key Area

The central key area is the thorax with its joints and muscular attachments to the head and neck, the shoulder girdles, and the pelvis. Especially important is the midthoracic area and the ribs with their costal attachments to the sternum and the musculature in this area. The functions of the central key area are first and foremost balance, postural control, and a stable reference for extremity function. Movement in three planes, frontal, transverse, and sagittal, allows for weight transference, interplay between right and left, and the ability to cross the midline with the extremities.

Some therapists classify the head and neck as an extension of the central key area, or as a proximal key area in itself. The function of the head and neck in movement (excluding communication or eating) is manyfold: important aspects are orientation to the world around us, being a stable reference for the eyes, keeping the eyes horizontal to receive and therefore perceive information as accurately as possible, and enhancing balance as far as possible.

▪   Proximal Key Areas: Shoulder and Pelvic Girdles

- *The shoulder girdle.* Caillet (1980) describes the shoulder girdle as consisting of seven components: the glenohumeral joint, the suprahumeral connection (the coracoacromial ligament; the coracoid process and the acromion process together form the coracoacromial arch, which supports the head of the humerus above), the acromioclavicular joint, sternoclavicular joint, sternocostal joints, costovertebral joints, and the scapulocostal attachment. The shoulder girdle cannot be viewed separately from other body segments. Through its attachment to the spine and the pelvis via the trunk musculature, the shoulder girdle influences and is influenced by alignment and neuromuscular activity of the pelvic girdle, trunk, head and neck, and extremities. The function of the shoulder girdle is to be a mobile yet stable reference (mobile stability) for arm and hand function and at the same time a functional part of balance.
- *The pelvic girdle.* The pelvis moves in relation to the lumbar spine and therefore the trunk, and to the hips. The pelvis comprises the two iliac bones and the sacrum, connected via the sacroiliac joints and the symphysis pubis. These joints are immovable, although they do allow for small rotational components to transfer stresses and strains. The pelvis moves between the lumbar spine above and the hip joints below. The

pelvis as a key area is, therefore, not the pelvis alone but the pelvis together with its proximal and more distal relationships. Functionally, the pelvis, with the lumbar spine and hip joints, is mainly responsible for translation of those forces that act down onto the base of support and up through the body, stability and mobility (mobile stability), and weight transference.

■ Distal Key Areas

The hands and feet are mobile and adaptable entities with lots of specific sensory receptors to allow interaction of the body with the environment.

- *Hands.* The human hands are unique in their ability to oppose the thumb to the other fingers, thereby allowing the whole range of movement from finely tuned and graded movement to strength and power grip. Many layers of small muscles within the hand make it possible to alter rotational components to change and adjust movement. Some areas are more stable, others more mobile, depending on the function. The lumbrical grip is based on extension of the wrist and is a foundation for reach and grasp and thus for both pinch grip and power grip. The functions of the hands are to explore the environment; to touch and feel and receive information; to underline expression and meaning (gesticulation); to manipulate objects and perform fine motor skills; as well as carrying, lifting, and moving things, and being an extension of the body in pushing, for instance, a wheelbarrow. The arms and hands have a role in balance, seeking environmental support when needed.
- *The feet.* The feet transmit forces between the environment and the body and between the body and the environment. They are resilient and provide springiness when walking in hilly environments or up the stairs, running, and changing direction. They improve the reach of the arm by their power in tiptoeing. The toes are important for turning around and changing direction. The function of the feet is to seek information from and about the environment, to adapt to the support base to balance and weight transfer.

Elbows and knees allow the change of patterns of movement through the change of rotation between the upper and lower limb segments in conjunction with the proximal and distal key areas. The sum of individual components within these areas enables vast variations to meet the requirements of a diversity of tasks. The interplay between the key areas allows for balance, weight transfer, and movement at the same time. No body segment functions in isolation.

Many muscles and joints converge in the key areas; for instance, in the hand alone there are 19 bones, combined with the wrist and lower arm there are 29; 20 muscles are intrinsic to the hand and ~19 are in the lower arm and act on the hand in some way, not counting the upper arm. The central key area comprises the ribs, sternum, vertebrae, and deep and superficial musculature. Specific receptors in muscles, tendons, joints, and skin pick up any change in activity and report to the CNS. This allows for an infinite variety of movement, stability, and adjustment. Clinical experience suggests that handling of one key area influences tone and activity of other body segments and key areas in two ways: (1) through skin, joint, and muscular attachments directly and indirectly; and (2) probably because handling influences many specific receptors and the transmission of information to the CNS. All information from the periphery converges in the spinal cord, and an abundance of interneurons transmit this information over many levels within the spinal cord and therefore spread information over a relatively large area, as well as to the brain.

> Many muscles and joints converge at the key areas. Therefore, the influence from proprioceptive and skin receptors on the CNS is substantial.
> Control of key areas and the interplay between them seem especially important for balance, selectivity of movement, adaptation to the environment and tasks, and, therefore, for function.

Treatment aimed at improving muscular interplay, alignment, and mobility in and between key areas may improve coordination and the relationship between stability and movement. As a result, patients may experience improved balance and selectivity and generally more control over their body.

In a treatment situation the therapist has to assess which key area (or areas) is most dysfunctional, whether this has to be treated in isolation first, or whether the patient will regain more control if there is interplay between more key areas in activity. This focus often varies during treatment. The choices must be directly related to the individual patient's movement problem and the functions that need to be regained first.

Selective Movement and Functional Activity

Berta Bobath described patterns of movement as "sequences of selective movement for function" (Bobath 1990). Selective movements are interdependent and interactive with the postural control mechanism (Raine et al 2009). The CNS needs to control for the effects of interaction torques in adjacent joints from motions at other joints when performing a multijoint action, such as reaching. Thus the ability to produce torque over one joint will influence and be influenced by the torques produced at other joints (Mercier et al 2005). Therefore, the recovery of selective movement is a necessity for efficient postural control, alignment, and function (Raine 2007). The focus of the Bobath Concept is on maximizing the individual's selective movement control (Graham et al 2009). This is achieved by analysis of movements and task performance to identify the most significant impairment(s) in that specific individual, leading to the given limitation in activity or function.

A functional task may be divided into short-term goals or components, which consist of the motor activity needed to reach the goal (the process)—movement strategies and patterns, selective movement, and neuromuscular activity—and must relate to the environment in which it is being performed (**Table 2.1**).

Few studies have focused on the relationship between body functions and structures, activity, and participation (WHO 2006). Normann (2004) showed that, even if the therapist spent most of the treatment time improving the patient's control of neuromuscular recruitment in relevant activities, the treatment showed observable changes in activity and the patients spontaneously reported improvement in participation. Smedal et al (2006) in their study of two patients with MS, demonstrated that it is possible to regain activity through training that focuses on body function and structures in conjunction with different activities, and that the effect lasts.

Brock et al (2011) compared the short-term effects of two physiotherapy approaches for improving ability to walk in different environments following stroke: (group A) interventions based on the Bobath Concept in conjunction with task practice, compared with (group B) structured task practice alone. The participants in group A received individualized interventions based on a detailed assessment of the individual's movement strategies and the neurological and neuromuscular deficits underlying motor dysfunction and ongoing clinical reflection based on the patients' response to treatment. Participants receiving intervention B undertook physiotherapy treatment based on structured task practice.

Table 2.1 Components of a functional task: from neuromuscular activation through selective motor control, patterns of movement, and motor activity to the goal of the movement with regard to the individual and the environment

Functional goal	For example, dressing, personal care, fetching a book, making a cup of coffee, going to the bathroom, walking to answer the telephone, or opening the door. Extended goals are instrumental activities of daily living, such as shopping
↑	
Motor activity	For example, turning around, weight transference for transfers, stepping, sitting down, and lying down
↑	
Patterns of movement	Movement over more than one segment or joint, the sequencing of selective movements, for instance, in reaching and grasping and stance and swing
↑	
Selective control	Isolated movement over one joint or key area based on stability in other parts
↑	
Neuromuscular activity	Depends on the postural set(s) chosen for the task; relates to the recruitment of neuromuscular activity necessary to move to reach the goal

The results of this study demonstrated short-term advantages for using interventions based on the Bobath Concept (group A) for improving walking velocity in people with stroke.

Clinical Example

The movement of the pelvis (pelvic tilt) in lateral and anteroposterior directions is essential to all weight transference and transfers and is therefore integrated in all functional activities. Pelvic tilt requires different neuromuscular activity in different postural sets and through movement from one position to another, for instance in sitting down, in supine to change position in bed, moving from one chair to another, or to wiping one's bottom in the bathroom (**Fig. 2.27a–c**).

Control of pelvic tilt in supine does not necessarily carry over automatically to the transfer from sitting to standing or walking. If, based on clinical reasoning, it is necessary to work on pelvic tilt in supine, for instance to improve the actual range of available movement, to enhance proprioceptive information for the awareness of the body part and

update of body schema, then pelvic tilt needs to be worked on and facilitated throughout the transfer from supine to sitting as well; moving through and controlling the different postural alignments in this function to gain carryover into sitting. The same applies from standing to sitting and vice versa. The relationship between stability and movement changes through the transfer and needs to be facilitated, controlled, and regained throughout the movement. Carryover to different situations may be enhanced if the treatment is varied, incorporating different alignments and rotational components and specific learning to control eccentric activity.

The hip abductors are important for the stability of the pelvis during locomotion (Grimaldi 2011; Shumway-Cook & Woollacott 2006). The hip abductors on the stance leg prevent a contralateral drop of the pelvis during swing phase of the opposite leg, (i.e., a functional [or physiologic] lateral pelvic tilt). Many patients have reduced recruitment of this activity during stepping and are therefore unstable during transfers or walking. Hip abductors may be recruited and facilitated in different ways:

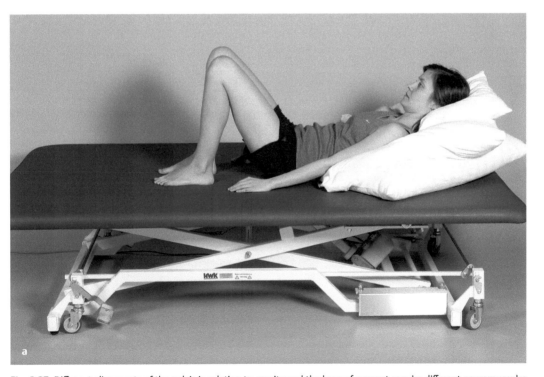

Fig. 2.27 Different alignments of the pelvis in relation to gravity and the base of support require different neuromuscular activation to move. **(a)** Pelvic tilt in supine. (*Continued*)

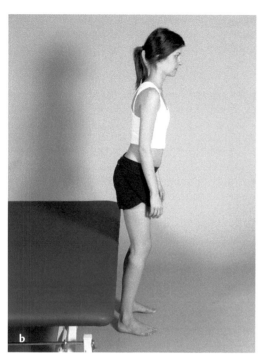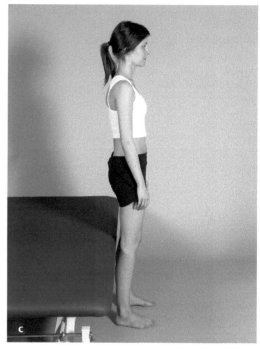

Fig. 2.27 (*continued*) **(b)** Pelvic tilt in the movement from sitting to standing. **(c)** Pelvic alignment in standing.

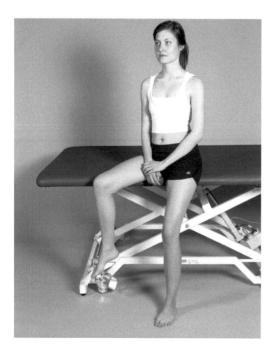

Fig. 2.28 Facilitating hip abductors, standing down from asymmetrical sitting to single leg standing.

stepping sideways, sitting asymmetrically on a high support (**Fig. 2.28**), walking from step standing, or improving specific strength in side lying. Stepping down from a high support requires recruitment of hip abductors on the standing leg and may facilitate the first step to walk, if the alignment is appropriate. Locomotion is initiated from many different postural sets, not just parallel standing or step standing, and we walk forward, backward, sideways, and turn around. All these variations need to be incorporated in treatment.

▉ The Relationship between Automatic and Voluntary Movement

Information, perception, and cognition are all important for action. Umphred (1991) states that motivation, challenge, and success are cognitive elements, even if we are not consciously aware of such feelings during everyday movement. She also states that visual and vestibular systems play an essential part in cognitive analysis and recall of previous experiences, and that these lead to learning and semiautomated movement. Whiting and Vereijken (1993) are of the opinion that the CNS is self-organizing and solves its motor tasks here and now as a response to environmental requirements, without cognitive attention. Cognition is a process that may be separated into several stages:

- Confronting the task.
- Assessing and evaluating the terms and components of the problem.
- Choosing a solution from many possible solutions.
- Choosing an appropriate way to solve the problem.
- Using the preferred choice.
- Operative stage (action).
- Comparison between the result and the original terms of the task.

The role of *cognition* in movement is undisputable, but the level on which cognition is most involved will vary depending on the requirements of the task. Luria and Umphred emphasize conscious thought in the planning of motor strategies when attention to the movement is important, whereas Whiting believes that cognition is an awareness of movement within the CNS without reaching a conscious level.

Motor learning seems to require the same CNS processes irrespective of the CNS being healthy or damaged (see Chapter 1.3 Motor Learning and Plasticity). The difference lies in the ability of the patient's CNS to receive information, to process the information, and to recruit the appropriate activity. There is a graded transition between movement that is most automatic (postural responses) and movement that is least automatic (volitional and conscious) because there are elements of cognition in all activities. The differentiation between conscious thought (least automatic) and awareness (more automatic) is clinically relevant, even if both these aspects have elements of cognition. We are more conscious when we learn a new complex task that demands precision than of the background activity of postural control and balance that allows improving precision. When learning how to play tennis we are consciously aware of the handgrip on the racket, the direction and rotational components of the strokes, and the visual feedback from the flight of the ball in time and space. Our conscious thought is not involved in all the background activity of the body, the actual and immediate adaptation and adjustments that need to be in balance to perform the skilled movement at the same time. We are more concerned with reaching the goal than in

the processes involved to be successful. When basic skills are learned, we develop the memory to recall the experience (i.e., how the movement *feels*). This feeling seems to be based on the comparison of expected performance (previous experience) and actual performance (i.e., perception) and seems to be closely linked to the feeling of success.

The CNS has a capacity for dual or simultaneous activity (i.e., to do two or more things at the same time). Walking on a busy street, jumping from one stone to another in the mountains, or shopping requires that we can receive and process many different types of information at the same time as we move and act appropriately. We are aware of the goal, of people around us, the complex environment, or things that happen around us, as long as we are in balance. We are normally able to perform two functions at the same time; both walk and talk, shop and move around to take things down from shelves at the same time as reading the shopping list, dress and undress while standing, shower and soap our bodies, and do mathematical calculations while walking. Our attention is not focused on walking but on the simultaneous functions. This is called *simultaneous activity* or *dual task* (Mulder et al 1996). Many routine and more automatic activities may, however, be brought to conscious awareness and controlled through focused attention, concentration, and willpower if the person deems it necessary. The CNS problem-solves tasks in different ways depending on the situation.

Following neurological damage or, for instance, lower limb amputation, the ability for simultaneous activity diminishes. When balance is threatened, the focus of our attention is pulled away from the task to how balance can be preserved to avoid falls. Many patients use conscious effort in an attempt to preserve balance. If their attention is disturbed—a ringing phone, a kettle boiling, other people moving in the vicinity, they are in danger of falling and may hurt themselves.

Postural control is one of the most automated functions of a healthy CNS (Mulder et al 1996; Mulder 1991; Dietz 1992; Massion 1992; Massion 1994; Horak 1997; Shumway-Cook & Woollacott 2006; Brodal 2010). Postural control is the foundation for selective activity of the extremities, and postural stability is a prerequisite for movement control and the ability to vary movement. Movement and postural control are closely integrated. Movement of the extremities requires adjustments of the postural mechanisms, both before (aAPA), during (pAPA), and in response to (feedback) the movement. Trunk adjustments are more automatic and are learned during childhood because movement and the position of the center of gravity have to be controlled simultaneously (Massion 1994). The hands and feet interact more directly with the environment and are classified as the least automatic elements of normal movement control. The movements of individual fingers for precision of movement are least automatic and mostly voluntary, whereas the posturing of the hand and wrist along with the postural control of the arm and body are mostly automatic and less voluntary.

Examples of skills are writing, throwing and catching a ball, cycling, and driving a car. All these are based on an appropriate postural background. Skills become more automatic as they are learned and require progressively less attention. Many (over) learned routine-based basic tasks, such as ADLs, walking, and reaching, need little or no conscious thought or attention. The term *overlearned* was used by Mulder et al (1996).

> Everyday activities, such as walking, reaching, and eating, are mostly automatic functions that normally require little attention and effort.

(Over) learned activities and balance seem to have a structural correlation (form–function; see Chapter 1.3 Motor Learning and Plasticity) in the CNS, developed through activity-dependent interaction with the environment (i.e., experience). *Structural* is *not* the same as *unchangeable* or *fixed*. The CNS is not stereotyped or rigid. The ability to vary is great and depends on the situation in which the motor activity is being performed. New skills, from the first attempt (willed, attention demanding) to initial control (semiautomated) to acquired skill (automated) exist in a landscape between functional and structural plasticity.

> Everyday activities have a structural correlation in the CNS, based on experience.
> The expression of activity varies depending on the individual, the goal, and the situation.

In situations where there are increasing demands for adjustment, for instance, when the base of support changes or is moving, when objects are in the way, when the shirt buttons are small or the button holes are too small, or when the sock on the foot is twisted, our attention is increasingly focused on the task until the problem is solved. Once solved, the progression of the activity is more automatic again. Cognitive regulation, visual information (eye–hand contact), and sensorimotor adaptation are all important to skill acquisition, especially to hand function. More and less automatic movements are closely integrated, and humans switch between these controls depending on how easy or difficult, known or new the task is.

> Automatic and voluntary control of movement is closely integrated and forms the basis for functional skills and balance.

Walking has both cognitive and more automatic elements. The initiation of gait; alteration of tempo, speed, and direction; attention to obstacles and people; and unevenness are the more cognitive elements. The cognitive elements are not focused on the actual motor strategies that are used; they are related to problem-solving the initiation of gait, the goal, and the environment. Walking is at its most automatic in unchallenging environments when there is no need for change (see Chapter 1.2 The Spinal Cord: Central Pattern Generators and Locomotion). After the initial step, the steps follow more automatically as the line of gravity falls in a controlled way outside the base of support and the person steps to regain balance. The trunk moves forward and up, the legs follow (i.e., a cranial to caudal recruitment of activity).

Walking may be consciously controlled if we so wish. Please follow the instructions below closely before you read on:
- Stand up.
- Place your feet parallel with each other.
- Flex the right hip and knee, lift the leg, and stretch out the leg.
- Place the heel down on the floor.
- Transfer weight on to the right leg and straighten the right knee.
- Flex the left hip and knee, lift the leg, and stretch out the leg.
- Place the heel down on the floor.
- Transfer weight onto the left leg, and straighten the left knee.
- Flex the right hip and knee, and swing the right leg through.
- Place the heel down on the floor.
- Then please go back to your seat.

The question is, did you use the same movement strategies when walking under instruction as when you went back to your seat? Usually people experience a big difference. Experience suggests that other motor strategies are used during verbal instruction than are used during normal effortless gait. The first step is mostly voluntary, and attention is directed toward the actual movement as well as the goal. Detailed instruction, either internally generated or externally generated by a therapist, increases conscious attention toward controlling components of movement that are not voluntarily controlled or directed in a normal situation. When movement is instructed, the sequence of components seems to be reversed (after the initial step); the leg moves in relation to the body, and the line of gravity lies behind the moving leg (normally the body moves in relation to a standing leg). The patterns of movement in the swinging leg are characterized by greater degrees and earlier initiated flexion over the swinging hip than during normal walking. In this example, the trunk moves after the legs, that is, a caudal to cranial recruitment. The recruitment sequence is reorganized, and the flexor activity increases, efficiency is reduced, it takes more time, and the physical and cognitive effort increase. The use of verbal instruction to recruit the activity of individual muscles, muscle groups, or isolated components may override automaticity and alter the recruitment sequence compared with normal function.

Postural control is based on vestibular, somatosensory, and visual information. The weighting of the relative importance of these sources of information depends on the actual situation. Patients who have a CNS lesion often have reduced, inappropriate, or limited APAs (feedforward) (Pereira et al 2014; Krishnan et al 2012; Dickstein et al 2004; Mancini et al 2009). Mulder et al (1996) studied improvement after CNS lesions and stated the following: "From the work performed in Nijmegen during the past 5 years, three principles of recovery can be distilled: (a) a decrease of cognitive regulation; (b) a decrease in visual dependency; and (c) an improvement in sensorimotor adaptability."

People with reduced balance become more dependent on vision and attention, even during more automatic functions, such as unchallenged walking. If visual information dominates, information via other channels equally important for balance—somatosensory and vestibular systems—is in danger of becoming neglected by the CNS. Vision is closely related to cognitive control through regulation and focusing of attention. The patient's CNS may stop listening to signals from the body; speed and balance reactions become reduced, and the sequence of recruitment of neuromuscular activity is reorganized.

Clinically, the factors mentioned by Mulder et al (1996) may be used as treatment interventions if the patient has some balance control but is too cognitively regulated:

- Distract the patient by giving him a cognitive task, and progress to mental tasks containing spatial elements (e.g., describing the interior of his house or flat in detail).
- "Blind" the patient by asking him to close his eyes or use non see-through glasses to improve perception.
- Improve the patent's sensorimotor adaptation by, for instance, specifically mobilizing the structures of his feet, improving flexibility and muscle length, improving alignment, and introducing gradual weight bearing combined with functional tasks working for dual task interaction.

During assessment, the therapist collects information through observation and handling and forms hypotheses about why the patient moves as he does. The reasoning process for the therapist involves deciding which are the patient's main problems: reduced postural control or more mobility problems. The focus may change as treatment progresses. If postural control is most affected, it might seem logical to facilitate regaining this through more automatic processes (i.e., not use specific verbal instructions to maintain balance). Appropriate interventions are specific choices of postural sets, nonverbal demands on the patient's postural control by introducing a dual task (throw a balloon, roll a ball, move a glass of water), free arms, especially facilitating or supporting the arms above shoulder level in standing, standing to sitting, and sitting, at the same time as alignment and muscle function are optimized (for individual examples, see Chapter 4).

If the patient has some postural control combined with normal cognition and therefore the ability to problem solve, but has problems in the recruitment and initiation of selective movement, other interventions may be more appropriate, for instance, the use of verbal instruction combined with facilitation of more optimal alignment during a relevant functional task. In some situations, specific focused attention toward detail, stimulation, and facilitation may improve the patient's awareness and body schema and result in better control of movement as a preparation for task acquisition.

Many patients with CNS lesions have reduced cognitive ability and/or perception. The interventions have to be made appropriate to the patient's ability—

to what she responds best. For instance, if a patient suffering from inattention or neglect makes spontaneous eye contact with a body part that is being moved or stimulated, it implies that this intervention raises the patient's awareness, and the possibility for integration of information from that body part is strengthened, improving the patient's body schema.

It is important for the clinician to determine what level of cognition to demand during treatment of the individual patient. Verbal instruction lifts the problem solving to a conscious level, which is not always appropriate. How much conscious thought should the patient put into movements and activities that in a healthy person would be more automatic? When should the therapist use verbal commands—and what type of commands? What about mental imagery and practice? These questions are relevant for the clinical reasoning process.

> The clinical challenge is to decide whether balance can be regained through conscious voluntary planning, or be facilitated on a more automatic level in functional situations. Tone, muscle dynamics, alignment, and sequence of recruitment must be optimized in both scenarios.

Handling

Handling refers to the physical contact between patient and therapist in a treatment situation and is not limited to the therapist's use of hands. Therapists have been interested in the influence that handling may have on the patient's development of independence in balance and movement. Some professionals claim that handling may hinder the patient's own development of movement strategies because handling may act as an external support. It is claimed that an external support, such as a brace, splint, walking aids, or personal support, may stop the patient in exploring her relationship with gravity.

Clinical experience underlines the importance of *appropriate* handling. The important question is *how* and *why* handling is used in the process of the patient's regaining and relearning of independence. Jeka (1997) and Jeka and Lackner (1994) studied the effect of external supports on patients' postural control The researchers found that, when the trial participants had fingertip contact with the environment, their postural activity changed. In these trials two different ways of using fingertip contact with a met-

al stick that stood firm were examined: (1) weight bearing or leaning on the stick; and (2) light fingertip touch. Weight bearing or leaning on the support reduced postural activity in the participants. Use of an external support causes sensorimotor reorganization of activity by, for instance, changing the sequence of muscle activation. If the participants touch only lightly, they receive information through their fingertips and increase their postural activity; light fingertip touch gives additional information to the CNS, more than vision alone. Touching the environment may orient the body and improve perception of the relationship between the body and space. However, postural activity was greatest when participants did not use any external support.

The influence of peripheral stimulation on movement has been studied both in animals and in people with spinal cord injuries (SCIs) (Lynskey et al 2008; Guertin 2013; Ferguson et al 2012; Hubli & Dietz 2013). During training it is important that movements are performed as normally as possible to train and modify spinal circuits for specific motor tasks. Increased peripheral stimulation through manual and electrostimulation techniques is also found to improve movements of the extremities after SCI. According to Hubli and Dietz (2013), "The aim of new neurorehabilitative approaches should be to optimize the use of task-specific sensory cues in order to facilitate locomotor pattern generation."

Many other studies stress the importance of somatosensory information for standing control (Meyer et al 2004; Kavounoudias et al 1998; Wang & Lin 2008; Maurer et al 2006), locomotion (Rossignol et al 2006; Prochazka & Ellaway 2012), reach and grasp (Mackay-Lyons 2002; Nowak et al 2004; Blouin et al 2014; Santello et al 2002), and postural control (Morningstar et al 2005; Levin & Panturin 2011; Peterka 2002; Lockhart & Ting 2007). MacKay-Lyons (2002) state that there are potentially three different roles for afferent feedback and that all involve adapting movement to the internal and external environments: (1) reinforcing the activities of the central pattern generator (CPG), especially those involving load-bearing muscles; (2) timing function, whereby the sensory feedback provides information to ensure that the motor output is appropriate for the biomechanical state of the moving body part in terms of position, direction of movement, and force; and (3) facilitating phase changes in rhythmic movements to ensure that a certain phase of the movement is not initiated until the appropriate biomechanical state of the moving body part has been achieved.

Handling provides somatosensory information to the patient and may therefore enhance, facilitate, or hinder the patient's development of postural and movement control, depending on how it is used.

The skin is our largest sensory organ. Skin, musculature, tendons, and connective tissue have abundant specific receptors that continuously inform the CNS of the state of the body. During handling, either through the therapist's hands or through other body parts (shoulder, knee, hip, etc.), a stream of information flows between the patient and the therapist. Physical contact through skin and musculature leads to intimate and intense communication between the two, which should not be misinterpreted. The therapist both receives and gives information through handling. When the patient moves or is facilitated to move, the therapist receives information about the patient's ability to respond, initiate, and move, and how he moves (i.e. recruitment of activity both locally and generally). If the therapist optimizes the patient's alignment locally to enhance muscle function, for instance by aligning the patient's pelvis more appropriately to the base of support in sitting, the therapist can assess the patient's response to handling in general.

The eyes and hands are two of the therapist's most important assessment tools. The most important part of handling is "listening" to the response. Figuratively, our hands may see around corners. *Stereognostic sense* means that we can identify objects through touch alone by picking up information about texture, temperature, and firmness and compare this information with previous experience to identify what it is (see Chapter 1.2 The Somatosensory system, Lateral Inhibition, The Sense of Touch). Therefore, the hands have the ability to both listen and see. Therapists need to improve and extend this skill for their interaction with patients. The hands and eyes provide the therapist with information about the following:

- Local aspects.
  - Weight distribution.
  - Alignment.
  - Muscle qualities, which may give rise to hypotheses about tone, flexibility, elasticity, activity, and adaptability or become the foundation for ideas about activity.
  - Quality of other soft tissues in the area.
  - Skin quality and temperature.

This information is received through the direct, local contact.

- General aspects.
  - Tone distribution.

  - Reciprocal innervation—interplay.
  - Patterns of movement.

The therapist's hands form part of the patient's base of support. If the patient is sitting, the therapist may adapt her hands to the patient's musculature in the hip/pelvic area. By using her hands, the therapist may gently move the patient in different directions: sideways, forward, and backward, and introduce rotatory components and assess the patient's ability to align his or her body in response to changes in the support base (the hands) and movement of body segments in relation to each other. The therapist observes, listens to the response, evaluates, and forms hypotheses about the characteristics of the key area and the interplay between key areas.

Touch may be one of the strongest direct influences on the patient, physically and psychologically/emotionally. Therapists therefore have to take great care in how they introduce handling to their patients, and what information they gives to their patients. Patients have to accept handling as well as respond to it for it to be effective. Through their hands and body language therapists must impart empathy, respect, and care. The use of handling is based on clinical reasoning, problem analysis, hypothesis formulation, goals, and which tools to use to help patients achieve their goals.

Many patients suffering from CNS lesions have paresis, weakness, altered or reduced somatosensory input and perception, and reduced coordination and dexterity, and are unable themselves to recruit appropriate activity in good alignment for task achievement. Malalignment may be in relation to the base of support, a body part in relation to other body segments, within a body segment, or between distal and proximal. If the patient is unable to create alignments that promote appropriate muscular activity or activate appropriate muscular strength, handling may be used to facilitate this. Specific mobilization of muscle and other soft tissues combined with enhanced somatosensory input in better alignment may improve the performance of the motor task. Handling is used to give patients information, perception of movement, and specific movement experience to strengthen their body schema, aiming to mimic how they used to move before the lesion, and thereby reawaken the memory of experiences and how they felt. Handling should cause a feeling of something recognizable by the patient and relate to familiar movements, activities, and functions.

Therapeutic handling is dynamic, specific, and varied; it may be mobilizing (musculature, joints), stabilizing, and/or facilitatory. In treatment, *handling* should never be static or stereotyped, and it is not the same as massage or stretching, but it may have elements of both. Occupational therapist Christine Nelson says the following about Berta Bobath, "I observed in her hands all the tissue mobilizing skills that have now become specialties" (Schleichkorn 1992).

Handling may be corrective, supportive, informative, leading, or stimulating, or it may demand movement. The hands are the most mobile parts of the body. The hand depends on inherent mobile stability, and the stable reference areas for movement vary depending on the task. For example, the neuromuscular activity in the thenar eminence and the metacarpal of the thumb; over the wrist and metacarpophalangeal joints as in the lumbrical grip; the hypothenar eminence and the index finger for the precision of the thumb and index in a precision grip; or a combination. The fingers are the mobile parts of the hand, the palm the more postural part. The postural activity and adjustment of the palm allow for variations in the use of the fingers. The therapist needs to explore and exploit these characteristics to invite the patient's neuromuscular system to be more appropriately active. The hands must shape themselves to the contact area and give comfortable, yet stimulating, information.

Handling is achieved not only through the therapist's hands. The therapist may use other body parts in contact with the patient to facilitate stability in one key area and movement in another to promote the relationship between stability and movement, and postural control and movement. The hand may function as a dynamic support and recruit stability in postural sets requiring postural activation. The hands should mimic the function in the area to be facilitated; if the patient has reduced hip stability, handling should impart activity to the abductors and extensors.

> The therapist's hands may touch, create friction, stretch, compress, and give information about muscle length and tension, direction, speed, and range. They may produce traction, compress or rotate, demand stability, and/or mobility depending on the problem and the functional goal. Information is specific to the desired activity.

The aim of using handling as a treatment tool is to recruit neuromuscular activity in a functional context. Clinical experience supports the theory that postural activity and control as well as the control of movement may be improved through handling.

Some patients do not accept handling. Sometimes, due to perceptual problems, they do not understand the information given and cannot relate to it, or they dislike the physical contact and may feel that it invades their personal space. Handling must then be on a minimal level and the patient clearly informed of why—for safety reasons, for instance. If the tone increases or there is tension as a response to what the therapist would deem as appropriate and relevant handling, it works contrary to its aim. This is quite rare, but it needs to be respected. If the therapist is professional, empathetic, explains everything, and is careful, most patients are receptive to handling, both as an assessment and as a treatment tool.

■ Facilitation

In the Bobath Concept the therapist aims to use afferent information to reeducate the individual patient's internal reference system to give the patient the possibility of more optimal movements or a greater movement repertoire. In the Bobath Concept, the use of afferent information to enable more optimal motor activity is described as *facilitation* (Graham et al 2009).

Berta Bobath stated that *facilitation* means "making easy," but in treatment it also means "making possible" and, in fact, making it necessary for a movement to happen (Schleichkorn 1992) (**Table 2.2**). Facilitation is about building the different body representations in the CNS. Facilitation involves, for example, hands-on stimulation to provide sensory information to maintain or update the body schema. The facilitation given is always related to the task; the therapist's aim is to provide the patient with appropriate sensory information normally experienced during the movement.

Table 2.2 The process of facilitation

- Make possible   (realignment, information)
  ↓
- Make necessary   (demands)   ⎫
  ↓   ⎬ (Facilitation)
- Let it happen   (activity)   ⎭

Facilitation means "making easy." The aim of the therapist is to handle the patient in such a way that movement feels easier for the patient because the patient's own activity is recruited. In this context, facilitation must not be interpreted to mean passive movements or passive techniques, such as the use of tapping over muscle or stimulation using ice.

To Make Movement and Activity Possible

To achieve this, the neuromuscular activity and biomechanical relationships have to be as optimal for the actual movement as possible. In this process the therapist works to improve the patient's underlying impairments. This phase of treatment prepares for facilitation, and contains all elements mentioned earlier in this chapter: choice of postural sets, key areas, selective components to functional activity, the relationship between automatic and voluntary activity, and handling.

An individual with a CNS lesion may develop secondary muscular and biomechanical changes that affect range of movement and flexibility, and thereby the patient's ability to balance, transfer, walk, and have functionally active and free limbs. The musculature is plastic and adapts to how it is being used. Many factors, including the following, influence muscle function:

- Tone.
- Positioning.
- Information to the muscle from the CNS and peripheral systems.
- Altered use or nonuse.
- Altered alignment.
- Circulation.
- Connective tissue adaptation (contractures or increased compliance/hypermobility).

"Shortened muscles are recruited more readily than their elongated synergists and as a result are stronger" (Sahrmann 1992). Shortened muscles, either because of viscoelastic properties, inertia, tonus, activation, positioning, contractures, or reduced ability to eccentrically lengthen, seem to be recruited first during activity. Handling seeks to improve these factors.

Many physiotherapists use the terms *inhibition of spasticity/associated reactions/increased tone. Inshibition* refers to neurophysiological processes (see Chapter 1, Inhibition — Regulation of CNS Activity) and should not be used with regard to movement or the control of movement. The aim of treatment is to regain a more

balanced interplay between excitatory and inhibitory processes in the CNS to improve coordination of muscle activation. Inhibition is an active neurophysiological process that requires excitation to release inhibitory neurotransmitters. A hypotonic muscle has decreased ability to eccentrically lengthen. Clinical experience suggests that specific handling of muscle may influence and enhance mobility, flexibility, contraction, and eccentric activity of muscle function. Handling is not classic stretching, whereby a muscle is stretched to its full length, but a treatment aimed at the intrinsic function of the muscle itself combined with facilitation of increased neural activation. Eccentric control is an essential element of this: the patient actively giving length. This form of mobilization is always combined with movement and is called *specific mobilization of muscle.* Treatment is combined with correction of alignment and leads into functional movement.

Clinical Example

Many patients suffering from neurological dysfunction spend a lot of time sitting.

Sitting may cause the thighs to roll into adduction and inward rotation. There may be a danger of developing shortening of adductors, inward rotators, and flexors of the hips (**Fig. 2.29**). Recruitment of abductors and extensors to stabilize the pelvis during transfers, for standing and walking, may therefore become limited. During treatment it may be necessary to mobilize shortened structures to improve alignment and facilitate muscular activity for muscle balance and stability.

As the range of movement, alignment, and muscle length improve, *in the same treatment session*; the transition to the next phase is made.

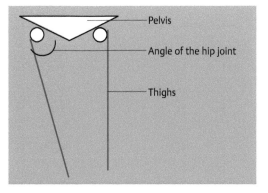

Fig. 2.29 Schematic drawing of the hip in sitting posture.

To Make Movement and Activity Necessary

The treatment moves into the activity phase, which implies that the patient begins activity exercises. The patient may be placed in a postural set that necessitates control of the muscles that have been mobilized, and their activation facilitated. The CNS is challenged into activity. The therapist's hands may facilitate key areas and stimulate activity to get a response. The situation is structured to allow the patient to move and respond without being afraid of falling. The aim is to gradually withdraw as the patient starts to take over, but the therapist may need to repeat input to increase the response to an appropriate level for the activity by facilitating neurophysiological processes of temporal and spatial summation.

When movement is possible, the patient is challenged to explore the possibilities during activity, for instance by being displaced through weight transference while standing to necessitate the initiation of a step. The therapist uses her hands to invite the patient's muscles to be active in sta-

bilizing the hip to free the opposite leg for the swing phase. Muscle function and alignment are facilitated, as well as interplay between key areas. Handling needs to be specific in placing, timing, and transmission of information, to enhance the patient's own activation to make movement easier. Therapeutic handling may involve facilitation of components of stability, mobility, and rotation through compression, traction, touch, or stimulation to move. The therapist's two hands have to give different inputs.

Facilitation is the bridge between assisting and stimulating the patient to recruit activity and his ability to take over and make the activity his own. *Placing* is a response to facilitation; it is the ability to automatically adapt to imposed movement and to support any movement by one's own activity. Placing is the automatic and active control in any phase of the movement, based on a response of an individual to enhanced proprioceptive and somatosensory stimulation (Bobath 1990) (**Fig. 2.30**). Placing may be stimulated through compression, distraction,

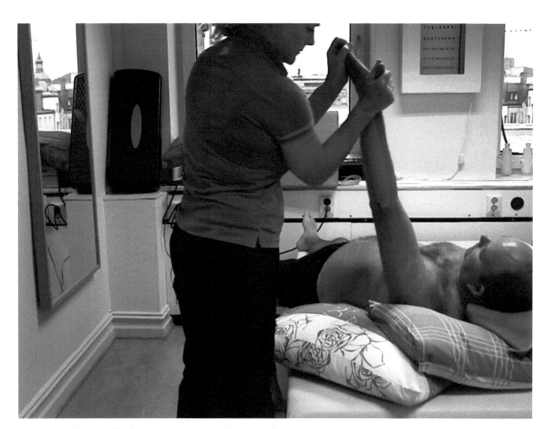

Fig. 2.30 Facilitation of a placing response in supine for reach and grasp activity.

rotation, movement, and touch, and it improves the proprioceptive intuitive knowledge of the position of the limb in the body schema (especially the length of the upper limb). As a result the patient may move more actively. If the therapist asks the patient to hold a limb in space, she asks for a response that is the result of cortical feedforward, that is, a voluntary movement.

Let It Happen

This is when the therapist allows the patient to respond to the challenge through his own activity by, for instance, taking a step. If the patient is unable to move his leg due to inactivity, another therapist may assist or facilitate the distal activity. Important factors are rhythm, tempo, and sequence of activation.

Facilitation has happened when the therapist removes her hands or reduces input significantly (there may still be weakness in the relevant muscles). It is important to recognize the right moment for taking off the hands. This is a very challenging part of the treatment. The aim is *hands-off*, to enable the patient to take over control. The patient has to be able to initiate movement without intervention to regain independence. By using her hands to give intermittent information, for instance intermittent light compression to facilitate stability, the therapist may feel and observe when the patient is ready to take over. There is continuous interplay between *hands-on* and *hands-off* as long as it is needed. When the patient takes over control, the therapist removes her hands or the input that the hands have given. The patient is encouraged to experiment with his regained control; the therapist may give intermittent stimulation as a reminder of where the patient is supposed to control, or to enhance and strengthen the response. Too much hands-on or static use of hands may make the patient passive.

> Treatment requires a continuous interplay between working on impairments and facilitating activity, making movement possible, demanding control, and encouraging action: Make possible → make necessary → let it happen.

The three stages *make possible → make necessary → let it happen* are closely integrated in treatment. The therapist does not wait for—or expect—alignment and muscle function to have normalized before the patient is required to activate and control. As soon as the patient acquires any level of control, the new

possibilities have to be used in a functional context to facilitate the patient's own experience through more appropriate recruitment of motor activity in function.

> The aim of handling is to enable the patient to be more active so that the therapist's hands can be taken away.

The therapist may use several different tools to aid the patient toward regaining control. Among the different tools and environments Berta Bobath used to facilitate patients were large balls. These soon became known as the Bobath balls. Berta Bobath did not like this, and said, "Once a Japanese doctor asked for permission to use the 'Bobath ball' in a publication. It is a beach ball, not a Bobath ball. What makes it Bobath is what you do on it" (Schleichkorn 1992). Later she expressed concern as to how the ball was used. "She still, however, has very valid concerns that people misuse and overuse the ball and associate it too closely with being her therapy, rather than just another tool to achieve specific aims" (Schleichkorn 1992).

Clinical Example Facilitating Stepping

During locomotion there is a constant change of activity during phase changes; the standing leg becomes the swinging leg, the swinging leg becomes the standing leg. The neuromuscular activity especially related to the pelvis, hips, and legs continuously changes from more stability during stance, to letting this activity go to allow swinging of the same leg (**Fig. 2.31**).

In walking forward on even ground, initiation of swing depends on several factors, including the following:

*   Postural control, which depends largely on the stability of the contralateral leg (i.e., the stance phase).
*   Quality of stance prior to the swing on the same side.
*   Speed, propulsion, direction of movement—momentum.
*   Ability to overcome inertia.
*   Ability to eccentrically lengthen the extensors and other muscles involved in creating stance.
*   Trunk stability to counteract the movement of the swinging leg.
*   Selective movement, acceleration, and deceleration.

Gravity and forward momentum assist the swinging leg, and the main neuromuscular activity in the leg during this part of swing phase is normally eccentric.

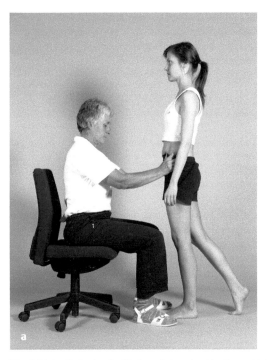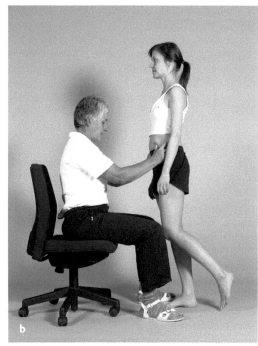

Fig. 2.31 (a–f) During facilitation of stepping the therapist has to ensure that she is not in the patient's way. The movements of the proximal and the central key areas are small and continuously changing and adapting. **(a, b)** Facilitation of the hips and pelvis on a model. The therapist's hands have to mimic the activity of the muscles that normally stabilize the pelvis over the standing leg in this situation. In stance phase, the pelvis moves in relation to the hip joint through extension of the hip. The therapist facilitates stability through light compression of the musculature together with a small input to lift, to gain height, over the standing leg to facilitate the movement of the hip in relation to the pelvis at the moment when weight transference is supposed to happen. The therapist's focus is on the stance leg to enhance stability and postural control to enable the patient to free the swinging leg. The therapist's hands are constantly changing. The swinging leg may be facilitated to eccentrically lengthen hip extensors. At the same time, the patient's center of gravity is slightly displaced in the direction of movement to necessitate the stepping through. (*Continued*)

The leg is not consciously and actively lifted through concentric flexion when walking. The most cognitive part is the initial step and the intention of walking; the steps that follow are more automatic. Bussel et al (1996) studied paraplegic patients attempting to step and walk, and found that the flexor reflex seemingly inhibited central pattern generation. This fits well with clinical experience with patients with other CNS lesions (MS, stroke), where initiation of swing too early or too actively seems to destabilize the standing leg. This could be caused by several factors:

• As many patients with CNS lesions sit for hours every day, their hip flexors may become short, hypersensitive to stretch, or lose the ability to eccentrically lengthen in the last part of stance as a phase transition is about to occur. The early swing would be initiated more as a reflex reaction in this case.

• Patients who have difficulties in walking often seem to be more preoccupied with lifting the leg to initiate swing. This strategy increases the cognitive aspect of walking, as well as reversing the recruitment order. Normally, the CNS is more concerned with sustaining stance than with initiating swing. We have to have a leg to stand on to be able to walk.

Treatment will be very different in these two examples. In the first scenario the therapist needs to mobilize the shortened (stiff and contracted) tissues, to desensitize the flexors, and facilitate the patient's control of eccentric activity, followed by relearning components of locomotion and the locomotor patterning. In the second example the patient has to unlearn lifting the leg too early; to learn to focus on acquiring a good stance on both legs (one at a time) to prepare for swing, and to learn the distal activation

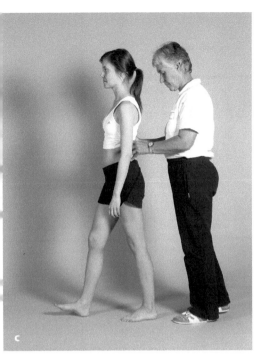
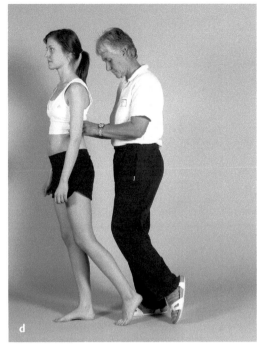

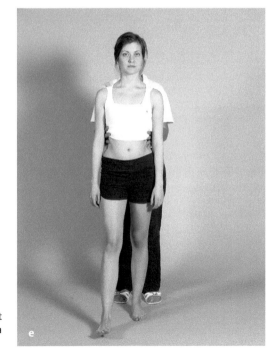

Fig. 2.31 (a–f) (*continued*) **(c, d)** Facilitation of stepping through the central key area. The therapist facilitates extension on the weight-bearing side at the same time as the thorax is stabilized bilaterally to allow the freeing of the swinging leg. The center of gravity is displaced in the direction of movement to facilitate pattern generation. The facilitation needs to mimic the patient's internal rhythm and tempo. **(e)** Facilitating a change of direction via the pelvis and hips. Extension through slight compression into the musculature and a small input to lift and gain height on the standing leg together with some rotation of the swinging side of the pelvis facilitate a change of direction of movement. As soon as the swinging leg has passed the stance leg and is approaching heel-strike, the therapist stops facilitating the stance leg to allow the heel-strike, getting the foot to the floor. The swinging leg is thereby ready to become a standing leg again.

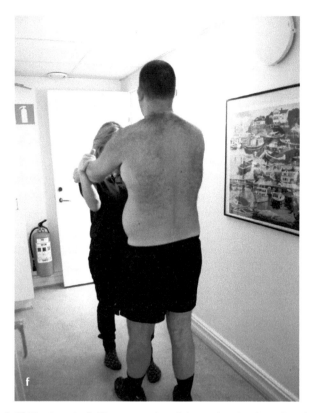

Fig. 2.31 (a–f) (*continued*) **(f)** The therapist facilitates extension of the trunk and reciprocal reach through the upper limb to facilitate rhythmical automatic movements of the legs. Recent research implies that lower and upper limb muscle activations are coupled during human gait (Sylos-Labini et al 2014). A central motor program, which excites motor neurons of leg and arm muscles conjointly during walking, may be generated by a spinal neuronal network. Based on this theory, research has demonstrated that automatic, alternating movements of the legs may be initiated by upper limb movements (Solopova et al 2015; Massaad et al 2014). Therefore, facilitation of leg muscle activity by active arm movements during locomotor tasks may be beneficial during gait rehabilitation.

of the foot: toes-off to lifting the toes to evolve swing, and then be facilitated through his individual rhythm to gain activation of the CPG. Treadmill training at a relatively fast speed may be useful for this patient to take away his increased cognitive regulation.

Experience suggests that it is possible to facilitate stepping even in patients who have severe neurological deficits and little or no volitional control of the most affected side, such as in the early stages after a stroke (**Fig. 2.32**) The facilitation of early stepping is strongly recommended to maintain the memory of walking and CPG activity, to facilitate postural control and the patterns of movement. The patient has to be facilitated through good alignment and with focus on stance initially. Bringing the patient early into a stepping rhythm may facilitate a responsive swinging of the opposite leg,

which provides the foundation for stronger perception and body schema of the most affected side and further volitional control of the leg in different situations. The prerequisites for this to happen seem to include the following:

- Help and facilitation to remain upright to oppose gravity (make possible).
- Mobile feet to allow weight transference onto and through the foot (make possible).
- Optimization of alignment to enhance appropriate muscular activity (make possible).
- Facilitation of selective hip stability on the stance leg immediately prior to destabilization (make possible → make necessary).
- Destabilization of the patient's center of gravity in the direction of movement (make necessary → let it happen).

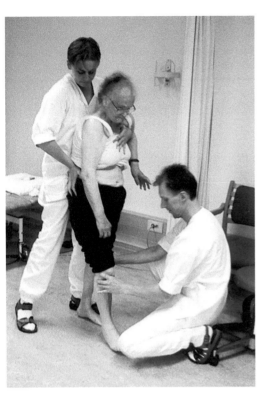

Fig. 2.32 The patient is being helped to achieve postural activation and to stay upright through the therapist's handling of her central and proximal key area. She has at this moment no stability or selectivity of her most affected side, and the assistant facilitates her stance phase first, then the transition to swing. The challenge is to coordinate the timing of the three people for rhythmical activation and phase transitions to facilitate central pattern generator activity.

- Allowing stepping (let it happen).
- Facilitation of rhythmical interchange without cognitive override (let it happen), as close as possible to the patient's own individual rhythm. If the stepping is too slow or too fast, the patient's CPG activity may not be facilitated.

Reduced interplay between the two halves of the body after a stroke generally has a strongly negative influence on postural control and also on the stance activity on the *least* affected side. The patient has problems in weight transferring, and stabilizing and balancing over the least affected side, which seems to influence the acquisition of swing on the most affected side. If stance activity is reduced, the patient may have to weight bear on both sides, and the release of swing may not be possible. Patients need to work on the stance phase on both sides to regain

postural control and stability to acquire CPG activity independently.

Active Movement; Learned Nonuse; Neglect; Passive Movement

"Motor activity is the tool of sensation" (Brodal, personal communication, 1998). Two aspects seem especially important for motor control: the memory of (1) how it felt to perform a specific movement or action and (2) the result. "The task is carried out and modified by adjustments, so that the sensations from the evolving movement match the memory of 'how it felt'" (Brooks 1986). Berta Bobath (1990) also said that, "The hemiplegic patient, just like a normal person, does not learn movements, but the 'sensation' of how the movement felt."

The peripheral nervous system (PNS) is still intact after a lesion to the brain or an SCI. The CNS receives all somatosensory information, which is integrated to a certain degree in the spinal cord, and the spinocerebellar tracts convey information from muscle spindles, tendon organs, and cutaneous mechanoreceptors going directly from the spinal cord to the cerebellum (Brodal 2010). This tract is still able to inform the cerebellum about movements even without conscious perception of sensation. The CNS therefore still "feels," although the patient may have severely reduced perception of sensation. Sensory deficits may be due to lesions to ascending systems, perceptual deficits, or learned nonuse.

Active Movement

Movement generates feedback from the body to the CNS from specific receptors and vision as well as information of the result. Active movement causes a diversity of information within the CNS. The length–tension relationship changes, and receptors in the skin and soft tissues and joints are stimulated to transmit information to the CNS. This information gives us something to feel and therefore perceive. Exploratory behavior, for instance, using the hands to touch our close environment and our own bodies, facilitates the perception of the body in relation to the environment and itself. According to Shumway-Cook and Woollacott (2006), "Perception is essential to action, just as action is essential to perception." These authors define perception as the integration of sensory impressions into psychologically meaningful information. Patients who are unable to move receive little or no information from their own body and are unable to explore their environment through their own body; perception may be disturbed as a result. Improved movement may improve perception, and improved perception may have a positive effect on movement control.

Yekutiel and Guttman (1993) describe a trial in which stroke patients with reduced sensation of the affected hand received a systematic training program more than 2 years poststroke. The patients were treated in their own homes—45 minutes each session, three times a week for 6 weeks. The patients had to identify touch to their own arm, find their affected thumb, discriminate between different objects placed in their affected hand, and draw with help from an assistant (document assisted). Compared with a control group, they showed significant improvement on all sensory tests. Some patients experienced functional improvement even if they were not encouraged to use their hand more in daily activities. This study demonstrates the close relationship between experiencing sensory stimulation, perception of sensation, and motor function.

■ Learned Nonuse

Learned nonuse or disuse is associated with conditions where reduced motor control, for instance of a hand, results in the patient not using his hand. Patients use what they are able to recruit; hence nonuse is a learning phenomenon involving a conditioned suppression of movement (Taub et al 2014). Body parts that function may compensate for loss of sensation or movement in nonfunctioning body parts. Stroke patients quickly learn to compensate by increasing the use of the less affected hand. If the affected hand is not used, it will not be stimulated, few or no impulses are transmitted to the CNS, and the arm is therefore not stimulated and becomes progressively more passive (Taub & Uswatt 2006). Loss of input to the CNS may result in a reduction of cortical representation area: hence the phrase "use it or lose it." This clinical phenomenon is directly linked to the postlesion plasticity that sets in a few hours after stroke (Oujamaa et al 2009). Research on stroke patients has shown area reduction in both the primary sensory cortex (SI) and the primary motor cortex (MI) representing the affected arm (Liepert et al 2000). Simultaneously, the least affected limb is substantially used and the sensory and motor representations for that body part increase in size.

Learned nonuse may also be implicated in a more negative process after neurological damage because it may be a contributing factor to interhemispheric imbalance (Takeuchi & Izumi 2012).

This development predisposes the patient to secondary soft tissue changes and learned nonuse because the arm does not experience stimuli (Ada & Canning 1990). Nudo & Wise et al (1996) state that the absence of rehabilitative training after a lesion may cause progressive area loss in relation to the functional representation of the affected body part. "In addition to the primary motor deficit, mechanisms of sensory inhibition are involved to varying degrees in the stroke patient's nonuse of the affected hand, whether this is due to central neglect or learned nonuse " (Yekutiel & Guttman 1993).

> Active movement provides a diversity of information to the CNS.
> Active movement is essential to perception.

■ Neglect

Neglect is described as inattention to a body part or space and may be defined as "a failure to report, respond, or orient to novel or meaningful stimuli presented to the side contralateral to the brain lesion when this failure cannot be attributed to either sensory or motor defects" (Heilman & Valenstein 2003). This definition does not identify the mechanism of neglect but suggests that this disorder is not solely due to sensory or motor limitations (Bowen et al 2013). Clinically, neglect is very heterogeneous in nature; it can vary in sensory modality (i.e., visual, auditory, or tactile neglect), spatial reference (i.e., egocentric [viewer based] vs. allocentric [object based]), and region of space (i.e., peripersonal [within reaching distance] vs. extrapersonal [beyond reaching distance]) (Nijboer et al 2013). Neglect may be observed in patients with CNS lesions, and most frequently in those with right hemispheric stroke. In the following, therefore, *left* will be used to describe the most affected side. In patients with neglect there seems to be an erroneous processing of multisensory input (Himmelbach & Karnath 2003). Several studies have tested the multisensory nature of neglect and demonstrated a reduction of neglect symptoms by using different sensory stimuli, such as proprioceptive-kinesthetic stimuli (Eskes et al 2003); visual stimuli (Harvey et al 2003), and somatosensory input (Lafosse et al 2003). Robertson & Eglin et al (1993) state that the most important aspect of treatment of *neglect* seems to be the regaining of active movement in the affected extremities in the field of neglect. Several studies on neglect (Lin 1996), sensation (Yekutiel & Guttman 1993), and motor function (Feys et al 1998; Sunderland et al 1992) demonstrate that active movement improves neglect. Sensory stimulation and intensive treatment improve neglect, sensation, and motor function. Increased motor activity and increased awareness are strengthened through positive feedback. It seems as if activation of the left arm in the left part of the room (in the field of neglect) changes lateral awareness and spatial representation (Robertson et al 1998). Experience supports that unilateral focus and stimulation of the left side in treatment of patients suffering from neglect enhance the patient's awareness of the neglect field (i.e., perception). Through specific mobilization and stimulation of muscles and soft tissues, the correction of alignment, stimulation of the hand by contact with the patient's face and body, or objects that she finds interesting, as well as facilitating the patient's postural control, the patient's concentration and perception of the neglected side may be strengthened. Clinically, intensive proprioceptive and tactile stimuli seem to have a positive effect.

Progression during treatment is indicated by increased interaction and interplay between right and left. Bilateral simultaneous activity, such as carrying a tray or using one hand to support the activity of the other (e.g., opening a water bottle, cutting a piece of bread, holding a bunch of grapes while picking one off to eat), may be introduced once the patient is able to shift her focus between left and right with little prompting. If the patient "forgets" her left arm during bilateral activities, the focus has to go back to the left again. The therapist must emphasize that the patient maintains her attention to promote bilateral simultaneous processing of stimuli. Rhythmical interaction between right and left may have a positive effect. Therefore, in some patients, the facilitation of locomotion may promote interaction between the two body halves and thereby perception.

The therapist needs to continuously evaluate the patient's response and change strategy if awareness fails.

> Facilitation of active movement through intense sensory stimuli seems to improve neglect. The patient's awareness increases during active movement.

In a clinical situation it is not possible to test and evaluate the degree and relative presence of somatosensory and perceptual deficits if the patient has severe motor problems as well. Only through treatment that focuses on sensation (feeling contrasts in different objects), perception, and facilitation of movement as well as observation of the patient in different situations over some time, is it possible to formulate a more accurate hypothesis.

■ **Passive Movement**

If the patient is unable to initiate any activity, it is important to give the patient the sensation and experience of movement through being moved, thereby to accomplish the following:
- Avoid the development of nonuse.
- Create awareness to the body part—stimulating a body part by moving it does cause some transmission of impulses to the CNS.
- Give to the patient a feeling of movement and interplay.
- Maintain motion, range, and circulation.
- Enhance motor learning.

Several studies have examined brain activity following passive movement of the upper limb (Lindberg et al 2004; Macé et al 2008). These studies have shown activity in regions such as the contralateral sensorimotor cortex, the premotor cortex, supplementary motor areas, and the inferior parietal cortex (Loubinoux et al 2003; Tombari et al 2004). Thus sensory stimulation by passive movements may even benefit motor learning. Wong and colleagues (2012) demonstrated that passive movement of the arm increases the extent of motor learning.

The therapist aims to facilitate and stimulate activity even if the body part has to be moved passively. The rationale behind using passive movements is to deliver a pattern of sensory input contextualized to that task to maintain or increase sensory representations in the brain, by which the motor system is facilitated in reestablishing a normative pattern of motor output. If the patient's attention to the movement or to the feeling of the movement does not improve spontaneously during treatment, the patient may be encouraged to create a mental image of the movement, or how the movement or activity was solved or used to feel. Mental imagery is the mental practice of motor tasks (Ietswaart et al 2011). Mental imaging in neurological rehabilitation activates brain motor areas and is thought to intensify brain plasticity. Mental imagery may strengthen or maintain connections in the CNS by activating the same regions of the brain that are activated when movements are actually performed (Decety 1996). However, a study done by Dijkerman and colleagues (2004) where the subjects were mentally reinforcing different physical tasks, demonstrated that mental practice gave improvement on the trained task only. Hence mental practice may reactivate only recently used motor representations and thus allow for an increased and sustained effect of physical practice. This has implications for clinical use; mental practice may be effective only in consolidating movement patterns that the patients have practiced physically.

In a comatose patient, verbal information may strengthen the input, although most information needs to be transmitted through the proprioceptive and tactile systems. The PNS and the spinal cord are intact in patients with CNS lesions. Handling aims to make the patient's CNS listen and respond as far as possible and is therefore not really passive. Passive movement is important also for circulation, muscle length, and range of movement, which may allow development of the patient's own activity.

> Passive movement is important if patients are unable to initiate movement of their own.
> Passive movement seeks to stimulate activity and requires the patient's attention.
> Handling through passive movement aims to make the patient's CNS listen to the input and respond as far as possible, and is therefore not really passive.

Clinical Example

A patient once said to me that *movement is the expression of the soul.* She had amyotrophic lateral sclerosis and was completely paralyzed. When a patient is unable to move by herself, her perception of her own body changes and diminishes. Patients who have a swollen, stiff, and inactive hand have a reduced feeling of contrasts in sensory input. The information they do receive about their hand is of an inactive weight, sometimes combined with pain. Some feel numbness, whereas others are unable to feel the hand at all, even if they are able to respond positively to classic sensory testing. The therapist needs to re-create the feeling of mobility and movement, to move the hand as it would have been moved when active. Specific mobilization of muscles and joints, tactile stimulation, shaping of the hand to the patient's own body parts and different objects

may enhance the perception of the hand as a part of the body. This way some of the prerequisites for more active movement are achieved.

▮ Control of Associated Reactions

Associated reactions and associated movements were discussed in Chapter 1.4, Consequences of and Reorganization after CNS Lesions. Associated reactions are well-known phenomena in CNS pathology. They are viewed as a result of an activity-dependent process of learning whereby the CNS makes new connections and strengthens or weakens connections depending on their use. The interplay between individuals and their environment informs behavior and CNS processes and function. Associated reactions may develop as a response to impaired stability or movement or to hypersensitivity to stimuli. In activities or situations demanding stability that the patient is not able to recruit, he may develop associated reactions as a pathological fixation (Lynch-Ellerington 2000). In our practical experience patients showing associated reactions always have a hidden weakness as their initial main problem. Over time, there is often a causal combination. Assessment and clinical reasoning allow the therapist to formulate hypotheses for both the main problem and the trigger for associated reactions. Therapy aims to treat the patient's main problem(s)—the negative signs—and should not focus primarily on the associated reactions. A one-sided intervention aimed toward the so-called positive signs will not improve the patient's underlying movement problem, and therefore not facilitate the patient's regaining function. If the main problems are targeted, and the patient's motor control improves, the associated reactions may gradually diminish by themselves because they are no longer required or triggered. Sometimes associated reactions may be so disturbing or destabilizing that the main problem is not accessible, and they need to be treated more directly. In these situations the associated reactions need to be changed or influenced to change, to access the patient's primary movement problem of, for instance, instability.

> It is essential to analyze and treat the cause of the associated reactions and not just attempt to dampen down the reactions.

■ The Role of the Therapist

The therapist should accomplish the following:
- Form hypotheses of the causal relationship between the patient's main problem (weakness, instability, perception, and others) and the presence of associated reactions through observation and handling.
- Choose a relevant and appropriate task for goal achievement.
- Recognize which movement components are missing, then make it possible to achieve the goal through as optimal control as possible (note the importance of input, alignment, and muscle function).
- Create an environment that is conducive to the patient's control.
- Enable the patient to control his own associated reactions and deviant motor behavior by finding the right level of challenge.
- Handle the patient to correct alignment and facilitate muscle activity to make the control of movement possible and necessary.
- Inform the patient by increasing his awareness and knowledge of himself in relation to possible causal relationships and the consequences of destabilizing associated reactions.

■ The Role of the Patient

The patient should achieve the following:
- If possible, prevent associated reactions by learning to control their triggers through focused attention. The patient needs to become aware that they are present and why. The patient's own control over her associated reactions is the first step in acquiring a wider movement repertoire and more selective movement control.
- Use the hand as a CHOR hand in functional activities like sit to stand and standing (see examples in Chapter 4).

Some patients move relatively efficiently with mild associated reactions. Clinically, these reactions seem totally automated and stable and may be an expression of an established and relatively appropriate behavior modification (sensorimotor). They may be a nuisance to the patient, or they may be embarrassing. To minimize them, the patient will have to be very motivated and focused during treatment, and even more so when she moves about by herself. During a learning phase the patient will have to slow down and become more aware of how she moves, which requires a reduction in tempo and efficiency. The therapist has to assess whether there is a potential for change and if this change would enhance the patient's efficiency.

■ Feedback

During training of healthy persons, feedback is used to detect errors in performance by comparing the actual movement to the expected goal, to improve the next attempt and thus facilitate motor learning (van Vliet & Wulf 2006). Intrinsic feedback may help to create an internal representation of the movement goal (van Vliet & Wulf 2006).

Feedback may give patient's information of and about their movement and may take many different forms:
- *Intrinsic feedback* is the information the patient receives through his own systems as a result of moving, vision, and somatosensory impulses:
  - Through the experience of movement and level of control.
  - Through one's own feeling and observation of the level of success—was the goal reached, or not?
  - Through handling from the therapist. This is both intrinsic and extrinsic because handling in itself is imposing movement and information to the patient from the outside at the same time that response and adaptation to the handling transmit intrinsic feedback to the patient.
- *Extrinsic feedback* is a supplement to intrinsic feedback. It is verbal and visual (e.g., the expression and body language of the therapist) and has different aims:
  - Motivating and encouraging.
  - Knowledge about the process of movement, that is, about the performance itself (KP).
  - Knowledge about the result (KR) of the movement.

There is no consensus on type and timing of feedback, and several authors have debated this (Shumway-Cook & Woollacott 2006; Ronsse et al 2011; Luft 2014; Taylor et al 2014; Shmuelof et al 2012). Most studies have been performed on healthy individuals; it is therefore difficult to extrapolate the findings to clinical settings and patients with neurological dysfunction (van Vliet & Wulf 2006).

■ Intrinsic Feedback

Individuals suffering from CNS lesions have different physical and neuropsychological deficits. Altered movement and perception of somatosensory information influence the patient's intrinsic feedback. After stroke, intrinsic feedback systems may be compromised (van Vliet & Wulf 2006). There may be deficits in ascending systems, altered muscle tone, altered sequence of recruitment and sensorimotor organization, altered alignment, or perceptual problems. Perceptual and cognitive problems affect the patient's planning, feeling of movement, and movement experience. Their ability to integrate feedback and use this constructively to find appropriate and optimal solutions for motor problems will therefore also be affected. In many cases patients themselves are able to evaluate how successful the movement was and may not need verbal reinforcement. The feeling that the patient gets when he feels that "this was right," or "this is what it used to feel like," may be more compelling than any verbal information.

Therapeutic handling provides the patient with feedback through touch and facilitation to move. Specific mobilization of musculature and correction of alignment allow the patient a better starting point for motor control. Through therapeutic handling the patient receives normalized information of the interrelationship between body segments and between the body and the environment. This may provide the patient with a better basis for successful goal achievement, which both reminds him of what it used to feel like and uses memory to strengthen the patient's own performance.

■ Extrinsic Feedback

The therapist frequently uses a combination of intrinsic and extrinsic feedback. The type of feedback depends on the patient's problems, motivation, and cognitive ability. KP and KR (Schmidt 1991; Shumway-Cook & Woollacott 2006) require the patient both to perceive and to integrate information and develop new strategies based on the feedback. Many patients do not have this ability because of perceptual or cognitive problems and cannot use KP or KR. Verbal feedback assumes that the patient is able to perform the activity differently through verbal information or commands. Many patients with a neurological deficit do not have sufficient or appropriate motor function to alter or adjust their movement and are unable to change strategies. Internal feedback provides the CNS with information that is different from before and therefore gives a different basis for movement production compared with before. Their ability to recruit movement is changed; their ability to solve motor problems will be difficult if their previous movement experience is very different from their movement ability now or if their body schema or perception is altered. Long or too detailed explanations are often confusing for patients and may hamper their ability to feel the activity.

Through extrinsic feedback, movement planning and production may be lifted to a level of cognitive attention that should not normally be there for the activity. Motivating feedback through words or sentences that are short and to the point may be more appropriate: yes, stop, no, good, excellent, or similar expressions may be enough to strengthen the patient's perception or provide the needed feedback. Positive feedback is motivating and must be objective and honest. KP is provided about the actual performance, the process of movement. Patients with sensory or perceptual dysfunction may find KP useful if they are able to understand and integrate the information for problem solving. This requires that the patient has few or no cognitive problems. KR is knowledge of the end result of the movement. Many patients are able to evaluate their own achievements; they observe or feel the result of their own actions and do not need verbal reinforcement. Some neuropsychological deficits may disrupt the patient's ability to analyze or understand the level of achievement; and such patients will need information about the results.

> The feedback varies and depends on the patient's movement ability, his perceptual or cognitive function, and the type of goal activity (more automatic or more voluntary).

■ Carryover

Transfer of task and *carryover* are terms used for the effect of training to be carried into practical situations and tasks at home or on the ward. In the literature effective learning is related to *context*; that the activity is goal oriented and used in different situations in the patient's daily life. Schmidt (1991) discusses the importance of varied training; the ability to perform the same skill in different contexts or situations. Carryover may be analyzed on different levels:

- *Generalization:* transfer of movement components to different movements and functional activities.
- *Performance:* the ability to maintain improved control from the beginning to the end of a treatment session.
- *Learning or retention:* the maintenance of improved control between treatment sessions.
- *Transfer or carryover:* from treatment to ADLs at home or in the ward.

■ Generalization

Movement is organized in relation to the individual, the task, and the environment (Shumway-Cook & Woollacott 2006). Action is organized in time and space to suit the task in the environment. Therefore, training needs to focus on variation, that is, varying the components of movement in different contexts, environments, and requirements for control through the evolvement of movement to ensure carryover.

Training may be practiced through *drill* or *varied repetition*. *Drill* is when the same component, movement, or activity is repeated many times in the same way.

Example ━━━━━━━━━━━━

The patient may practice standing up repeatedly in the same way from the same chair. Although a person never performs the same activity in exactly the same way, there is very little variation in the combination of different movement components. If the person has very little problem-solving capacity, and therefore a reduced ability to carry over, drill may be necessary. One patient suffered a severe stroke, which caused complete expressive and receptive problems, severe apraxia, memory and problem-solving deficits, as well as severe motor problems. He was able to stand up from sitting in his wheelchair and to walk with personal assistance after several months of training. He was not able to transfer this ability to standing up from his toilet at home and had to be drilled in his own bathroom to succeed. Too much variation, even within the same task, may be too complex for some patients. Generalization is not possible through drilling. The patient improves his performance only in what he practices on, in the context he practices in.

Varied repetition is when the movement, postural set, and activity are varied with regard to the neuromuscular component trained.

Example ━━━━━━━━━━━━

Hip stability may be trained in supine, in different ways in supine using equipment, and in different supine postural sets; through the activity of sitting to standing combining different alignments, different supports, and different heights; in standing, step standing, single-leg standing; in stepping down from a high seat; in different transfers and ADLs; and during personal care. The focus is on facilitating hip stability, but the contexts are varied to create a wide repertoire of movement experiences, which may strengthen the patient's ability to carry over. Through variation, the internal model of the activity or component may be learned, thereby strengthening the transfer between tasks (see Chapter 1, Body Schema and Internal Models).

Varied repetition in treatment allows the patient to develop a wide repertoire of movement and movement experience, which she may use in different functional contexts.

■ Performance: Transfer of Control from the Beginning to the End of a Treatment Session

Treatment is goal oriented toward improvement of the patient's control of movement. The therapist evaluates her clinical reasoning and treatment in the same session. If the patient shows improvement in a component or activity level from the beginning to the end of the session, that is, improvement in performance, he has achieved this level of carryover. If carryover has not occurred, the therapist has to reevaluate her clinical reasoning, her hypotheses, and the intervention.

■ Learning or Retention: Maintaining Improved Control between Treatment Sessions

If the patient's movement control remains the same from one treatment session to the next, he has not retained what he learned. The therapist has to consider the following aspects:

- Her clinical reasoning and choice of intervention.
- Has the patient been allowed and encouraged to practice enough? A certain level of repetition is necessary.
- Whether the patient is being met with conflicting demands: is he doing one thing in treatment while his daily life requires something different?
- Whether health professionals and carers emphasize conflicting components.
- Whether the patient is compliant; is he able to understand and integrate information and follow advice?

Berta Bobath is reported to have stated the following:

- If the patient is unchanged, change the treatment. It has had no effect.
- If the patient is worse, change the treatment. It may be inappropriate.
- If the patient has improved, change the treatment. The patient is no longer the same.

The change needs to be appropriate and not just for the sake of change.

> Patients should always feel that specific treatment leads to functional improvement within the same treatment session. They should not feel that the training does not meet their needs.

■ Transfer or Carryover from Treatment to ADLs at Home or in the Ward

As Berta Bobath said in 1988 (Schleichkorn 1992): "Our treatment does not consist of a number of exercises. We are preparing the child for daily life and this in functional situations. For instance, we treat him while he is being fed or when he feeds himself, while he dresses or undresses himself, or is being dressed or undressed. We treat the child while he plays, while he stands or walks, and so on. This is necessary to obtain direct carryover of the treatment into daily life." The same principles apply to adult rehabilitation.

In our society it is a reality that most people suffering an acute CNS lesion are admitted to the hospital. Many will be transferred to rehabilitation wards or centers after a short time. This environment is dramatically different from the home situation in terms of layout, furniture, objects, size, and people whom the patient may have to share rooms with. If variation and generalization are attended to, it may be possible to achieve carryover to the patient's own home. It is a challenge to use the available facilities for the benefit of the patient: training in a gym, on a ward, in the patient's room on the ward, on the stairs, and other environments inside and outside. Some patients may be motivated by staying in an institution for some time, because they meet other people in a similar situation to their own, and they may motivate, advise, and help each other. Treatment aims at improving the patient's control of movement in functional activities, such as during dressing and undressing, transfers, walking, and using the arms, as well as directly improving missing components. Variation is ensured during the following:

- Use of different supports: chairs, plinths, stools, mats, walls, objects, tables.
- Exploration of movement through different postural sets.
- Different activities and different environments inside and outside.

As well as specific therapy, the training needs to be made clear to helpers and carers with whom the patient interacts throughout the day. Multidisciplinary communication and cooperation between different health professionals is therefore necessary.

It takes time to learn, to change synaptic connections, to reorganize established and damaged systems, to learn new and to unlearn inappropriate things. Clinically, significant changes may be achieved in treatment (functional plasticity), but these are not always transferred into the patient's daily activities (structural plasticity). If this happens repeatedly, the therapist has to reevaluate her analysis and approach. Treatment should have reached a certain level of intensity and performed for a certain time before it is possible to state that treatment is not working. In the acute stage following a stroke, new functions are learned very quickly, more so than at later stages due to the increase in neurotrophic factors (see Chapter 1, Neuroplasticity). If the patient has learned strategies that might have seemed appropriate at the time but not any longer, it may take time to unlearn the strategies to allow the learning of new ones. Neurophysiologically, learning and unlearning involve the same process because they involve synaptic changes—both are learning. An important factor is how much and how often the synapses are stimulated in one specific direction.

> Learning and carryover take time to be established.

2.3   Other Interventions: Some Key Points

■ **Strength Training**

As we grow older, most of us experience the loss of strength. The quadriceps of a 70-year-old person has only 60% of the strength of that of a 20-year-old. This is the same for men and women (Macaluso & De Vito 2004): the process of losing strength is attributed to a quantitative loss of muscle mass (sarcopenia), a selective atrophy of type 2 fibers due to a progressive loss of motor neurons in the spinal cord that causes an initial denervation of fast-twitch fibers. These fibers are reinnervated by type 1 motor units through collateral sprouting. Strength training in elderly people improves their muscle strength and function.

An upper motor neuron lesion causes weakness (see Chapter 1.4.1, Upper Motor Neuron Lesions, Weakness). Many people suffering from a CNS lesion are elderly and may have experienced considerable weakness even before their lesion. Current evidence suggests that, generally after stroke, the negative impairments, weakness, loss of dexterity, and fatigue limit recovery of function more than the positive impairments (Canning et al 2004). In a longitudinal study of 22 patients suffering a first stroke, Canning and colleagues (2004) found that strength and dexterity in total contributed significantly to function throughout, strength made a significant separate contribution to function at all test times, and the combined contribution of strength and dexterity was greater than that of either alone.

Historically, strength was not thought to be relevant in patients with upper motor neuron lesions. According to Bobath (1990), "Weakness of muscle may not be real, but relative to the opposition of spastic antagonists," and "Weakness of muscle may be due to sensory deficit, either tactile or proprioceptive or both." This last statement still holds as one reason for weakness. Berta Bobath strengthened patients by using their own body weight in opposition to gravity; like stepping down, sitting down, and one-legged standing.

Research has demonstrated, however, that weakness is a significant problem in CNS lesions, but the exact mechanisms behind the muscular weakness are not fully understood. Insufficient activation of the motoneurons (MNs) results in weak or absent muscle contractions. With time, the reduced descending signals lead to alterations in motor unit recruitment, firing patterns, muscle fiber type, muscle length, and length–tension relationships and results in disuse atrophy in stroke patients (Garland et al 2009; Garland et al 2014) are probably all significant contributors to the muscular weakness in CNS lesions (Bowden et al 2014).

The musculature contralateral to the brain lesion is often most affected; however, muscles ipsilateral to the brain lesion, the side often referred to as nonparetic, or maybe more correctly as least affected, may also be impaired. Muscle strength ipsilateral to a brain lesion tends to be more impaired proximally than distally (Bohannon & Andrews 1995), and may affect both balance and function because varied degrees of trunk, leg, and arm impairments are observed on the ipsilesional side (Kitsos et al 2013; Suzuki et al 2011; Bae et al 2013). Therefore, the problem of weakness on both sides of the body has to be addressed in treatment.

Many patients may be able to recruit strong muscle activation in total patterns but are unable to recruit muscle activation selectively to enhance functional stability, for instance, in moving from sitting to standing, in stance, and for locomotion. Strength training therefore needs to be selective and in functional patterns. Heel-strike is recognized as being one of the most important signals to the CNS to activate a selective stance phase. Information about unloading, heel-strike, and weight transference is critical for the control of stepping (Maki & McIlroy 1997). Important components of heel-strike are postural control and core stability, selective activation of the proximal hamstrings to bring the heel in contact with the floor, selective extension of the knee, eccentric lengthening of the distal hamstrings and of the posterior compartment of the lower limb, and active dorsiflexion and extension of the toes. As the body moves forward over the ankle, which acts as a pivot, the muscular activation patterns change, but knee and hip extension are maintained throughout stance to varying degrees and with different combinations of muscle coordination. Strength training requires focused attention on the part of the patient and may enhance the patient's awareness and perception of the relevant body area.

> Strength training needs to be selective and functional. Strength training requires focused attention on the part of the patient and may enhance the patient's awareness and perception of the relevant body area.

Clinical Examples

Clinically, some muscles seem specifically important to strengthen:

- Abduction of arm for deltoid and triceps to facilitate separation of trunk and arm: abduction will challenge scapular stability, core stability, and facilitate a functionally free arm movement.
- Triceps as a selective antagonist to biceps for coordination of arm and hand function.
- Thumb abduction for wrist extension.
- Toe extensors for heel-strike.
- Ankle evertors for heel-strike.
- Soleus and gastrocnemius for propulsion in gait.
- Proximal hamstrings and distal quadriceps for the different stages of stance phase.
- Proximal hamstrings that stabilize for the selective extension of the knee in swing, as well as acting with the quadriceps to maintain and evolve extension through stance.
- The gluteus medius is important for generating both forward progression and support, especially during single-limb stance.
- Hip extensors, abductors, and external rotators for hip stability through stance.
- Hip extensors for propulsion in walking.
- Core stability as a basis for strength and selectivity distally.
- The intrinsic foot muscles for "core stability" of the foot for improvement of foot posture; an active foot facilitates the GRF for loading and weight transfer.

In the lower limb, muscle weakness may be seen as caused by the loss of excitation of the CPG due to disruption of excitatory commands to reticular pathways. Approximately 18 million fibers run from the brain to the reticular pathways, which are the biggest pathways in the brain. These provide strength, and they control all CPG activity. A lesion to these pathways causes weakness of CPG activity.

Vestibular augmentation seems to be mostly lacking; therefore to strengthen the lower limb for stance and swing phase the therapist needs to focus on strengthening from the foot upward so that the exercise is based on the context of the vestibular system (Mary Lynch-Ellerington, personal communication, 2005).

▨ Treadmill Training

Treadmill training is used for many different neurological conditions, and it is based on two basic princi-

ples: (1) facilitation of CPG activity and (2) repetition to consolidate new learning. Treadmill training has been extensively researched, especially in stroke and SCI as well as in healthy subjects; the results regarding its efficacy are still debated (Mehrholz et al 2014). In a recently updated Cochrane review (Mehrholz et al 2014) the conclusion was that people with stroke who receive treadmill training with or without body weight support are not more likely to improve their ability to walk independently compared with people after stroke not receiving treadmill training. In other words; body weight support did not increase the chance of walking independently compared with people after stroke receiving other interventions. However, people after stroke who are able to walk at the start of this intervention appear to benefit most, improving walking speed and endurance.

Some essential factors need to be taken into consideration when treadmill training may be indicated for an individual patient, and that treadmill training may be used as an option but not as stand-alone treatment to improve the walking speed and endurance of patients who are able to walk independently.

Aaslund (2008), in her study of 28 healthy people walking on the ground and on a treadmill with and without body weight support, found that gait is significantly influenced when walking on a treadmill using a harness and ~30% body weight support.

- Treadmill alone.
  - Increased cadence.
  - Increased forward tilt of the trunk.
  - Increased vertical acceleration.
  - Increased variability of anteroposterior trunk acceleration.
- Treadmill with harness and body weight support.
  - Restricted the mean acceleration in all directions.
  - Increased variability in trunk acceleration in anteroposterior and vertical directions.
  - Caused stereotypical trunk acceleration in the mediolateral direction.

Aaslund concluded that, based on these results, task-specificity of treadmill therapy is questionable.

Several studies suggest that, to regain the ability for independent walking, a patient needs to be able to rise independently from sitting (Lee et al 1997; Cheng et al 1998), and that getting the heel down to stand up is an essential factor for this function. Heel-strike is also important for facilitating the phase shifts during locomotion.

Clinically, treadmill training seems to be effective for some patients. If patients have used treadmill training in a sports studio before, they seem to adapt more easily after a CNS lesion. Patients who already have an independent walking ability seem to gain improved speed and rhythm over ground, but they need time to get used to the treadmill before finding it useful. However, several studies have demonstrated that body weight–supported treadmill training has not led to better outcomes than a comparable dose of progressive over-ground training for disabled persons with stroke, SCI, MS, PD, or cerebral palsy (Dobkin & Duncan 2012). Some patients who have problems with mild dyssynergic movement patterns seem to normalize their movement patterns as speed increases to a level probably more like their own internal speed (CPG rhythm). However, some patients suffering from severe neglect and low tone do not seem to benefit from the use of body weight–supported treadmill training; some seem to be facilitated into inactivity and use the harness as a swing, but respond more positively to facilitation of walking over ground.

Constraint-Induced Movement Therapy

Constraint-induced movement therapy (CIMT) is an intensive treatment program aimed at overcoming learned nonuse in stroke patients. This treatment approach was first introduced in long-term stroke patients by Taub et al (1999).

Following the research by Nudo et al (1996), it is hypothesized that the neural mechanisms underlying the adaptive changes seen in the patient's cerebral cortex are related to the unmasking of existing but previously inactive connections: "The short time course of 12 days makes the formation of new anatomic connections by means of sprouting as a major mechanism unlikely because clear evidence of axonal growth has not been found until months after a lesion occurred. A more likely mechanism is a reduction in activity of local inhibitory interneurons, thus unmasking pre-existing excitatory connections. An alternate and possibly complementary mechanism would be the enhancement of the synaptic strength of existing synaptic connections" (Liepert et al 2000). Studies on CIMT have shown that deficits in motor function following damage to the CNS can be considerably enhanced, even in the chronic phase many years after the injury. There are strict inclusion criteria for this treatment program. The patients must have the following (Kim et al 2004):

- A certain level of balance that is not dependent on the less affected arm.
- Twenty-degree active wrist extension and at least 10° active extension at the metacarpophalangeal joints of two fingers and the thumb.
- No severe spasticity or pain.
- Good cognition.
- A high level of motivation.

It is worth noting that these criteria make this program relevant to only 4 to 6% of all stroke patients; 95% will not seem to benefit from this treatment. The program itself consists of inactivation of the patient's less affected hand by fitting a specialized glove with a hard plastic plate extending beyond the palm. This prevents the patient from using the hand in any manual dexterity tasks, but at the same time allows the hand to act as a support in two-hand activities. The patient should wear the glove at least 6 hours a day and up to 90% of their waking hours, but for shorter periods if used early after stroke. It may also be used to promote weight transference to the most affected lower limb by the use of an inflatable splint or back splint to the less affected leg. Caution should be exercised if the constraints are used in the early rehabilitation phase. Patients should not be enrolled in this program until at least 1 to 2 weeks poststroke due to the vulnerable penumbral zone surrounding the infarcted area. Training consists of a structured program with coarse, fine motor, and general ADLs for 6 to 7 hours a day as well as using it outside the treatment area. The patients are allowed 10 minutes off every hour, as well as during hygiene activities (going to the bathroom, showering).

This training intensity after a neurological injury is often in sharp contrast to the amount of therapy time given to most patients in a hospital or rehabilitation setting. Comparing conventional therapy time of at the most 1 to 1.5 hours (physiotherapy and occupational therapy together) a day (7.5 hours per week) to CIMT of at least 6 hours per day (30 hours per week) demonstrates the importance of the treatment intensity to enhance the patient's potential because the amount of practice has been put forward as a crucial factor in determining outcomes in physical rehabilitation for stroke survivors (Ada et al 2006). In their meta-analysis of augmented exercise time, Kwakkel (2004) found that increased intensity in the form of more treatment improved outcomes related to ADLs and walking. Although optimal doses of daily repetitions have not been determined from animal models or human studies we *speculate* that required doses to facilitate neural reorganization associated with improved functional recovery are probably much higher than normally provided to the neurological population.

■ Robot Training

Robotically based systems for neurological rehabilitation are technologically based interventions. There is an increasing interest in robotic training for both upper limb (Lum et al 2002; Casadio et al 2009) and gait (Bharadwaj et al 2005), which aims to promote motor performance and function through repetition, rhythm, and facilitation of relevant muscles as well as to enhance or maintain range of motion at relevant joints. A recently updated Cochrane review (Mehrholz & Pohl 2012) concluded that electromechanically assisted gait training combined with physiotherapy may improve recovery of independent walking in people after stroke. Specifically, people in the first 3 months after stroke and those who are not able to walk appear to benefit most from this type of treatment. However, the robotic gait training was not associated with improvements in walking velocity or walking capacity, which implies that patients who already have an ability to walk do not benefit from electromechanical and robotically assisted gait training. The results must be read with caution due to the fact that some of the trials included in this systematic review did include individual ambulant walkers at the beginning of the studies. In addition, there was a difference between the trials with respect to duration and frequency of treatment, and the use of equipment type and added stimulation in some devices, such as functional electrical stimulation (Mehrholz & Pohl 2012).

A robot can never replace the individual approach and the multilevel interactions between the patient and an experienced physical therapist (Poli et al 2013). Thus robotic training is meant to be an adjunctive tool to increase the intensity of training for the neurological population.

■ Multidisciplinary Teamwork

As long as the patient is an inpatient, she probably needs some physical assistance to achieve ADLs. All these activities are relatively complex physically, requiring balance, weight transference, alterations in rotational components, alterations of stability and movement components and areas of references, variations in movement strategies, and problem solving. The most complex activity is supine to sitting; at the same time, this transfer is the one transfer many carers expect the patient to perform independently very early on.

If the patient is to regain control of movement, all personnel should have the same understanding of the treatment plan. This is to ensure that the patient is not given conflicting messages. The cornerstones of teamwork are each professional's general and specific knowledge, expertise, and role. Multidisciplinary teamwork challenges all parties and is difficult to achieve. The individual professionals need to understand and respect each other; be loyal to the patient, to the goals, and to the interventions; strengthen each other's roles; and follow each profession's interventions as closely as possible. At the same time, the different professions have their specific roles that cannot be replaced by others. The patient is exposed to the specific interventions from different professionals and receives the sum of the multidisciplinary teamwork. This is the environment in which the patient learns anew. The rehabilitation process is discussed in Chapter 3.

Example

The *24-hour concept* is multidisciplinary teamwork put into practice and relates specifically to the carrying through of treatment principles in daily activities. The multidisciplinary team agrees on which movement components are most important to facilitate, repeat, and consolidate during different activities in the patient's daily life. The 24-hour concept strengthens the patient's learning process because of the following:

- The activity is varied and repeated during the day and possibly the night (bathroom).
- Repetition is varied.
- The activity aims at a known performance for the patient.
- The activity is adapted to suit the individual's needs and movement problems.
- The effect of carryover increases when treatment interventions are transferred to the everyday context.
- Teamwork requires good multidisciplinary communication, both formally and informally, follow-through, and loyalty toward the patient and goals, as well as a common basic understanding and competency.

It is the responsibility of the involved professionals to ensure the treatment is carried through. Often, this is made easier if they see the patient together in practical situations: the nurse, occupational therapist, and physiotherapist may see the patient together in the morning during personal care, during transfers in and out of bed, and during dressing or at meal times, and agree on a strategy to help the patient improve and regain independence if possible. The use of photos from practical situations may aid this process. Cooperation between the patient, carers, and health professionals needs to be stimulating for learning. Good multidisciplinary teamwork gives motivation and learning to the whole team.

Assistive Devices

Many patients do not recover fully after a lesion to the CNS. The sensorimotor problems may vary from slightly reduced balance and dexterity to severe loss of function causing a need for assistance with all ADLs. It is therefore not possible to put forward general guidelines on the use of compensatory aids. Several aspects need to be evaluated:

* Timing for giving an assistive device.
* Positive and negative aspects of different aids within the same group, such as walking aids and wheelchairs.
* Evaluating how the aid is used in relation to its effect on the patient's function over time and adapting or changing the type of aid as needed as the patient progresses.

Timing

The therapist may need to decide on the use of aids. Important things to consider are whether the aid accomplishes the following:

* Reduces the patient's effort while allowing him to explore his environment.
* Enhances or improves the patient's motor problems over time.

How the patient moves and the degree of associated reactions express his movement ability at that time but do not necessarily reflect the extent of the lesion. The patient's motor problems are a result of the lesion itself; cognitive, perceptual, and sensorimotor deficits; the immediate restitution process; and use-dependent plastic changes in the CNS, together with muscular changes and compensatory motor strategies. The aim is for the patient to compensate as little as possible while being active and participating. The patient's movement abilities change with time; therefore any assistive device needs to be adapted and altered in different phases of recovery. In the early stages after stroke, in some patients suffering from MS, head injury, or incomplete SCI, the use of a wheelchair may be appropriate and necessary to allow patients to explore their environment and be more independent. A walking aid may be appropriate for some patients during different stages and in different situations, but it may be disadvantageous for other patients. The different types of assistive devices are discussed in the next section.

Positive and Negative Aspects of Different Aids within the Same Group

* Wheelchairs.
* Walking aids.
* Orthotics.
* Other.

Wheelchairs

Some patients may need a wheelchair temporarily or for different purposes, such as transport over longer distances or shopping trips, whereas others may need a wheelchair for daily use. There are some important aspects that need to be considered when fitting a wheelchair:

* *Sitting posture and comfort.* The patient needs to be seated in proper alignment to enhance postural activity.
* *Use.* The chair needs to be appropriate for the patient's and the carer's needs.
  - Ease of transfers into and out of the wheelchair for the patient and carers.
  - Temporary, periodical, or constant use.
  - Active or supporting (comfort), or a combination.
  - Environment inside, outside. Terrain?
  - Manual or electric? Does the patient need more than one type of chair, for instance an active manual chair, a chair with standing function, an electric chair for inside or outside use?
  - Carer-driven or self-driven? Some patients are unable to drive their own wheelchair, either due to the extent of motor problems or due to cognitive or perceptual dysfunctions. Generally, the neuropsychological problems of severe neglect, inattention, some apraxias, decreased problem-solving abilities, and uncritical behavior may prevent the use of a self-maneuvered wheelchair. Clinically,

however, some patients with neglect or inattention learned to use the wheelchair independently. Sometimes, the confrontation with the problem seems to cause an intellectual compensation in otherwise cognitively able patients. Therefore, if appropriate, these patients should be allowed to explore independent wheelchair maneuvering in controlled circumstances.

– Transportation generally (in and out of cars and so on).

If the patient is driving the wheelchair manually, it needs to be as light as possible. Depending on the patient's need for stability and his balance ability, the position of the centerline of gravity in relation to the drive shaft is important. The closer the center of gravity of the patient is to the drive shaft, the easier it is to maneuver the wheelchair; however, it is more unstable.

Patients suffering from stroke may need to drive the wheelchair using the less affected arm and leg. Ashburn and Lynch (1988) and Cornall (1991) have pointed out the disadvantages of asymmetric and static use of one side of the body, which may work against recovery and treatment and enhance the development of associated reactions. One-hand-driven wheelchairs may strengthen use-dependent plastic changes toward the patient's less affected side and induce learned nonuse in the more affected body half. Therefore, it is of primary importance to evaluate the patient's use of a wheelchair and what it may do to the patient in the longer term. Therapists should experience themselves the effect of a manually driven wheelchair inside, outside, and up an incline, using one hand and leg, and two arms.

An electric wheelchair may be an appropriate tool in a rehabilitation phase or for permanent use for some patients. The patient is able to participate to a greater degree socially and in different activities, such as going to appointments or to the shop without undue effort or a feeling of being dependent on carers.

Walking Aids

Walking aids may be sticks, crutches, rollators, high walking frames, or other devices. Any walking aid alters the person's relationship with the base of support, increases the base, and changes the line of gravity. Patients need to learn new postural and motor strategies if they have not used a walking aid before. The type, the height, and the way in which it is being used will influence the patient's postural activity. If a walking aid is chosen for the patient, the therapist needs to teach the patient how to use it appropriately.

Treatment should focus on the patient regaining as much independent control as possible. The use of a walking aid may be appropriate to allow the patient to move around safely and be exposed to gravity to enhance postural activity if it is used as a reference more than as a support. Many patients who receive a walking aid early in their rehabilitation as a compensation for balance problems weight bear on the aid and so increase flexor activity in their trunk, pelvis/hips, and arms. Increased flexor activity may hamper development of stability as a basis for balance. Therefore, treatment should aim at improving the patient's postural control and movement, and the patient should not be given a walking aid before this is explored.

Motivation is important to recovery. For some patients the ability to ambulate as soon as possible is a major driving force, even if the balance and movement prerequisites are not sufficiently developed to allow them to walk safely. The challenge is to inform, motivate, and, at the same time, teach patients to improve their postural control and movement patterns, and teach them to use the walking aid as well as possible. The patient needs to experience taking steps through therapeutic facilitation as early as possible. Stepping may enhance balance and rhythm through CPG activation, not allowing the CNS to "forget" walking by increasing cognitive control. Seeing that the aim is to walk again may motivate the patient. The timing of when the patient may walk in the department with or without assistance or supervision is a decision that depends on the patient's safety and motor control as well as on the competency of the carers.

Bilateral Aids

Bilateral aids (sticks, crutches, rollator, Zimmer frame, and high walking frame) may invite the patient to lean or pressure bear on the aid, especially if the aid is too low. A rollator, Zimmer frame, or high walking frame allows little variation and flexibility because rotation is not needed. With severely disturbed stability, as in ataxia, a bilateral walking aid may be appropriate.

One-Handed Aids

One-handed aids (stick or crutch) displace the patient's line of gravity laterally toward the aid depending on how it is being used. Despite the frequent prescription of walking aids to improve patients' mobility and help them maintain balance while performing ADLs living after a lesion in the CNS, few studies have focused on the effects of different walking aids on postural control, weight-bearing patterns, and gait of patients with hemiplegia. However, if the patient is able to use the walking aid more as a reference for balance and movement than a support to weight bear upon, the patient's postural control may in some cases be facilitated (Jeka 1997; Boonsinsukh et al 2009); a light touch cue may be used to improve stability in walking using a walking stick. The contribution of haptic cues from the hand suggests that walking aids may be useful in providing additional spatial orientation information for the control of balance. When the patient is holding the walking aid, the CNS receives augmented somatosensory cues from the hand and arm that may provide information about spatial orientation to improve balance control; therefore the use of a cane in the light touch contact fashion may improve stability (Boonsinsukh et al 2009). However, in a study of early gait rehabilitation following stroke where light touch cues by a stick was used, the researchers found that some patients with subacute stroke could not control the amount of force on the cane to achieve the light touch cue (Boonsinsukh et al 2011); the larger amount of contact force on the cane produced by the patients suggested a greater need for mechanical support during gait; thus the use of light touch cues with a cane is not suitable for all patients. The use of walking aids for ambulation following neurological injury may change the strategies of the legs and arms in balance control (Marigold & Misiaszek 2009). A walking stick may hamper development of the patient's balance control if he leans on it and increases asymmetry. In addition, the involvement of a secondary task, such as holding an object in the hands, may have a negative effect on the upper-limb balance reactions preventing the ability to involve the arms in compensatory balance reactions (Bateni et al 2004). Also, engaging the arms by the use of walking aids may direct the balance strategy toward the arms and away from the legs (Misiaszek & Krauss 2005). For compensatory stepping reactions (change of support strategies), holding on to a walking aid could potentially obstruct lateral movement of the legs and consequently limit the capacity to execute compensatory stepping reactions during lateral loss of balance (Bateni & Maki 2005). When using a walking aid one might have to use additional cognitive resources, which may lead to impaired ability to maintain or recover balance especially in older people (Bateni & Maki 2005).

A high stick may be used to enhance extension and interplay between body segments if it is used as a balance aid without pressure. Sometimes it may be appropriate to use a stick outdoors, during shopping, or in other circumstances when balance is especially challenged, but the patient might not use it in her own home.

Shoes and Orthoses
Studies by Mulder et al (1996) and Geurts et al (1992) demonstrate that orthopedic footwear influences the size of the base of support and sensory feedback.

Shoes
Shoes that support the ankle reduce the proprioceptive feedback from the ankle and lower leg, influence postural control, and may reduce the degree of automatism in balance as demonstrated in a study by Geurts et al (1992), which included patients with neuropathies and amputations; however, some of the results may extend to CNS disorders. Heel-strike is important for transfers and walking. A shoe with a good heel support, a firm sole, and a firm heel may promote feedback about loading and unloading of the heel. This is supported by Hijmans and colleagues (2007), who concluded in their systematic review article that "insoles with tubing or vibrating elements may improve balance, whereas thick or soft soles may deteriorate balance." The effects of these different types of insoles or soles are consistent with theories about somatosensory mechanisms that play a role in control of balance. Furthermore there are results from studies demonstrating that barefoot walking strengthens intrinsic muscles more than training with heavy footwear (Rose et al 2011) and also potentiates reception of sensory inputs (Kavounoudias et al 2001; Shinohara & Gribble 2009).

Ankle/Foot Orthoses
Ankle/foot orthoses are used to stabilize this area during transfers, in standing and walking, and to facilitate the lift off of the foot during the swing phase. The cause of the instability must be assessed and treated. Orthoses that enclose the ankle and lower leg may give distal support to allow patients to explore their postural control. At the same time, external fixation may provoke loss of range of movement, flexibility,

and movement. Pressure on muscles and joints may cause a sensorimotor reorganization, which leads to the development of new strategies for balance and movement. Instability of the foot and ankle is rarely an isolated problem in CNS lesions and needs to be viewed together with alignment, tone distribution, recruitment pattern, and sequence of muscle activation in the body as a whole.

Most orthoses aim to maintain the ankle slightly dorsiflexed. This may cause increased flexion of the hip and knee and alter alignment throughout (**Fig. 2.33a–d**). Hip stability may be negatively influenced by this increased flexor activity, which affects the patient's ability to transfer and walk. A general disadvantage of the use of splints is the immobilization of the foot, which loses its adaptability, flexibility, and varied feedback. The ability to use the foot and ankle as a mobile and stable base for the body may be compromised.

A lower limb support may be indicated in some cases. There are several different types available, and more are being developed. The patient needs to try different types and evaluate them over time. There are different plastic splints for covering the posterior aspect of the lower leg and the sole of the foot (**Fig. 2.33a,b**), toe-off types of different materials, ankle supports of soft materials with Velcro fastenings (mostly used in orthopedics), ankle orthoses that support the ankle medially/laterally (**Fig. 2.33c, d**), and arrangements fastened to the patient's shoe (e.g., a Klenzak splint) with or without a T-strap— there are several orthoses available and more are developed all the time. All of these influence alignment and support the ankle and foot to varying degrees. Only evaluation over time may determine if this influence is positive or negative.

It is important to decide whether a potential splint should be used all the time that patients are on their feet, or whether it should be used for specific situations. The foot has an increased tendency to twist in situations in which balance is perceived to be threatened, such as outdoors, in a throng of people, on uneven ground, in traffic. If the splint is used only at certain times the adaptability of the foot and ankle may be maintained, thereby allowing the patient to experience weight bearing through extension. Patients should stand and move in their bare feet regularly and receive varied input.

Knee Orthoses

Some patients experience hyperextension of the knee, which might be painful and cause destabiliza-

tion. During normal walking, the hip and knee move forward over the foot in the stance phase. The knee is rarely fully extended but is at its peak of extension at midstance and just before toe-off. Reduced mobility of the foot and ankle in dorsiflexion prevents this forward movement of the lower leg and brings the knee into hyperextension as the body continues its forward direction. This may be caused by increased tone in the posterior crural muscles; reduced eccentric control of the gastrocnemius, soleus, and deep posterior muscles of the lower leg, the medial hamstrings group, or hip adductors; as well as malalignment of the rotational components between the different segments of the leg, pelvis, and trunk. If the hip flexes in stance, hyperextension of the knee ensues. Mobility and stability of hip/pelvis and ankle/foot as well as of the trunk are essential for dynamic knee function. Reduced coordination of hip-stabilizing activity and ankle/foot mobility catches the knee in the middle. Therefore, a splint to reduce hyperextension of the knee is rarely necessary if the underlying cause is treated.

Shoulder Orthoses

Shoulder subluxation is a frequent problem after stroke and may be a risk factor for the development of pain and additional functional impairment. Glenohumeral subluxation (GHS) is an increase in the space between the humerus and acromion altering the alignment of the joint that allows the weight of gravity to pull caudally on the flaccid arm. Paci and colleagues (2005) define GHS in hemiplegias as a "non-traumatic, partial or total change of relationship between the scapula and the humerus in all directions and in all planes, as compared with the non-affected shoulder, that appeared after stroke." GHS can cause shoulder pain and should always be treated early after stroke onset. There are several factors contributing to GHS. The position of the scapulae on the trunk affects the length–tension relationship in the muscles working as force-couples to stabilize the scapular–thoracic and glenohumeral joints. After stroke, reduced trunk activity with poor trunk alignment influences the position of the scapulae. In addition, the muscles stabilizing the scapula may be weak or of low tone, causing altered scapulae alignment on the thorax. Without normal tone, the rotator cuff can no longer maintain the integrity of the glenohumeral joint. Factors contributing to development of pain in GHS include inappropriate positioning of the upper limb in supine and sitting,

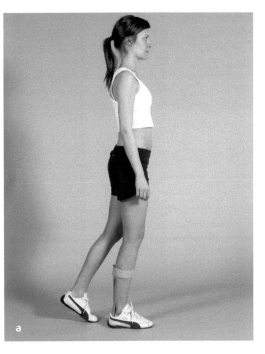

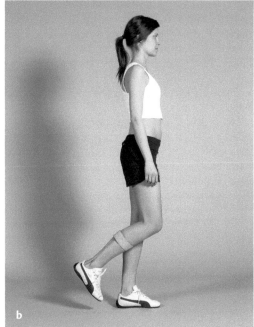

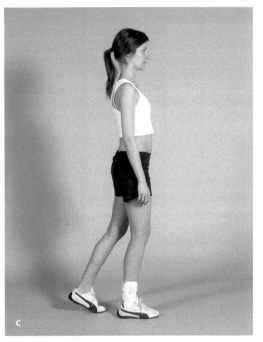

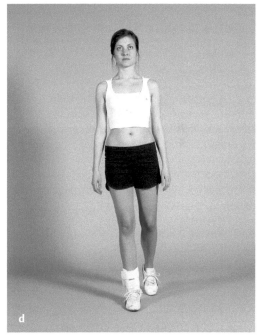

Fig. 2.33 Two different orthoses. **(a, b)** The model is wearing a splint of polypropylene. Notice the change of alignment in the two pictures; in **(b)** she is more flexor dominant and her left hip seems to be more inactive as compared with **(a)**. **(c, d)** The model with a different type of splint, called an air cast. This stabilizes the ankle mediolaterally without compromising dorsal and plantar flexion. It takes up a lot of room in the shoe and is not good for continuous use, but may allow facilitation of postural activity in better alignment when standing early after a central nervous system lesion.

lack of support of upper limbs and the trunk in the upright position, as well as pulling on the hemiplegic arm during patient transfers. The use of arm slings is controversial but has been shown to reduce subluxation in some cases. There are many different types that influence alignment to varying degrees. Some of the disadvantages are that some of these maintain the arm in a fixed flexed pattern and hamper movements at the shoulder, and patients need help by qualified staff to put them on. A Cochrane meta-analysis (Ada et al 2005) concluded that there is insufficient evidence of the effect of orthosis and slings in preventing subluxation and pain, and that there was a potential for restricting shoulder range of movement. Also, discomfort and unpleasant odor discouraged many patients from using the orthoses and slings. Most slings give proximal supports, and some patients feel that their balance improves during the use of an arm sling and that the arm is supported in a position of less pain. Yavuzer and Ergin (2002) studied the effect of a single-strap sling on postural control and gait parameters in 31 patients and found that this type of sling improved gait as measured by three-dimensional gait analysis and video recordings (**Fig. 2.34a–c**).

Patients who are unable to take care of their arm due to neglect, inattention, or cognitive deficits, and who have a severe subluxation of the shoulder or are starting to experience pain, may benefit from using a shoulder orthosis. There are many different types that need to be tried in conjunction with patients and their carers to ensure proper use. Few of these seem to be very accurate in reducing subluxation because subluxation of the shoulder joint is caused by a combination of different factors: reduced postural control, reduced stability of the shoulder girdle complex, altered alignment of the scapula to the thorax, as well as paresis. The orthosis may, however, protect against trauma caused by the arm falling heavily by the patient's side, and thus signal to carers that handling of the shoulder and arm must be performed with care.

Electrical Stimulation

Using electrical stimulation to produce movement is not new. In 1790, Luigi Galvani (Cambridge 1977) applied electrical wires to leg muscles of the frog and was the first to observe the effect of electrical stimulation on muscles. Electrostimulation has been used as a tool in neurorehabilitation to improve voluntary movement control, functional motor ability, and ADLs.

Functional Electrical Stimulation (FES)

FES is the process of combining electrical stimulation with a functional task, such as walking, cycling, or grasping objects for several rehabilitative purposes and across differing diagnoses (Doucet et al 2012). Foot drop stimulators (FDSs) are a special class of FES devices that specifically deal with the challenge of foot drop during walking. The most usual way to apply FDS is through small portable units that attach to the upper calf. Most FDS stimulates the common peroneal nerve, which causes contraction of the muscles responsible for dorsiflexion (e.g., tibialis anterior, extensor hallucis longus, etc.) to assist with ambulation skills (Thrasher & Popovic 2008).

A meta-analysis examining the effectiveness of FES demonstrated a statistically significant improvement in gait speed. However, studies have not yet shown an improvement in overall functional ability with FES treatment (Robbins et al 2006). Although electrical stimulation has the capacity to produce movement, it has been demonstrated to be less efficient than normal human movement and compromises the natural rate of fatigue resistance in the muscles because the Henneman's size principle is reversed (where smaller motor units are recruited before larger motor units during voluntary contractions) (Doucet et al 2012). In addition, FES typically activates only one or two muscles groups and often demonstrates limitation in range of movement due to the fact that a full range of movement involves a coordinated activation of several muscle groups.

Other Aids

Aids that aim to help with daily activities at home or at work need to be evaluated on an individual basis. A home visit or workplace visit together with the patient and her carers may expose problem areas where assistive devices may be of help (e.g., specially fitted work chairs, kitchen appliances). The physiotherapist and occupational therapist may work well together to ensure that the patient's functional needs are met and balance and movement are optimized.

■ Evaluation and Adaptation

All aids should be evaluated with regard to how they are used and their positive and negative effects on the patient's function, postural control, and movement. They will need to be modified as the patient's condition changes over time, either through improve-

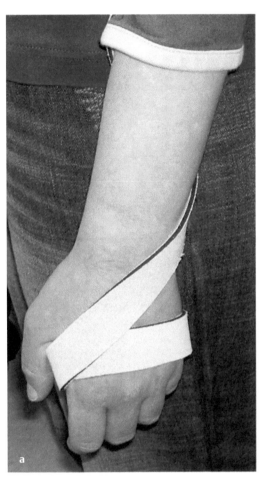

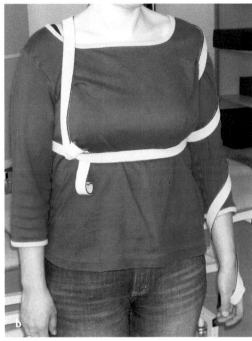

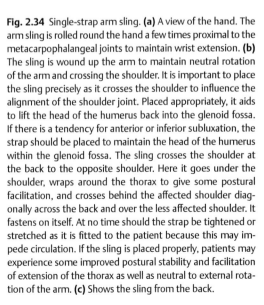

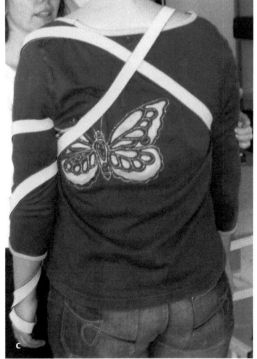

Fig. 2.34 Single-strap arm sling. (a) A view of the hand. The arm sling is rolled round the hand a few times proximal to the metacarpophalangeal joints to maintain wrist extension. (b) The sling is wound up the arm to maintain neutral rotation of the arm and crossing the shoulder. It is important to place the sling precisely as it crosses the shoulder to influence the alignment of the shoulder joint. Placed appropriately, it aids to lift the head of the humerus back into the glenoid fossa. If there is a tendency for anterior or inferior subluxation, the strap should be placed to maintain the head of the humerus within the glenoid fossa. The sling crosses the shoulder at the back to the opposite shoulder. Here it goes under the shoulder, wraps around the thorax to give some postural facilitation, and crosses behind the affected shoulder diagonally across the back and over the less affected shoulder. It fastens on itself. At no time should the strap be tightened or stretched as it is fitted to the patient because this may impede circulation. If the sling is placed properly, patients may experience some improved postural stability and facilitation of extension of the thorax as well as neutral to external rotation of the arm. (c) Shows the sling from the back.

ment in function or through some deterioration. The patient needs to be followed up as long as needed to assess, adapt, and evaluate the type of aid used and to determine whether the patient is benefiting from its use or if the type of aid needs to be changed.

Summary

Human movement is varied, without inappropriate effort, efficient, effective, precise, and successful, developed through the interaction between the person, the task, and the environment. See page 91.

Muscle synergies may be a mechanism by which the nervous system activates repetitive and correlated multijoint coordination. See page 92.

Voluntary movements are exposed to two antagonistic constraints: (1) to move the focal segment(s) toward a goal, and (2) to stabilize the "postural" segment(s) to maintain balance. See page 91.

The ability to maintain balance is described as "the acts of maintaining, achieving or restoring the body repetitive of mass (COM) relative to the base of support (BoS)." See page 91.

Postural control and anticipatory and protective reactions are elements of balance. See page 93.

The postural control system includes all sensorimotor and musculoskeletal components involved in maintaining balance. See page 92.

The control of posture can be divided into two different but interacting systems: the anticipatory or feedforward system where postural corrections are made prior to movement, and the feedback or reactive system where corrections are made in response to perturbations. See page 93.

Several modalities of sensory information are available for the CNS for postural control. See page 98.

Human postural control has to be adaptable and stable under many different conditions, which require a process of reweighting of multisensory stimuli . See page 97.

The recovery of trunk control thus seems to be a prerequisite for more complex functional abilities. See page 101.

In a functional context, the sensorimotor and perceptual interaction between the body and the base of support is more important for the level of postural tone than the size of the base of support. See page 103.

Mobility is essential for stability, as is stability for movement. See page 104.

Inappropriate compensatory strategies—alternative behavioral strategies—may delay or hinder the development of balance and selective motor control in patients with CNS lesions. See page 108.

Standing seems to improve both trunk positional sense and overall function. See page 109.

The Bobath Concept is a problem-solving approach to the assessment and treatment of individuals with disturbances of function, movement, and postural control due to a lesion of the CNS. See page 116.

Postural sets describe the interrelationship between body segments at a given moment. See page 116.

Movement may be described as continuous change of postural sets. See page 116.

A selective movement in one postural set requires a different neuromuscular activity in a different postural set. As the biomechanical alignment changes, so does the neuromuscular activity. See page 117.

Many muscles and joints converge at the key areas. Therefore the proprioceptive influence—as well as information from the skin—on the CNS is substantial. See page 139.

Control of key areas and the interplay between them seem especially important for balance, selectivity of movement, adaptation to the environment and tasks, and therefore for function. See page 139.

Everyday activities, such as balancing, walking, reaching, and eating, are mostly automatic functions that normally require little attention and effort. See page 144.

Everyday activities have a structural correlation in the CNS, based on experience. See page 144.

The expression of activity varies depending on the individual, the goal, and the situation. See page 144.

Automatic and voluntary controls of movement are closely integrated and form the basis for functional skills and balance. See page 144.

The clinical challenge is to decide whether balance can be regained through conscious voluntary planning or be facilitated on a more automatic level in functional situations. Tone, muscle dynamics, alignment, and sequence of recruitment must be optimized in both scenarios. See page 146.

The therapist's hands may touch, create friction, stretch, compress, approximate, and give information about muscle length and tension, direction, speed, and range. They may produce traction, compress or rotate, demand stability and/or mobility, depending on the problem and the functional goal. Information is specific to the desired activity. See page 148.

Facilitation means "making easy." The aim of the therapist is to handle the patient in such a way that movement feels easier for the patient because the patient's own activity is recruited. In this context, facilitation must not be interpreted to mean passive movements or passive techniques, such as the use of tapping over muscle or stimulation using ice. See page 149.

Treatment requires a continuous interplay between working on impairments and facilitating activity, making movement possible, demanding control, and encouraging action: Make possible → make necessary→ let it happen. See page 151.

The aim of handling is to enable the patient to be more active so that the therapist's hands can be taken away. See page 151.

Active movement provides a diversity of information to the CNS. See page 156.

Active movement is essential to perception. See page 156.

Facilitation of active movement through intense sensory stimuli seems to improve neglect. The patient's awareness increases during active movement. See page 157.

Passive movement is important if patients are unable to initiate movement of their own. See page 158.

Passive movement seeks to stimulate activity and requires the patient's attention. See page 158.

Handling through passive movement aims to make the patient's CNS listen to the input and respond as far as possible, and is therefore not really passive. See page 158.

It is essential to analyze and treat the cause of the associated reactions and not only attempt to dampen down such reactions. See page 158.

The feedback varies and depends on the patient's movement ability and perceptual or cognitive function, and the type of goal activity (more automatic or more voluntary). See page 160.

Varied repetition in treatment allows the patient to develop a wide repertoire of movement and movement experience that may be useful in different functional contexts. See page 161.

Patients should always feel that specific treatment leads to functional improvement within the same treatment session. Patients should not feel that the training does not meet their needs. See page 162.

Learning and carryover take time to be established. See page 162.

Strength training needs to be selective and functional. See page 163.

Strength training requires focused attention on the part of the patient and may enhance the patient's awareness and perception of the body part. See page 163.

3 Assessment

Introduction

In different phases and stages of a patient's rehabilitation, health care professionals may assume different roles according to the patient's changing needs: fellow human being, supervisor, guide, informant, professional, helper, or care provider. These roles depend on the patient's rehabilitation process and current needs. Health care professionals diagnose, treat and inform, adapt, plan, and structure the rehabilitation together with the patient, factoring in the patient's potential and limitations as a person, as a whole.

Multidisciplinary teamwork brings together each profession's general and specific competencies and roles, and patients have their own competencies as well. Taken together, these can provide insight into the potential challenges in an individual's rehabilitation process. The health care professional's most important task may be to find possibilities and potential—the positive building blocks within the patient and his or her care network—that may enhance the patient's progress. The patients' needs are central to the choice of interventions. This chapter discusses the following broad areas:

- The International Classification of Functioning, Disability, and Health (ICF).
- Physiotherapy assessment and clinical reasoning.
- Outcome measures.

3.1 The International Classification of Functioning, Disability, and Health

The International Classification of Functioning, Disability, and Health (ICF) is a tool used to classify different aspects and factors that influence a person's life. It is a classification of health and health-related domains that describes body functions and structures, activities, and participation. The domains are classified from the body, the individual, and societal perspectives; thus the ICF is a biopsychosocial model. Because an individual's functioning and disability occur in a particular context, the ICF also includes a list of environmental factors.

The ICF is useful to understand and measure health outcomes. It can be used in clinical settings, health services, or surveys at the individual or population level. Thus it complements the *International Statistical Classification of Diseases and Related Health Problems*, 10th edition (ICD-10) and looks beyond mortality and disease. By using the ICF, there is also the hope that health care professionals will communicate in the same language. *Functioning* refers to all body functions and structures, activities, and participation and is a positive term, whereas *disability* refers to impairments, activity limitations, and participation restrictions.

- *Body function* is a classification of the physiological and psychological systems of the body.
- *Body structure* classifies anatomical parts of the body: organs, extremities, and their components.
  - *Impairments* are problems of body functions and structures.
- *Activities and participation* covers all activities performed by individuals.
  - *Limitations* are problems the individual may experience in the performance of activities.
- *Participation* classifies the involvement in life situations by the individual in relation to health, body functions and structures, activities and relations.
  - *Restrictions* are problems that an individual may encounter in the way or level of participation in life situations.
- *Environmental factors* refer to the physical, social, and attitudinal environment in which people live and conduct their life.

  As well as these sections, the ICF involves another area that is not classified:
- *Personal factors* encompass the particular background of an individual's life and living and comprises features of the individual that are not part of a health condition or health states, which may be age, sex, experiences, personal beliefs, religion, lifestyle, and the like.

The interaction between these factors is illustrated in **Fig. 3.1**, and interventions at one level have the potential to modify other related elements. ICF may be used to ensure that all aspects of a person's situation have been evaluated as a basis for the rehabilitation process.

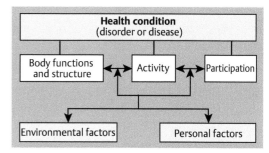

Fig. 3.1 The interrelationship between the different factors of the International Classification of Functioning, Disability, and Health (ICF). (Adapted from: ICF, WHO 2006.)

physical function to the patient's full potential, thereby enabling him to participate as actively as possible in his life again. The assessment should indicate which functions have been spared in relation to the regaining and learning of activities, postural control, and movement; which functions have been damaged or are dysfunctional; and what the consequences are for the patient. Assessment leads to information that allows the therapist to formulate hypotheses as to cause and effect of the patient's problems, and to evaluate which systems within the central nervous system (CNS) seem to be functional or dysfunctional. The therapist can then use this as a foundation for treatment interventions. Knowledge of components of movement that are important for balance and extremity function is a basis for both assessment and treatment. The ultimate goal of assessment is to define the patient's potential and how he can reach optimal function within the limits of available resources.

> Evaluating the patient's potential is an important goal of assessment.

3.2 Physiotherapy Assessment

All aspects of motor, sensory, cognitive, and perceptual functions are important for action as illustrated by a model first presented by Shumway-Cook and Woollacott (2006) (**Fig. 3.2**).

The physiotherapist has a specific and important role in the regaining, learning, and maintenance of physical function. The aim of assessment is to understand the patient's situation. The therapist has to come to know who the patient is, how she lives, her networks and family relations, her work situation, and her resources, and at the same time analyze her movement function. Assessment is therefore both resource and problem oriented. Physiotherapy is used to improve

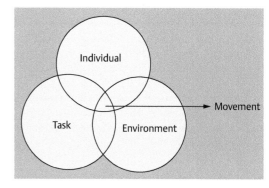

Fig. 3.2 The figure illustrates how movement is influenced by factors within the individual, the individual's environment, and the goal of his or her actions.

Neuropsychological dysfunction and sensory loss have in many cases been used to decide on the patient's rehabilitation potential in the acute phase after a stroke. These early symptoms are not a sign of the patient's real prognosis: perception and cognitive dysfunctions in most cases do improve as the patient becomes oriented to her environment. Thus focus on sensory, perceptual, and cognitive problems alone may lead to a more negative view of the patient's potential. The patient must be allowed time for the acute effects—chaos—of the lesion to settle before conclusions are drawn about the prognosis and thereby the level of rehabilitation effort the patient needs or is offered. The physiotherapist assesses *what* activities the patient is able to do, *how* the patient solves her movement tasks and reaches her goals, and *why* she moves as she does.

Occupational therapist Christine Nilson said the following about Berta Bobath in 1991 (Schleichkorn 1992): "She encouraged my creativity and taught me to see each patient as an individual. She offered problem-solving skills that led so logically to treatment intervention." Observational analysis of movement during activity is the most important tool of the assessment and leads to appropriate handling of the patient followed by clinical reasoning and treatment interventions.

Handling is both an assessment tool and an intervention, and it leads to a response from the patient. During handling the aim is to influence the patient's ability to move and his response to being moved. His response is important to determine the level of his response and his ability to learn; evaluation of the response is therefore important for the assessment. In this way, assessment and treatment are interlinked, inseparable processes. During assessment, the therapist collects information and starts a process of clinical reasoning to form hypotheses about *why* the patient moves as he does—hypotheses about the patient's *main problem* regarding activity and function. Treatment interventions are started, the results are continuously evaluated, hypotheses are discarded if treatment does not improve the patient's motor control, and new hypotheses are formulated as the treatment progresses. In general, the assessment proceeds as follows:

- History.
- Functional activity.
- Body functions and structures.
- Clinical reasoning.
- Outcome measures.
- Evaluation and documentation.

History

This part of the assessment aims at getting to know the patient and viewing her as a whole in the knowledge that rehabilitation is a process that often takes many years. The patient is assessed in relation to ICF domains: participation, activity, and body functions and structures—both as she previously functioned and how she presently functions. The therapist has in mind the patient's likely potential, resources, and problem areas. It is essential to form a relationship founded on respect and trust, and to gain information on social aspects, her roles, medical history, present situation, needs, and wishes. In a team setting, the different members of the team can decide whether they wish to interview the patient and her carer together or separately. Preferably, they should divide the interview in a way that saves the patient from having to repeat the same story to members of the whole team.

Social Aspects

- Marital status, family, and close social network.
- Social roles, the patient's needs and wishes.
- Housing.
- Hobbies and leisure activities.
- Work situation.
  - Profession, type of position/work, tasks.
  - Unemployed or pensioner? Reasons.

Medical History

- Previous level of function.
  - Physically: vision, hearing, problem areas, use of aids or assistive devices (walking aids, wheelchair, orthopedic shoes, orthotics, etc.), level of activity.
  - Mental function.
  - Other diseases.
  - Medication.
- Previous treatments.
  - Physiotherapy. For what reason? Effect of treatment?
  - Other.
- Previous contact with the health service.
- Present illness or disorder.
- Results from medical examinations and tests, such as computed tomographic scans, magnetic resonance imaging scans, X-rays, neurophysiology tests, among others.
- Any contraindications or any aspects of treatment that may need special attention.

- Factors that may exacerbate or improve the patient's motor control and why—as the patient sees it. The patient is often able to verbalize or express her experience of how different things may influence each other, for example, stress and tone.
- The patient's perception of his own situation: frustrations, hopes, needs, goals.

If the patient is unable to communicate, this information needs to be collected from his carers, who can often provide good information.

A person who suffers from acute illness or trauma undergoes catastrophic changes in his life, which may last for a short or long time or may even be permanent. The therapist needs to find out where he is in his own rehabilitation process: Is he in shock or have he and his carers started a process of reorientation? Time and information are of the essence and may be the most important intervention besides specific treatment and empathy. It does take time to realize and understand what has happened and to obtain an overview of the extent and consequences of the lesion.

■ Communication

During the interview and observation of the patient's general condition, the therapist forms an impression of her verbal and symbolic understanding: does she understand words? Does she understand nonverbal instructions given through the use of gestures?

■ Functional Activity

This part of the assessment builds on interview, observational analysis together with the patient's response to hands-on interaction (handling).

The aim is to clarify *what* the patient is able to do; his degree of independence; and his ability to cooperate and interact.

During the interview the patient is asked what activities of daily living (ADLs), personal hygiene, instrumental ADLs (IADLs, e.g., going to the store), and leisure activities he is able to do that are relevant to the current situation. His capability for activities informs the therapist of the following:
- General condition and general level and ability of movement.
- Communication function.

- Functional activity:
  - Quantity: *What* the patient is able to do.
  - Quality: *How* the patient moves.
  - Clinical reasoning process: Why does he move in this way.
- Use of aids.

If the patient is in an acute phase after a CNS lesion, both the level of activity and movement control will alter quickly due to spontaneous recovery and increased learning potential. The therapist needs to evaluate the patient's condition and abilities continuously to adapt and change interventions appropriately to enhance the patient's recovery.

■ General Condition

Observation of the patient's general condition provides the initial impression of the patient's status and how she feels:
- General condition and respiration.
- Stamina.
- Comfort and feeling of security.
- Effort.
- Ability to relax.
- General autonomic function.

■ What? How? Why?

Berta Bobath said, "See what you see and not what you think you see" (Schleichkorn 1992). Observation of the patient's activity starts when the therapist sees the patient for the first time, and before any form of intervention, such as transferring to a plinth, and before he is asked to change his clothing if appropriate. The patient's movement repertoire is analyzed through functional activity (**Table 3.1**).

If he has the ability to stand or walk, transfer, dress and undress when sitting and standing, these functions are analyzed first, as appropriate. The patient is met at the level he functions at; if he is unable to do any of the aforementioned activities, his ability to accept the base of support, to maintain a position and move within it, his ability to be placed are assessed. A general observation informs the therapist of the following:
- Feeling of security.
- Effort.
- Time, efficiency, appropriateness.
- Posture.
- Balance.
- Patterns of movement, sequence of activation and alignment.

Table 3.1   International Classification of Functioning, Disability, and Health (ICF) sections

- Interaction with the environment	– The patient's ability to interact with the environment. – The patient moves in relation to the environment. – The environment, people, and objects move in relation to the patient. – Gives information on the patient's perceptual and dual task capacity and how automatic the patient's balance is.
- Transfers	– For example, in a wheelchair or walking depending on the patient's functional level, weight transference in different postural sets of sitting and standing, in the transfers standing–sitting/chair–bed or other chair/in and out of bed, i.e., the patient's ability to control and vary movement. The key words are postural stability and orientation, eccentric and concentric control. – What is the patient able to do by himself, what does he need help for, and why? – The transfers from sitting to supine and vice versa are possibly the most complex and demanding tasks a person performs in daily life. – This transfer requires that we are able to eccentrically grade the movement from sitting to supine through a continuous changing relationship with the base of support, rotational components to align the body to the new base, eccentric work combined with aspects of specific concentric activity to lower the body down. Sitting up from supine requires a selective, graded, varied recruitment of motor activity through rotation to align the body in sitting on the edge of the bed. Both these transfers need the combination of flexion, extension, and rotational components, and a controlled recruitment of motor units for selective eccentric/concentric activation based on postural control from one position to another. The relationships with gravity and the base of support are very different in the postural sets of sitting and supine, and therefore require different muscle activation to achieve and maintain. – There is a conflict between the complexity of this task and the expectation from health personnel that the patient should be able to achieve this function as soon as possible for the sake of independence. – For most patients, the transfer from sitting to standing, standing and walking is easier than getting in and out of bed.
- Dressing and undressing	– Dressing and undressing require postural control to enable patients to weight transfer in sitting or standing and free their arms for function (see Chapter 2, Figs. 2.15 a-d and 2.17 a-g). For most patients dressing and undressing will also require learning, as many must find new strategies or even wear different clothes to master this task.
- Personal hygiene	– Is the patient able to manage visits to the bathroom by herself? Is she continent, does she participate in washing herself in the morning? Is she used to taking a shower or bath, and can she manage this? Is she able to get out of bed, to sit, or stand for any of these functions? If not, what help does she need? – Why?
- Eating/drinking	– Does the patient eat or drink by himself? Does he spill food/drink, why? – Sensation in his face may be poor, his motor control around his mouth may be decreased, or there may be perceptual/cognitive dysfunctions. If the patient coughs when he drinks or eats, he may have dysphagia. This is often a problem that is overlooked if the problems are small, but may cause complications for nutrition or for the patient's lung function and be an important social factor.

Table 3.1 (*continued*)

- Perception and cognition (see also Body Function and Structures)	– How does the patient interact with her own body and with the environment? Is she able to avoid obstacles; is she attentive to people, furniture, objects? Is she able to vary her movement repertoire in relation to the room and what is in it? – If in a wheelchair, how does she relate to it? Can she maneuver it herself, how? How does she problem solve footplates, brakes, and table. If she is able to dress and undress or participate in this activity, is she able to cross her body to undress sleeves, does she find her arms and legs? How does she solve the task? Is she focused, attentive—to what degree? Does she finish what she has started? If the patient has suffered a stroke, how does she take care of her affected arm during these tasks? – If the patient has problems understanding or responding, either to verbal information or to problem solving a "new" situation, he may have cognitive deficits. The therapist needs to find out if he has organic deficits (vision or hearing) or cognitive problems. His ability to problem solve may be assessed in all practical situations: use of wheelchair or walking aids, during transfers or any other relevant activity. – If the patient seems to have perceptual or cognitive deficits, a multidisciplinary assessment is of special importance. Nurses, assistants, carers may inform the team about how the patient problem solves and masters different situations through the day, and about his concentration, attention, moods, insight, self-interest and interest in his environment. Neuropsychologists and occupational therapists may assess the patient more specifically and give advice on how the patient should be helped in daily activities to enhance his perception and cognition. The patient's perceptual and cognitive function should be assessed and reevaluated over time for appropriate treatment and to evaluate the consequences for the patient's function and daily life.

- Selective function of the extremities: ability to vary and change.
- Tone.
- Compensatory strategies.
- Associated reactions.
- Sensation.
- Perception: attention to and experience of one's own body in relation to the environment.
- Cognition: attentiveness, understanding, focus, problem-solving abilities, memory, concentration, and insight.

What functional activities is the patient able to perform? Is she sitting passively in a chair or lying in a bed without the ability to move? How does she respond when facilitated or helped? Can she transfer, stand, or walk, and how safe is she in those situations?

The analysis is both resource and problem oriented. It should give answers as to what the patient can realistically perform independently, when she needs support, and how she solves tasks through movement. It is important to talk with the multidisciplinary team and the patient's carers to form as full a picture as possible, as well as to observe the patient when she is not aware of being observed.

■ Use of Aids

Does the patient need aids, such as a wheelchair, walking aids, other technical or orthopedic aids? Why?

Information from other health professionals working with the patient gives a more complete picture of the patient's strengths and weaknesses.

■ Body Functions and Structures

This part of the assessment involves observation, handling, and analysis and includes these important factors:
- Quality of movement, movement patterns, stability, and mobility.
- Sensation, perception, and learned nonuse.
- Pain.
- Autonomic function.

Observational Movement Analysis

Observation informs about visible and invisible aspects of function: spatial relationships, perception of one's own body and its relationship to the environment, aspects of perceptual and problem-solving abilities, concentration, attention, motivation, mood, and orientation, as well as sensation and movement ability. Therapists tend to assess the patient in different positions, and because we move *between* different postures and positions normally, the patient is assessed in relation to dynamic activity. Assessment in supine may give additional information about tone, alignment, and range of movement, if appropriate. If the patient experiences increased problems with hypertonia during the night or in the morning before or as he is getting out of bed, his sleeping patterns and positions need to be assessed specifically.

Handling

During handling the therapist assesses how movement is performed—initiation, recruitment, sequence, alignment—and gains information about muscle activity, stability, and movement within and between key areas. The therapist then forms hypotheses about which key areas seem to be most affected, unstable or fixed. Through an invitation to move through handling and facilitation, quality of movement and muscle activity as well as range of movement are assessed further. Assessment is not passive; the patient's ability to recruit activity and move is important. Through correction of components that seem deviant or malaligned, the therapist again invites the patient to move through handling. Has anything changed, positively or negatively? In this way, the therapist forms an impression of tone distribution, stability, postural control and balance, tempo and selectivity, and the patient's ability to vary and adapt.

Analysis

Observational movement analysis is a process of detailed description of human movement. This can involve one aspect of a task or the performance of a whole task within daily life (International Bobath Instructors Training Association 2008). Analysis of movement and task performance enables the therapist to identify activity limitations as well as underlying problems of impairment. It involves the analysis of movement sequences during task performance by which the therapist determines how the movement differs from typical motor behavior and analysis of the compensatory strategies used. The Bobath therapist considers task fulfilment, the assistance required, and the quality and efficiency of task performance (Levin & Panturin 2011). It is important to recognize that the Bobath therapist acknowledges that movement within the "normal" population of individuals (i.e., persons without a neurological deficit), varies within a wide range of efficiencies and compensations (Raine et al 2009). Thus movement within the neurologically able population is not always efficient and without compensations. A recent survey by Raine (2007) (Raine & Phys 2007) established that, rather than aiming to promote "normal" movements, the Bobath therapist promotes efficiency of movement to the individual's potential.

Aspects of movement that are analyzed are muscle activity: interplay, alignment, patterns of movement, all of which may have consequences for the patient's ability to regain and learn movement. Observation and handling are not performed satisfactory without the patient being adequately undressed, preferably wearing short trousers (with a bra or sun top for women). If the patient is unwilling to undress to this level, even if other people are not around and after being given information on the importance of being adequately undressed to allow the therapist to properly analyze movement, the patient's wishes must be respected.

Assessment of body functions and structures requires the therapist to have a thorough knowledge of human movement and to be specifically competent to analyze the interplay of movement. This part of the assessment is qualitative as well as resource and problem oriented.

The therapist needs to gain insight into *how* the patient moves, *what* he is able to perform, and *how* movement is being performed. This requires an analysis of body functions and structures in the activity domain (ICF). Handling allows the formation of hypotheses of which *neuromuscular interplay* brings the patient to where he is. The musculature changes alignment and moves joints under the influence of gravity. Component analysis is the analysis of neuromuscular activity.

Knowledge of human movement and prerequisites for balance and movement in normal situations allows the analysis of deviations from normal movement. The patient's way of moving is analyzed in relation to hypotheses of how he moved before the CNS lesion.

■ Quality of Movement

The therapist needs to have a picture in mind of how the patient might have moved before the CNS lesion, and view the movement deviations in this light. It is complicated to analyze how the patient is moving, the underlying neuromuscular activity, and the consequences this may have for the patient's function simultaneously. It may be easier to divide this part into phases: What neuromuscular activity does the patient recruit to maintain a posture or to move (**Fig. 3.3**)?

The following qualities are evaluated in relevant postural sets and activities:

- *Midline orientation*: Does the patient move in all planes and seem to have a perceptual relationship to his own body and the environment?
- *Ability to move to and from the physical base of support*: It is evaluated through observation and handling. Is the patient able to adapt his tone and neuromuscular activity to be where he is, to maintain the postural set, and to move through weight transference to another postural set? For example, if the patient is sitting, the therapist may place her hands over his greater trochanters, sense the hips, the position of the pelvis, his ischial tuberosities, and the muscle activity in the area. The patient is facilitated to move in different directions and the therapist observes, senses, and analyzes the adaptive movements of the related key areas during weight transference in different directions. The therapist observes and handles the feet and the hands to assess their adaptive abilities: to transfer weight onto the feet or to shape the hand to different objects; reach, grasp, and let go.
- *Interplay and interrelationship between different key areas*: The key areas are assessed both individually and together to see how they adapt to each other through movement. Neuromuscular activity is analyzed in the specific postural sets the patient adopts and moves within (i.e., the patient's relationship to gravity and the base of support).
  - The interplay between the trunk, head and neck, and the pelvic and shoulder girdles gives information about the patient's postural control, especially core stability, and her ability to align her body in relation to the environment.
  - The ability to maintain postural stability during self-generated movement of the extrem-

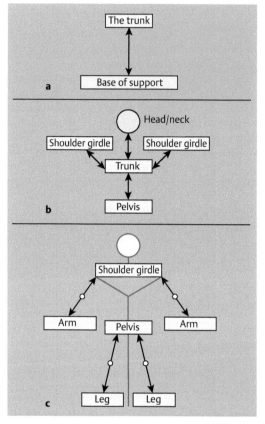

Fig. 3.3 (a) Observation and analysis of the patient's line of gravity in relation to the base of support. Where does it fall, and which neuromuscular activity must the patient recruit to be where she is and to move from there? The trunk, head, and neck are central to balance and require coordinated movement in three planes. Analysis of this relationship gives information on holistic function and balance; midline: symmetry/asymmetry; weight distribution: active/passive (weight). (b) Analysis of the interrelationship and interplay between the central and proximal key areas: interplay, selectivity, variation and change, mutual influence. (c) Analysis of patterns of movement within the extremities and the distal–proximal relationships: adaptation to the environment, patterns, selectivity and mutual influence.

ities (or as they are moved for her); or is the patient displaced or dependent on fixation through the arms/legs to maintain balance?
  - The interplay between the hands/feet and the proximal key areas informs of postural control, selectivity, patterns of movement, and the ability to vary in relation to the goal (task). Also, is the patient able to support herself using arms and legs and move her trunk in relation to her extremities?

- *Patterns of movement, sequence of activation, and biomechanical factors*: Joint position and range, rotatory components, and alignment inform as to which neuromuscular activity the patient has used to get where she is and is currently using. Does the patient recruit anticipatory postural activity to maintain stability for movement? Does this background activity vary with different tasks? Is selectivity present in all parts or are some movement components missing or inadequate?
- *Selective control of movement*: The individual movement and neuromuscular activity within the key areas. Is there freedom of movement and activity in all planes? *Selectivity* is controlled activity of one body part based on stability in another. Does the trunk rotate too early or too little during arm movement? Is the head free to scan the environment? Are the scapulae free and stable? Does one shoulder girdle glide too early when the other is moved during tasks?
- *Muscle quality*: Flexibility, length, and elasticity. Does the musculature exhibit qualities needed for interplay of eccentric and concentric activity? Is compartmentalization maintained (see Chapter 1, The Neuromuscular System).
- *Tone*
  - Appropriate, adaptable tone that varies in relation to different postural sets and activity.
  - Hypotonia: less tone than would seem appropriate or expected for the activity. Is there an increased sense of *weight* (limpness or flaccidity, inactivity, weakness) during movement or when moving and handling the patient?
  - Hypertonia: more tone than would seem appropriate or expected for the activity. Is there resistance or increased assistance to movement in one direction? Where? Which qualities does this express?
  - The presence of associated reactions: when are they expressed? In which situations? Is it possible to facilitate the patient's postural control and movement so that the associated reactions are diminished?
  - Spasticity and/or secondary problems of soft tissue changes?
- *Compensatory strategies*: Which strategies does the patient employ to solve motor tasks? Appropriate or inappropriate? Is it possible to facilitate the patient to gain control and make inefficient strategies superfluous?

- *Does the patient respond to facilitation*? Is it possible to facilitate the patient to take over and make the movements his own (placing)? If not, why not? Is there resistance to movement? If so, where? Is there little, or no, muscular activation? Is the stimulation strong enough? What are the consequences? If the patient does respond, where is the initiation? How is the pattern?

The patient's response to being handled gives important information about how the patient may be facilitated; if he tolerates the closeness of the therapist and if he interprets the information and demands that she transmits through handling. This requires that the therapist is precise in her handling and facilitation.

■ Sensation, Perception, and Learned Nonuse

Observational analysis gives the therapist an impression of whether information is integrated in the patient's CNS or not, and if this information is being used in relation to the patient's ability to move. Sensory testing may be performed to assess the patient's *conscious* awareness of sensory impulses, which is important, especially for stereognosis and dexterity of the hand (see Chapter 1, The Somatosensory System). Testing shows how sensory information is transmitted and processed within the CNS. Poor sensation may be due to lesions of the ascending systems directly or due to alterations in sensory perception (i.e., association areas). If sensory perception is affected, the CNS does not interpret the information that it receives, which is a problem with sensory integration and not reception. Therefore, results from sensory testing should not be used to decide on a patient's rehabilitation potential. If appropriate, sensory testing should be performed both before and after a period of intensified sensory stimulation to the most affected body part. Sensory stimulation aims at improving both transmission and the patient's attention toward the body part that is being treated: improved focus often implies that the patient's CNS starts to interpret and integrate sensory information to a higher degree. The therapist should attempt to discriminate whether the sensory problems are organic (sensory pathways) or perceptual because this is important for therapeutic intervention.

■ Lesions of the Ascending Systems

Sensory processing involves many somatosensory networks and many different areas of the CNS, thus sensory impairment in CNS diseases after lesions can result from a lesion located anywhere from the spinal cord to the cortex. Impairment of body sensations is a significant loss in its own right and has detrimental effects on exploration of the environment, safety, identification of sensory features of objects through touch, use of hands, and motor recovery. Loss of discrimination involves impairment of one or more of the following: localization of tactile stimuli; two-point discrimination; texture discrimination; appreciation of size, shape, and form of objects through touch; discrimination of limb position; discrimination of direction and extent of limb movement; and weight discrimination (Carey & Matyas 2011). Assessing the severity and type of sensory loss is important for the process of rehabilitation.

Sensory Testing

In sitting, the patient should place—or be helped in placing—both hands behind her body with the palms up. In this way she is not able to see what the tester is doing, and tonal influences are often neutralized as the arms are in flexion, adduction, and internal rotation with flexion at the wrists. First the therapist needs to gain a general impression of whether there are differences in superficial sensation between the patient's two hands, using her own hand to touch.

Finger Discrimination

Finger gnosis is tested by the therapist touching one finger at a time and asking the patient to name which finger without seeing. Recognition of the individual fingers is important for discrimination and informs the therapist if the fingers have maintained their cortical representation:

- If the patient is aphasic, she may move the same finger on the opposite hand to indicate which one she thinks it is.
- If recognition is weak, but mostly correct, there is some connection to the cortex.
- If there is no recognition, the patient has *finger agnosia*: the cortical representation of the individual fingers is not aroused.
- The patient may have receptive problems and may not understand these instructions, in which case this testing inappropriate.

Intense sensory stimulation may improve this to some degree, but the patient's prognosis for discriminative hand and finger function may be reduced.

Localization of Touch

Two-point discrimination (TPD) is defined as the smallest separation between two stimulations placed on the skin at the same moment in time that can be discriminated as two separate points (Kim & Yi 2013). TPD is performed to test the ability to locate stimuli precisely. The therapist uses two equal and sharp objects (needles or similar) and starts by testing the patient's index finger, because this finger is most densely packed with sensory receptors. The therapist pricks the patient simultaneously with the two objects. The therapist needs to test for different distances between the two points at different locations on the finger to find where the patient is able to discriminate the two points. The smallest distance for two-point localization is measured for future reference.

Joint Position Sense

Joint position sense is defined as the ability of an individual to identify the static location of a body part (Proske & Gandevia 2009).

The therapist moves the joints of the index finger or the thumb and asks whether the patient can describe the position or copy with the other hand. If he is not able to do so, the therapist may test his wrist and gradually more proximal joints of the arm. It should be noted that this form of testing is very limited:

- Joint position sense depends more on input from active muscles and compression/stretch of skin than joint receptors alone.
- Only the patient's conscious awareness is tested, not how the CNS receives, interprets, and integrates the information that it actually receives (see Chapter 1, Somatosensory System); therefore, if results are deviant, firm conclusions should not be drawn

Conscious awareness of sensory information is more important for hand function than for walking. In people with CNS lesions there is no primary damage to ascending systems at the level of the spinal cord. Sensory impulses are received and integrated to some degree in the spinal cord and transmitted to the cerebellum and other higher centers. This information may therefore be used for pattern generation and interlimb coordination through the cerebellum. The patient's fine tuning of balance will be impaired to some degree if sensory information from the soles of the feet is diminished (Kavounoudias et al 1998; Meyer et al 2004).

Perceptual Function
Patients with CNS disorders may exhibit perceptual dysfunctions that cause decreased attention or neglect toward the most affected side. Neglect is obvious in patients who do not turn to the affected side; do not take care of, or dress their most affected extremities; or walk or wheel into objects, people, door frames, or furniture on the most affected side.

Some patients do not integrate information from the most affected side when they receive information from their less affected side at the same time. The therapist may suspect this form of inattention if the patient has some movement in the most affected arm but does not attempt to use it. This may be assessed through *simultaneous bilateral touch*. The prerequisite for performing this test is that the patient does have sensation when the most affected side is tested alone.

Simultaneous Integration
In sitting, the patient should place—or be helped in placing—both hands behind his body with the palms up. In this way he is not able to see what the tester is doing. The therapist stands behind the patient and touches one arm at a time, asking the patient to say which arm/hand is touched (right or left). At intervals she touches both arms or hands at the same place at the same time. If the patient still only says the less affected side, this implies that information from the most affected side is suppressed (i.e., not integrated). Dysfunction in simultaneous integration is called extinction—when the patient is in situations that require integration of stimuli from both sides at the same time, such as in traffic, among people, in many daily situations, he may be in danger of causing damage to himself.

Learned Nonuse
Patients may exhibit sensory problems as a result of inactivity or nonuse. Usually this applies more to the distal body parts, hands, and feet. Learned nonuse may be overcome by stimulating, mobilizing, and facilitating the patient's activity. If the patient expresses that she can feel her hand or foot better after treatment, this implies that there is a degree of learned nonuse.

Pain
Pain may limit the patient's recovery and learning processes and lead to depression, loss of motivation, and social isolation. The patient may experience pain when the arm is being moved, for instance, during dressing and washing, and this may lead to withdrawal from daily activities and treatment, and deterioration of functional ability.

Possible Causes
- *Increased tone:* malalignment and possible fixation of joints in unnatural postures, static activation of muscles and decreased circulation, or sudden pulls (cramps, spasms).
- *Trauma:* due to poor handling, falls, or instability of joints.
- Altered sensory awareness/perception.
- Other causes (e.g., disuse over time, swelling, inflammation, degenerative conditions).

The physiotherapist must assess the cause of pain; where the pain is, which situation exacerbates or improves it, and when the patient experiences pain (day, night, during activity, at rest), and thereby get an impression of causal factors and severity. History and movement analysis (observation and handling) as well as information from other examinations (X-rays, ultrasound, etc.) and from carers as well as using a *visual analog scale* (VAS) may be helpful. Pain is always a priority of treatment.

Clinical Relevance
Chronic poststroke pain is common and occurs in 11 to 55% of all stroke patients (Klit et al 2009). However, several types of pain can occur in the same patient simultaneously. It is important to identify the origin and type of pain to find the relevant treatment for the patient.

Central neuropathic pain is defined as pain arising as a direct consequence of a lesion or disease affecting the CNS (Treede et al 2008). Central poststroke pain (CPSP) belongs to central neuropathic pain (Klit et al 2009). CPSP refers to pain resulting from a lesion or dysfunction of the CNS after a stroke, and it is characterized by pain and sensory dysfunction involving the area of the body that has been affected by the stroke. It has been shown that stroke in the brain stem and thalamus is more frequently associated with central pain than other locations (Klit et al

2009). The exact prevalence of CPSP is not known, partly owing to the difficulty in distinguishing this syndrome from other pain types that can occur after stroke (Klit et al 2009). Patients suffering from CPSP present with diverse sensory symptoms, and the pathophysiology is poorly understood; but central disinhibition, imbalance of stimuli, and central sensitization have been suggested (Kumar et al 2010).

Hemiplegic shoulder pain (HSP) may cause a lot of discomfort and suffering for the individual. Lindgren and colleagues (2007) reported that, in 327 patients with stroke, almost a third of the subjects developed shoulder pain (Lindgren et al 2007). HSP is usually diagnosed when pain is located in the affected shoulder region or arm, with an onset poststroke (with no direct relation to trauma or injury), and is present during rest or during active or passive movement. The literature is rife with inconsistent reports about the epidemiology, risk factors, and etiology. However, HSP may be related to the resting position of the scapula and humerus, and/or deviating movement of the scapula or humerus (Niessen et al 2008). Effective shoulder position, movement, stability, muscle performance, and motor control are heavily dependent on scapular performance (Kibler 2012). Moreover, the scapular position and activity are dependent on the activity in the trunk. Thus, when addressing the hemiplegic shoulder complex, the first area to be assessed is the alignment and activity in the trunk. If the trunk muscles are not working to ensure the optimal alignment of the trunk, the position of the scapulae on the thorax will be compromised (De Baets et al 2013). The coordinated coupled movement between the scapula and humerus, the so-called scapulohumeral rhythm (SHR), allows for glenohumeral alignment to maximize joint stability and therefore for efficient arm movement (Kibler 2012). Precise SHR is needed to preserve the suprahumeral space and prevent impingement of the soft tissue when abducting and forward flexing the arm. Proper coupling of the humerus and scapula includes upward rotation and posterior tilting of the scapula and external rotation of the humerus (Braman et al 2009), which is important during both active and passive movements of the arm. Stabilization of the scapula is provided through the scapulothoracic musculature by approximating the scapula to the thorax. Muscles such as the *m. trapezius, m. levator scapulae, m. rhomboideus minor and major,* and *serratus anterior* are responsible for maintaining scapular position on the thorax. If the strength of these muscles is diminished, the positioning of the

scapula can be affected. Variation of the dynamic pattern and of the resting position of the scapula on the thorax has been called scapular dyskinesis. *Dys* (alteration of) *kinesis* (motion) is a general term that reflects the loss of appropriate control of scapular motion (Kibler 2012). In addition to influencing scapular position and movements, altered scapular muscular activity is suggested to contribute to the development of rotator cuff impingement, and consequently to the development of shoulder pain (De Baets et al 2013; Vasudevan & Browne 2014). Shoulder impingement has been defined as compression, entrapment, or mechanical irritation of the rotator cuff structures and/or long head of the biceps tendon, either beneath the coracoacromial arch (subacromial) or between the undersurface of the rotator cuff and the glenoid or glenoid labrum (internal) (Ludewig & Reynolds 2009). Limitations in scapular upward rotation and posterior tilting during arm elevation might reduce the available subacromial space, thus contributing to development or progression of impingement as well as a poorer environment for tissue healing (Ludewig & Reynolds 2009).

Soft tissue tightness of muscles or structure restricting normal scapular motions during arm movements is another potential mechanism for HSP. Humeral external rotation is believed to be advantageous to the subacromial space, allowing improved clearance for the greater tuberosity (Flatow et al 1994) and reduction in shoulder external rotation have been linked to subacromial impingement. Furthermore the pectoralis minor muscle, based on its attachments from the coracoid process to the upper ribs, is capable of producing scapular internal rotation, downward rotation, and anterior tilt. Thus excessive active or passive tension in this muscle can lead to prevention of the normal scapular movement that should occur during arm elevation (Ludewig & Reynolds 2009).

The muscles acting on the glenohumeral joint working as dynamic stabilizers are mainly the m. deltoid and the rotator cuff muscles. Weakness of the deltoid puts more tension on the rotator cuff muscles, especially the supraspinatus tendon, where prolonged tensile overload can lead to mechanical fatigue, loss of elasticity, and, eventually, potential tearing of the tendon (Yi et al 2013).

HSP impedes rehabilitation and may also interfere with balance, walking, transfers, self-care activities, and quality of life (Turner-Stokes & Jackson 2002).

Complex Regional Pain Syndrome 1 (CRPS1) (Pertoldi & Di Benedetto 2005) is the more recent term used when referring to shoulder–hand syndrome (SHS) or reflex sympathetic dystrophy. These disorders are most common in the limbs and are characterized by pain, active and passive movement disorders, abnormal regulation of blood flow and sweating, edema of skin and subcutaneous tissues, and trophic changes of skin, organs of the skin, and subcutaneous tissues. The condition is not unique to stroke patients and is also associated with phantom limb pain. It is prevalent among patients with head injury, spinal cord injury (SCI), and even mild injury to the extremities. In a systematic review by Geurts et al (2000) both SHS and poststroke hand edema are described. Geurts et al came to the following conclusions:

- The shoulder is involved in only half of the cases with painful swelling of the wrist and hand, suggesting a *wrist–hand syndrome.*
- Hand edema is not lymphedema.
- SHS usually coincides with increased arterial blood flow.
- Trauma causes aseptic joint inflammation in SHS.
- No specific treatment has proved advantageous over any other physical methods for reducing hand edema.
- Oral corticosteroids are the most effective treatment for SHS.

In the author's experience, careful but persistent mobilization combined with correction of alignment and sensory stimulation may improve this problem.

▪ Autonomic Function

A CNS lesion may cause altered autonomic function, both locally and more generally. Local changes are present in many patients with CNS dysfunction and may be caused by dysfunctions in central regulation or as a result of inactivity and immobility. Altered autonomic function often manifests as a more distal problem, in the hands or feet:

- Altered circulation: The skin color is more bluish, reddish, or pale.
- Changes in temperature follow changes in circulation: The extremity is cold to touch. If the patient has an infection, such as vasculitis, the area will be warmer and more red.
- Swelling is observed and palpated and is fairly common in the hand or foot of a patient who has had stroke or has multiple sclerosis. If chronic, it may cause further circulatory, movement, or pain-related problems. If there is a generalized

stiffness or swelling in a patient's leg or thigh combined with pain or tenderness, or the pain increases when the foot is dorsiflexed and the big toe extended (Homan's sign), the patient has to be examined for possible deep vein thrombosis.

Skin Quality

There may be changes in the skin due to inactivity, immobilization, and decreased circulation. Inactivity may lead to thick and hard skin and may cause further immobility of the affected area. A hand that is not used becomes drier with increased skin thickness because the dead skin does not rub off during use.

General Symptoms

These are more common in SCI, especially complete SCI. The symptoms may vary in intensity and character:

- Sweating above trauma level.
- Increased heart rate.
- Headaches.
- Increased blood pressure.
- Reddened skin.

> **What? How? Why?**
> These are the three most important questions in the ongoing assessment of the patient.

▪ Clinical Reasoning

Clinical reasoning is the decision-making process involved in the diagnosis and management of patients' problems (Edwards et al 2004). It is central throughout the whole process of assessment, intervention, and evaluation. Clinical reasoning has been defined as the "thinking and decision making associated with clinical practice that enables therapists to take the best-judged action for individual patients."

History, observation, and handling form the foundation for the process of clinical reasoning as well as the therapist's special and general competency and information from others. Activity and participation are assessed in combination with the patient's problem-solving ability and motor behavior in relation to the tasks and environment:

- Resources and restrictions in participation.
- Resources and limitations of activity.
- Deviations or loss of functions and structures

of the body as a direct result of neurological lesions or as a consequence of the lesions. Quickly learned compensatory strategies may be difficult to separate from the direct impairments. Compensatory strategies may lead to further deviations. In this context, deviations from body functions and structures relate to those problems that change the patient's prerequisites for normal human movement control.

- Changes in tone will influence the patient's ability to remain upright and interact with gravity, and may cause malalignment or alterations in muscle length, muscle flexibility and elasticity, range of movement, changes in noncontractile tissues, and the ability to vary eccentric and concentric activity.
- Changes in reciprocal innervation may disrupt the muscular interplay between agonists, antagonists, and synergists and alter the recruitment sequence of motor units and the interplay between stability and mobility in movement.
- Changes in patterns of movement and their ability to vary according to the goal disrupt the sequence of muscular activation and cause altered alignment and thereby altered working relationships for muscles.

Problems with body structures and functions cause reduced balance and movement and influence the patient's ability to transfer and to perform daily activities (**Fig. 3.4**). Therefore, the therapist's specific knowledge of movement and analysis are important tools in assessment and treatment, and for the process of clinical reasoning to improve the patient's ability to act and interact; an in-depth understanding of human movement is crucial to the clinical reasoning process (Raine et al 2009).

An exact assessment is fundamental to, and inseparable from, the clinical reasoning process (Raine et al 2009). Clinical reasoning is based on the therapist's general and specific knowledge and experience, both professional and personal. Clinical reasoning is the mental process by which decisions are made, based on the ability to identify critical cues from the assessment process using theoretical and professional knowledge and life experience. The therapist needs to evaluate all findings from interview, observation, and handling to gain a picture of the individual patient. Clinical reasoning is a process of problem solving whereby the therapist

formulates a *main problem* or *hypothesis* based on the collected data, causal relationships, and the patient's expressed problems; it is the interpretation of the information gathered. This leads to goal formulation, interventions, and evaluation of interventions (**Fig. 3.5**). Clinical reasoning requires an ability to analyze the interaction between the various ICF dimensions.

The following are required of the therapist:
- Understand the patient's needs and expectations.
- Gain an impression of the patient's resources and limitations in all three ICF domains.
- Formulate hypotheses about the factors that seem to be most important and limiting for the patient's level of activity, movement ability, and manner of movement.
- Choose goals, both short and long term, preferably in cooperation with the patient.
- Choose treatment interventions: tools.
- Evaluate treatment interventions and develop further hypotheses. Is the hypothesis appropriate? Judged on the results here and now and over a longer period of time.

The Aim of Assessment

The aim of assessment is twofold:
- To create a hypothesis about the patients potential.
- To create hypotheses of *why* the patient moves as he does.

What is the patient able to do? Which resources does he have? If function fails or if there is lack of function, the question arises: *Why?* or *Why not?*
- Is it due to balance or movement problems?
- Is it due to somatosensory and/or perceptual dysfunction?
- Are there cognitive problems?

Causes Based on Balance or Movement Problems

- Which neuromuscular activity is recruited and is not recruited in different situations?
- Is activity that should normally change between different activities missing or not changing?
- Is tone low because the patient uses compensatory strategies elsewhere and thereby does not allow efficient recruitment of muscle activity?

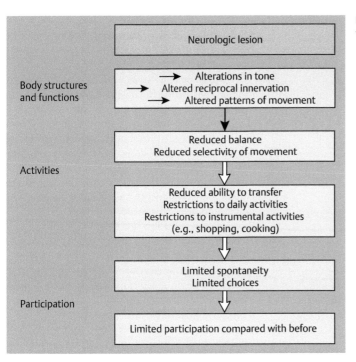

Fig. 3.4 Consequences of a lesion to the central nervous system.

- Are there primary sensorimotor problems, or a combination of these and inappropriate compensatory strategies?
- Does the patient display reduced postural control and balance?

Generally the somatosensory, vestibular, and visual systems have important roles in postural control and orientation.

Are there direct or indirect dysfunctions in any of these systems? In stroke, the vestibular nuclei are seldom affected directly, infarction or bleeding is rare at this level in the brain stem; also the vestibular nuclei are not under direct cortical control. A reduction in the patient's ability to move may lead to altered somatosensory information to the vestibular system, and the vestibular nuclei may become dysfunctional. Visual problems are frequent in many neurological conditions, such as nystagmus, hemianopia, and other visual field deficits, as well as visual neglect or inattention. All of these can influence the patient's postural control.

- Does the patient display reduced postural tone or areas of associated reactions that cause reduced postural control and balance? If so, the corticoreticulospinal and corticorubrospinal systems may be dysfunctional. These systems are partly responsible for postural tone and proximal stability.

Clinical experience suggests that balance dysfunctions may be caused by changes in tone (more or less than normal), reduced or altered movement control, and interplay between segments and/or perceptual dysfunction. Balance is one of the more automatic functions in human movement. If balance is reduced, the therapist needs to choose interventions (functions, activities, postural sets, handling, etc.), which enhance balance and movement on a more automatic level.

- Does the patient have any selective control in her arms or legs?

Selective control is understood as controlled and coordinated movement of one body part or one joint based on postural stability. Is there any sign of movement in the fingers or toes? If not, why not? Could it be that the postural components are not activated, thereby not allowing stability and selective interplay between key areas? Is there true paresis and therefore severely reduced neural activation due to the lesion itself? With true paresis especially distally, the corticospinal system would be partly damaged to varying degrees. The cortical systems are the most voluntarily activated (least automatic) systems in human movement control. Enhanced demands for selective attention combined with voluntary activation may be appropriate when selective movement is primarily affected.

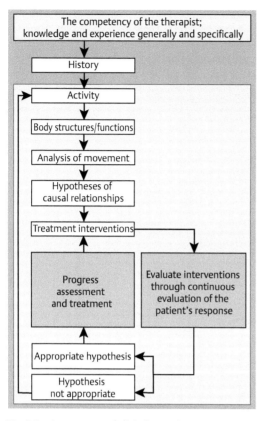

Fig. 3.5   Assessment and clinical reasoning.

Examples

Some patients have a problem with hyperextension of their most affected knee during loading of their leg. This may be caused by several factors:

- Incoordination between agonists and antagonists around the knee or reduced interplay between the hip/pelvis and the ankle/foot as a direct result of the lesion (body domain).
- Overreaction due to hypersensitivity to sensory/proprioceptive input (stretch or cutaneous hypersensitivity) as the foot meets the floor to bear weight (body domain).
- As a consequence of the patient "stiffening" her knee to be able to stand and walk (activity domain), that is, a compensatory strategy.

The neuromuscular activity in the hip region should vary in different phases of stance and swing. Does the patient's neuromuscular activity vary as it

should? Is extensor activity recruited appropriately at heel-strike and through stance? Is there eccentric lengthening of hip flexors and adductors to allow hip/pelvic stability?

If hip extension is not recruited appropriately, the therapist needs to facilitate/strengthen this activity. Lennon (2001) demonstrated through two case histories that recovery of more normal movement patterns for walking and functional ability can be achieved through physiotherapy poststroke. Hesse et al (1998) demonstrated a more balanced walking pattern with facilitation according to the Bobath Concept during therapeutic intervention. Facilitation enhances a more optimal recruitment (body domain) during functional activity (activity domain). Brock and colleagues (2011) showed in their pilot study that, for patients with moderate to severe stroke, interventions based on the Bobath Concept in conjunction with task practice may be more beneficial than structured task practice alone for improving gait velocity.

If the flexor musculature does not eccentrically lengthen to allow for hip extension, the therapist needs to mobilize and facilitate the eccentric control (body domain) and place demands on the hip extensors (make necessary—let it happen) during activity (see Chapter 2, Handling).

The activity around the shoulder girdle is an important component in all transfers (activity domain). The neuromuscular activity in the interplay between the shoulder girdle, the arm, and the trunk should vary depending on the activity to be performed (body domain). If the shoulder girdle is fixed, for instance, in elevation, the trunk on the same side is kept elongated and cannot shorten for stability or weight transfer. The therapist needs to hypothesize *why* the shoulder girdle is kept elevated:

- Is there reduced stability in the thorax or between the thorax and the scapula? Why?
- Is the instability due to reduced intercostal activity (body domain)?
- Is tone too low/too high and causing malalignments and poor coordination (body domain)?
- Is distal activity reduced (body domain) and causing the patient to attempt moving the arm from the shoulder to be active and task oriented (activity domain)?

Hypotheses on cause and effect lead to goals for treatment and possible interventions. The treatment will differ depending on which hypothesis is most probable, and the continuous evaluation of the patient's response to treatment.

- In which way does the patient compensate? Why?
- What components of movement is he missing that drives him to compensate in the way he does?
- Does he seem afraid or insecure? The patient needs to feel safe to explore his own movement abilities with less compensatory strategies.

The patient's compensatory strategies change according to the different activities he attempts to perform, whereas the main problem will be a dysfunctional component (or more than one) throughout. If the patient moves more appropriately with less compensation after intervention, the hypothesis is strengthened.

- Where and why are there associated reactions? In which situations do they occur? As the patient is attempting to balance, or move her arms or legs? How is the patient's postural control? How much effort does she use just to stay where she is?

Two aspects seem especially important when assessing and treating patients displaying associated reactions:

1. Analyze and formulate hypotheses as to the reason why:
   - Do the associated reactions seem to be a response to balance demands? The reason may then be reduced postural control.
     (Reduced interplay between stability and mobility between key areas; reduced stability more specifically related to the hip/pelvic area or the trunk; reduced stability and equilibrium control distally and therefore inefficient ankle strategy.)
   - Do the associated reactions seem to be related to movement of the extremities? What is the quality of the patient's movement ability, sequence of recruitment, selectivity, variation? Is tempo, initiation, or strength reduced?
   - Do the associated reactions increase with effort? Why does the patient increase her effort in situations that normally are not strenuous?
2. Does the patient display any control over her associated reactions? Is she aware of them and does she herself hypothesize on why they happen?

Many patients have good body awareness and may sense and verbalize causal relationships. These hypotheses are frequently correct, and the therapist needs to explore this in assessment and treatment.

■ Causes Based on Somatosensory or Perceptual Dysfunctions

Sensory information reaches the spinal cord and is modified and integrated to a certain degree at this level. In stroke, there is a small probability of a patient experiencing sensory deficits at this level. The spinal cord "senses" even if the patient cognitively does not. Sensory loss in stroke is caused by lesions to the ascending pathways or structures (e.g., internal capsule, thalamus, or cortex). Decreased sensation may be caused by learned nonuse or lesions to the perceptual systems causing inattention or neglect to the more affected side. In multiple sclerosis, information may be disrupted at the spinal cord level as well as in other areas of the CNS.

It may be difficult to differentiate between sensory loss and reduced sensory perception. Treatment aimed at drawing the patient's attention and ability to feel through improved mobility may reveal some answers; if the patient's sensation of the body part improves during treatment, it is possible that the problem is due more to a reduced sensory perception than to a true sensory loss. Learned nonuse may be improved through specific therapy as well as activating the extremity in all functional contexts. Perceptual dysfunction is seen in most ADLs; the patient may display reduced attention in relation to his own body and to his environment. It is important to develop a good working relationship with other health professionals to assess these dysfunctions and make a plan for interdisciplinary intervention. The patient's attention must be stimulated and demanded in all activities.

Balance and movement require the ability to perceive where the different body parts are in relation to each other and the environment. If the patient has perceptual dysfunction, this may influence his perception of the midline, and thereby interplay and balance. Treatment aimed at orienting the patient to his own body improves the interplay and coordination between body segments, which may lead the patient to be more oriented to his own body in the environment.

■ Causes Based on Cognitive Deficits

Does the patient understand what he is doing or is being asked to do? What about his hearing? Is he aphasic? Is he depressed or uncritical? Does he display insight and is he able to problem solve new situations? Is he concentrated and focused? Are there impairments that may have consequences for his functional ability?

Answers to all these questions are primarily hypotheses as they guide treatment and the choice of interventions related to the patient's movement problem.

> Choice of treatment follows a process of clinical reasoning. Observation and movement analysis in activities form the basis for hypotheses of which systems seem to be more affected and which ones seem more intact.

Clinical Example 1

The patient, Sissel, is asked to remove the wheelchair footplates **(Fig. 3.6)**.

Observation
- Sissel looks to her right (more affected side), weight transfers to her right, and reaches down to find the release mechanism to the footplate. She takes hold of it and adjusts her grip. She lifts her right leg off the footplate, taking a little help from her left arm. She then removes the right footplate.

Clinical Reasoning
- **Cognitive function:** Sissel remembers the instruction. She is attentive to her right, realizes where the release mechanism for the footplate is, integrates the information, and problem solves how to remove the footplate. She is focused and concentrated on the task. In this way, Sissel demonstrates that she understands, remembers, and solves the task. Her cognitive ability is good in this context.
- **Perceptual function:** She demonstrates adequate perceptual function through her attention to her more affected side. She receives, perceives, and integrates information from her more affected body part adequately for this situation.
- **Sensation:** Probably her sensation is good, because she is able to adjust her grip on the release mech-

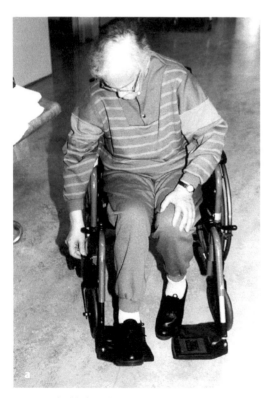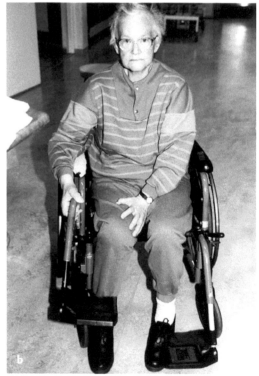

Fig. 3.6   (a, b) Clinical example 1.

anism even if she does not lean over far enough to make direct eye contact with it.

- **Balance:** Sissel's balance may be reduced because she uses her left arm to seek support on her right thigh and does not rotate her body far enough to gain eye contact with the release mechanism.

Clinical example 2

Sissel reaches for a tissue with her least affected arm (**Fig. 3.7**).

Observation

Sissel's posture is flexed both in the trunk and in the head and neck. It seems like her trunk is pulled down with the movement of her arm.

Clinical Reasoning

- Why are the trunk and head/neck kept in flexion as the arm reaches forward (activity domain)? Reduced trunk control affects the ability to coordinate forward displacement of the trunk and head with recruitment of arm activity. The anticipatory interplay between orientation and stability of trunk segments and arm function seems to be reduced (body domain).

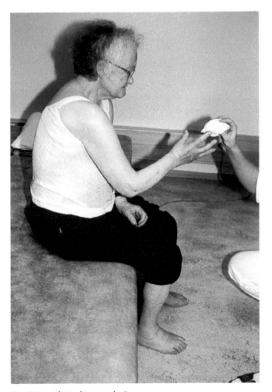

Fig. 3.7   Clinical example 2.

- She is dominated by flexion. Are the pectorals and latissimus dorsi muscles recruited excessively and/or too early to compensate for the reduced trunk control? Are the superficial neck flexors fixating to prevent her from falling? Do these compensatory strategies prevent her from recruiting more appropriate activity?

The therapist needs to sense and understand the differences in quality of movement and evaluate why these differences occur, to form hypotheses about causal relationships. Clinical reasoning follows through into treatment, which is continuously evaluated by the therapist. The therapist needs to assess physical and neuropsychological problems and decide on how these affect each other. Frequently there are combinations of dysfunctions. The therapist needs to analyze and interpret the data to inform or request supplementary examinations and treatments by the doctor, speech therapist, neuropsychologist, or others as needed.

Assessment and treatment are integrated in a continuous process.

3.3   Outcome Measures

The use of formal, validated, and reliable outcome measures to document change in neurological rehabilitation is necessary and also increasingly demanded. Most of these measures assess the patient's activity, and few focus on the assessment of impairments and how these may affect the patient's function. Most rehabilitation centers and hospitals have chosen some outcome measures that they prefer in their working context. The therapists need to decide on the best measurement tools to use. The measurement properties of reliability, validity, and responsiveness must be considered.

- Reliability: can the results be trusted?
- Validity: does the instrument measure what it is supposed to measure?
- Responsiveness: does the instrument detect changes in performance?

Detailed description of outcome measures is beyond the scope of this book, and only a few specific measures are mentioned.

▬▬▬   Measures: Body Domain

- The Trunk Impairment Scale (TIS) was originally developed by Verheyden et al (2004), and was further developed by Gjelsvik et al (2012) and called Trunk Impairment Scale–Modified Norwegian Version (TIS-modNV) (also available in English) (Gjelsvik et al 2012). The scale aims at measuring quantity and quality of trunk stability and movement in sitting, and is used to evaluate trunk function in two main domains: dynamic sitting balance and coordination, scoring 0 to 16 (16 max). Studies indicate that dysfunction in trunk control is a significant problem after stroke, traumatic brain injury, multiple sclerosis, and Parkinson's disease (Verheyden et al 2006; Verheyden et al 2007; Verheyden et al 2005). Verheyden et al (2005) and Hsieh et al (2002) refer to studies that demonstrate impaired trunk muscle activity and a correlation between paretic trunk muscles and limitations in everyday activities in patients with stroke. Postural and trunk control is a significant predictor of motor and functional recovery after stroke. Several authors recommend interventions aimed at improving trunk control in stroke (Cabanas-Valdés et al 2013; Hacmon et al 2012; Jandt et al 2011; Karatas et al 2004; Reisman & Scholz 2006; Ryerson et al 2008; Winzeler-Merçay & Mudie 2002).

- The Rivermead Visual Gait Assessment (RVGA) (Lord et al 1998) consists of two observations of the arms at swing and stance phases of gait, and 18 observations of the trunk and lower limb: 11 observations during the stance phase and 7 during the swing phase of gait. A four-point scale is used to quantify the degree of abnormality for each of the component items. A global score is calculated by summing the total numbers of scores, ranging from 0 (normal gait) to 59 (grossly abnormal gait). The RVGA can be used to measure change over time for patients with neurological disease and is sensitive to gait impairment (Lord et al 1998). There is indication of reasonable reliability and validity (Lord et al 1998). Our clinical experience suggests that the therapist needs time to learn this test, and that it is valuable to test intertester reliability between colleagues to ensure that they agree on how to evaluate the different items for scoring. In a test situation, the patient needs to be able to walk for 10 minutes but may take shorter breaks.
- GAITRite is a mat (5 m long) connected to a portable software tool for automated measurement of different gait parameters that are registered when people walk on the mat (e.g., maximum gait velocity, step-length, single- and double-stance phases). It is recommended that the person walk at many different speeds (as slow as possible, a little faster, normal preferred speed, faster than normal, and as fast as possible) to gain a reliable picture of the patient's walking ability and to compare with changes over time. By interpolation, a point estimate can be calculated for each of the variables at a normalized speed representative for that subject. Thus comparisons between test occasions can be done without the confounding effect of walking speed (Moe-Nilssen 1998). Results from the GAITRite have shown strong test–retest reliability and concurrent validity for healthy adults (Bilney et al 2003).

▧ Activity Measures

- The Postural Assessment Scale for Stroke Patients (PASS) (Benaim et al 1999) has been validated for stroke patients. It consists of two main domains: (1) maintaining a posture in sitting without support, sitting with support, standing without support, standing on paretic leg, and standing on nonparetic leg; and (2) changing posture through seven transfers including turning over in supine, supine to sitting, transfer between sitting, and standing and mobility in standing. These different items are measured on a four-point scale (0–3). Nearly 40% of the assessed stroke patients in Benaim et al's study (1999) scored 36/36 on day 90 poststroke. It is therefore recommended that more difficult items be added.
- The Berg Balance Scale (BBS) (Berg et al 1992; Finch et al 2002) consists of 14 standardized subtests scored on five-point scales (0–4), with a maximum (best) score of 56 (Berg et al 1992). Reliability and validity have been demonstrated in elderly people (Berg et al 1989; Berg et al 1992; Berg et al 1995), and scores below 45 may indicate increased risk of falling for elderly people (Bogle Thorbahn & Newton 1996). A recent systematic review concluded that the BBS alone was not useful for predicting falls in older adults with or without pathological conditions (Neuls et al 2011). The test has shown to be reliable, valid, and responsive to change in stroke patients (Mao et al 2002; Blum & Korner-Bitensky 2008). However, the BBS has floor and ceiling effects, thus it may not detect meaningful changes when used to

evaluate patients with severe balance impairment or those who have mild impairment (Blum & Korner-Bitensky 2008).

- The timed single-leg-stance test, or Single Leg Stance (SLS), measures, in seconds, the patient's ability to stand on one leg without falling. Normal values have not been decided, but the test seems to be relevant to demonstrate problems in activities where a one-legged stance is necessary (gait, stairs, turning around in standing and dressing). Many different ways of performing this test are described in the literature—it is not standardized (e.g., with or without shoes, eyes open or closed, etc.). Therefore, it is necessary to standardize it for the individual or the clinical setting in which it is being used. Its validity has been demonstrated by its relationship with other important variables, such as gait performance (Ringsberg et al 1998) and fall status (Vellas et al 1997). Several authors have suggested an upper limit of 10 seconds as a criterion standard for SLS times (Jacobs et al 2006; Morris et al 2000). For example, Jacobs and colleagues (2006) reported that an SLS cutoff of around 10 seconds provided the best sensitivity and specificity related to fall history in Parkinson's disease.

- Functional Reach (FR) (Duncan et al 1990) is a balance test that seems to have a strong correlation with ADLs. The person stands and reaches one arm forward at 90° forward flexion at the shoulder without changing her base of support. A mark is set on the wall at the tip of the patient's finger. She then reaches forward as far as possible without falling. A new mark is placed, and the difference between the two marks is measured in inches. The test should be repeated three times, and the median measure calculated. The measured distance demonstrates a relative risk of falling:
  - Not willing to try: 28 times greater risk of falling.
  - 1 to 6 inches (2.5–15 cm): four times greater risk of falling.
  - 6 to 10 inches (15–25 cm): two times greater risk of falling.
  - >10 inches (25 cm): very low probability of falling.

Measures of Walking

Walking speed (m/s) is calculated from timed walk tests.

- Timed Up and Go (TUG) (Podsiadlo & Richardson 1991; Finch et al 2002) was originally designed as a screening test for fall risk in the frail elderly and has been used extensively in people with neurological conditions. Time is measured as the patient stands up from a standard arm chair, walks 3 m, turns, walks back to the chair, and sits down again. The test has been found to be reliable and valid and responsive to change over time in elderly people (Barry et al 2014), as well as for patients with stroke (Persson et al 2014). TUG has been shown to be valid and to identify the risk of falling for community-dwelling older adults as well as for patients with stroke (Persson et al 2011). Patients who perform the test in < 20 s are assumed to be independently mobile.

- 10 m timed walk (10mTW) and 5 m timed walk (5mTW) are used to measure walking speed; however, the 10mTW has been validated with a wider range of conditions than the 5mTW and is thereby more generalizable (Tyson & Connell 2009), and has been shown to be a reliable and valid measurement tool in stroke patients (Tyson & Connell 2009).

- The six-minute walk test (6MWT) (Enright 2003) is used to measure the distance covered when subjects are instructed to walk as fast as possible for 6 minutes (Lord & Menz 2002). Standardized phrases should be used to instruct the patient to avoid the effect of encouragement and enthusiasm, which can make a difference of up to 30% in the 6MWT (Enright 2003). In older people, the 6MWT appears to provide a measure of overall mobility and physical functioning rather than a specific measure of cardiovascular fitness (Lord & Menz 2002). The 6MWT is believed to better reflect ADL performance than other timed walk tests of shorter duration (Solway et al 2001). The minimally clinically important difference (MCID) for change in walking distance is defined as 50 m (Lacasse et al 1996) and 30 m (Guyatt et al 1987).

▪ Self-Report Measures

A neurological disease or disorder affects emotion, memory and thinking, communication, and role function (ICF, social participation) as well as physical function. Hence, self-reported measures provide additional insights into the clinical status beyond what is provided by the physical measures:

- The Stroke Impact Scale (SIS) is a psychometrically robust, stroke-specific self-report measure developed to assess several dimensions of quality of life (Duncan et al 1999). It consists of eight domains (59 items in total). The SIS is a validated measure that enables a quantification of the patient's perspective on the impact of his or her condition (Jenkinson et al 2013).
- Borg's Rating Scale of Perceived Exertion (RPE) (Borg 1970; Finch et al 2002) is used to estimate the patient's experience of exertion on a 15-point graded scale from 6 (no exertion) to 20 (maximal exertion) after being active (e.g., 6MWT). According to Borg's range principle, a judgment of 50% of maximal exertion would have the same perceptual meaning for two people, even if it represented different absolute exercise intensity for each person (Buckworth & Dishman 2002). The scale values correlate well with exercise variables such as heart rate, ventilation, %VO$_2$ max, and workload (ARCM 1988).
- Visual analog scales (VASs) (Wewers & Lowe 1990) or numeric rating scales (NRSs) may be used to measure the patient's experienced gait problem, ADL problems, as well as pain. The patients are asked to estimate their perceived amount of problem on a scale from 0 to 100 mm, where 0 is no problem and 100 is the worst imaginable problem.

▨ Objective Goal Setting

A recognition and evaluation of patient-specific treatment goals is important in client-centered care (Stevens et al 2013); patients' active involvement in goal setting increases their motivation, participation, and satisfaction with regard to their therapy (Baker et al 2001; Hazard et al 2012). Specific, Measurable, Achievable, Realistic, and Time limited (SMART) (Monaghan et al 2005) is a valuable multidisciplinary tool that actively involves patients and their carer. In a physiotherapy setting, the therapist chooses a short-term goal together with the patient, after assessment and clinical reasoning. The goal should be task related and relevant to the patient's problems, resources, and needs, and achievable in a few days. The therapist decides the prerequisites for the goal achievement: quality, environmental factors, relevance for daily activities, and what kind of assistance, if needed. Preferably the patient should achieve the goal independently, but this may not always be possible. Individual goal setting in rehabilitation practice often proves to be challenging and is not always as patient centered as it should be with regard to people with severe language or cognitive impairment, poor insight, or a low state of awareness.

Patient-specific measures, such as Goal Attainment Scaling (GAS) is a method for quantifying progress on personal goals and used as a tool to encourage patients and professionals jointly to participate in goal setting with a client-centered perspective. The use of GAS depends on defining goals that are measurable. It is based on predicting an expected outcome, accompanied by two levels above and two levels below the expected outcome; thus creating a five-point scale (Ertzgaard et al 2011). By use of GAS, the team and patient are made aware that sometimes the patient achievement exceeds expectation, whereas at other times achievement is lower than expected (Bovend'Eerdt et al 2009). GAS is not a measure of outcome, per se, but a measure of the achievement of expectation; hence it cannot replace standardized measures, but it may be used alongside them to assist interpretation (Turner-Stokes 2011). For more examples on how to use this scale, the reader is directed to the book *Bobath Concept Theory and Clinical Practice in Neurological Rehabilitation* (Raine et al. 2009).

▨ Assessment Diagram

In the clinical reasoning process, it might be helpful to draw a body diagram to illustrate the interaction between body segments, the distribution of tone, selectivity, and specific problems (pain, altered sensation, edema, muscular shortening). The diagram can help give a quick overview of the sensorimotor problems and assist in the clinical reasoning process.

The diagram would *not* inform of causal relationships or about the patient's total situation, but it would sum up the findings of the assessment. It might be useful to make two or three illustrations: from the back, the front, and the side (**Fig. 3.8**). Associated reactions may be marked down on the diagram on the patient's more affected side in stroke. The symbols may demonstrate the degree of compensatory increased activity or fixation. The patient compensates in areas of the body that he can voluntarily control; therefore these may have to be used bilaterally. It may be appropriate to illustrate the difference between voluntary activation and pathology with different colors.

There may be a gradual transition between associated reactions and compensatory evoked strategies, and therefore difficult to decide which is which. The number of plus signs indicates the degree of increased tone in affected body parts:

- + Mild increased activity. Therefore variable in their expression depending on the activity requirements—what the patient attempts or is asked to perform. At rest they are not present.
- ++ Moderately increased activity. Quickly apparent when balance or movement is required, beyond the patient's control. Beginning of stereotypical patterning in associated reactions. The compensatory strategies vary with the activity to be performed.
- +++ Strongly increased activity. The associated reactions and/or compensatory strategies are fairly stereotyped even if the patient is not very active.

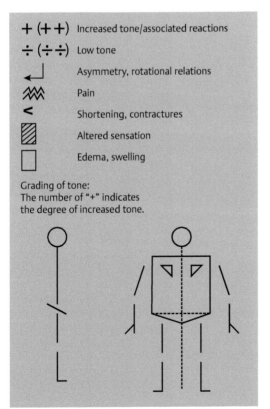

Fig. 3.8   Example of a drawing that can be illustrated with symbols.

The number of division signs indicates the degree of reduced tone in affected body parts:

- ÷ Mild reduced tonus or stability.
- ÷÷ Moderate paresis.
- ÷÷÷ Paralysis, that is, *no* tone or activity.

The diagram gives a visual impression of the patient's sensorimotor problems and does not reflect one position or situation. Free text may be added to highlight the following:

- Patient's main problem (primary neurological problem/negative signs).
- Patient's compensatory strategies (secondary feature).
- Patient's associated reactions/spasticity (secondary features/positive signs).
- Patient's clinical reasoning.

▄▄▄ Evaluation and Documentation

The assessment must be documented and serves many purposes: to document the assessment and treatment given, for communication between professionals, to evaluate one's own practice, and to give information to the patient. Documentation needs to include the following:

- Assessment.
- Clinical reasoning.
- Goal setting:
  - The patient's own goals (short term and long term).
  - Multidisciplinary goals (short term and long term).
  - Physiotherapy-specific goals.
- Outcome measures, which should encompass measures in the different domains of the ICF (body and activity domains). It may not be possible to set more than very general goals for participation if the patient is in the hospital or rehabilitation unit.
- Treatment intervention, both physiotherapy specific and multidisciplinary.
- Progression of treatment.
- Evaluation, including test results of the chosen outcome measures.
- Recommended further treatment or controls.

▄▄▄ Conclusion

The physiotherapist is the one professional on the multidisciplinary team who knows the most about movement and therefore is able to analyze specific movement in activities. Therefore, physiotherapists have a special responsibility to focus not only on the patient's activity performance but also on *how* the patient performs these activities, and *why* in this way. The hypotheses formed as a result of the assessment process are based on clinical reasoning, and view the patient in all ICF domains, although physiotherapy specifically aims at improving the patient's control of function, postural control, and movement. Clinical reasoning is the link between assessment, goal setting, and interventions and is a continuous process.

Summary

*Evaluating the patient's potential is an important goal of assessment. See page **178**.*

*What? How? Why? These are the three most important questions in the ongoing assessment of the patient. See page **189**.*

*The choice of treatment follows a process of clinical reasoning. Observation and movement analysis in activities form the basis for hypotheses of which systems seem to be more affected and which ones seem more intact. See page **194**.*

*Assessment and treatment are integrated in a continuous process. See page **195**.*

4 Case Histories

4.1 Chronic Stroke: Assessment, Treatment, and Evaluation

Social History and Activities

HS is a 45-year-old sales manager in an international company. He is married and the father of two. He used to work a full schedule and was physically fit. His hobbies included carpentry and football.

Medical History

In 2011, HS suffered an intracerebral hemorrhage, which was evacuated. He was in a coma for 1 week. When he regained consciousness he had no active movements of his left side and was subsequently wheelchair bound. Following a period of inpatient rehabilitation, he returned home, walking with a cane as a balance aid. He had an ankle–foot orthosis (AFO) on his most affected left ankle.

Initial Assessment

HS's foremost concerns were his balance and walking ability; he wanted to be able to walk independently to his summerhouse from his car. There is no parking near his summer house, so he has to park his car and walk to the house over varied terrain. His left hand and arm are stiff, and he has received repeated Botox (Allergan) injections for the last two years.

Table 4.1 summarizes HS's problems according to the International Classification of Function, Disability, and Health (ICF).

Initial Sitting Posture

HS's initial assessment included the following detailed description of his posture while seated (**Fig. 4.1**):
- Lateral flexion of head toward left.
- Reduced axial extension.
  - Thoracic spine toward flexion.
  - Posterior pelvic tilt.

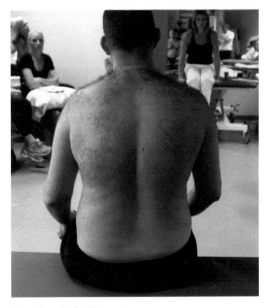

Fig. 4.1 Initial sitting posture.

Table 4.1   The problem list for HS according to the International Classification of Function, Disability, and Health (ICF)

Health condition	Lesion of the right hemisphere
Body functions and structures	Impairments • Weakness in ipsilateral (right) side of the trunk • Paresis of the left upper limb • Proximal weakness of the left hip and pelvis • Paresis and malalignment of left ankle Compensations • Compensates with right upper and lower extremities • Fixates left shoulder girdle • Retracts left pelvic half • Malalignment of head and neck
Activity dimension	See pictures and analysis of sitting, sit to stand, and gait Limitations • Walking independently in the terrain • Fast walking • Using his left hand in any activity
Participation dimensions	Restrictions • Social eating; needs help in cutting food • Does not go out as often as he would like • Joining family in activities

– Retraction of left pelvic half with the left side lower than the right.
• Retraction of left scapula and left chest wall.
• Left upper limb lower than right.
– Distance of elbows from body shows asymmetrical rotation of the glenohumeral joints and asymmetrical heights of elbows in relation to the trunk.

Two activities, sit to stand and gait, are analyzed in detail here for HS's case.

Introduction to Sit to Stand

The ability to stand from sitting is an important functional task that we perform several times every day. Sit to stand is essential for functional activities, such as transfers, ambulation, and walking up and down stairs (Lomaglio & Eng 2005). The sit-to-stand movement involves the whole body; different parts of the body are influenced and influence each other during the task. To stand up from sitting, the body mass must be transferred over the feet, which requires forward and upward displacement of the center of mass (CoM) of the body. Therefore a great demand is placed on both leg muscle strength and trunk control. The ability to perform sit to stand is an important predictor of fall risk and a main indicator of functional ability in stroke patients (Cheng et al 2004; Chou et al 2003). A person's balance, weight distribution through the lower limbs, and time taken to rise into standing are all important features to the efficiency of the sit-to-stand movement (Cheng et al 2004; Chou et al 2003). Neurological patients performing sit to stand often demonstrate compensations in different parts of the body, such as altered displacement of the CoM and asymmetrical lower limb weight distribution, as well as requiring more time to rise (Lomaglio & Eng 2005). The asymmetrical loading of the lower limbs and motor patterns influence the performance of activities that require interactions between the two sides of the body (Roy et al 2006). Asymmetrical sit to stand may affect the ability to stand upright and to gain midline control-negatively. As a consequence, the appropriate alignment between the vertebrae may be impaired as well as selective movement between the trunk and extremities (Chung et al 2013). Asymmetrical standing has been found to be associated with significant asymmetrical patterns of anticipatory postural adjustments (APAs) (Aruin 2006). During sit to stand, activation of the tibialis anterior (TA) muscle is an important

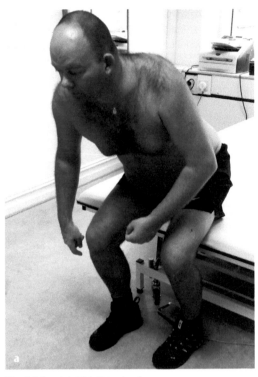
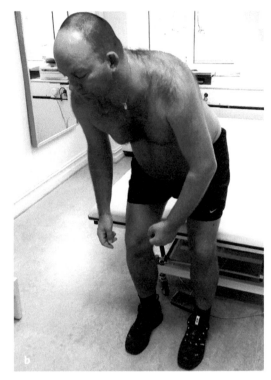

Fig. 4.2 (a–c) Initial sit to stand.

factor for APAs (Goulart & Valls-Solé 2001) because this muscle is active prior to the initiation of the forward motion of the trunk (Silva et al 2013). This activation is important for stabilizing the foot on the ground during forward trunk flexion and in setting an adequate stability level to allow the movement to happen without perturbations (Silva et al 2013). The lack of appropriate APAs combined with muscle weakness might be the reason why associated reactions are often elicited in the upper limb during this task.

The Bobath Concept considers independent sit to stand an essential goal for rehabilitation because it underpins independent locomotion and is connected with functional recovery of the upper limb and hand.

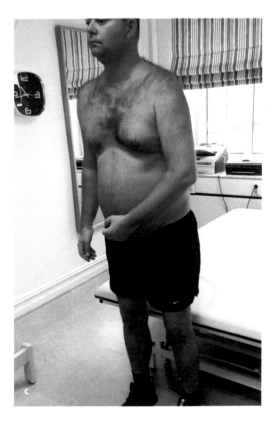

■ **Sit to Stand for HS: Movement Analysis and Clinical Reasoning**

HS was able to perform sit to stand without assistance, which was a positive indicator for his functional ability and placed him at a low risk for falls (**Fig. 4.2a–c**).

- HS initiates sit to stand through compensatory strategies of fixation through his right side, which leads to an asymmetrical movement.
- He shows excessive trunk flexion in the early stage of sit to stand, probably in an attempt to overcome the combination of trunk and lower limb muscle weakness. The degree of trunk flexion influences the coupling of trunk/hip flexion to potentiate lower limb extension; hence a greater degree of trunk flexion results in greater demands for and duration of lower limb extensor forces (Shepherd & Gentile 1994). Lack of core control further affects the ability to coordinate forward displacement of the trunk and head.
- HS uses excessive hip adductor activity, increased hip flexion, increased anterior pelvic tilt, and retraction of the left pelvic half, all of which further increase the difficulty in rising into extension.
- He has malalignment within the left foot and ankle compartment, which interferes with active interaction with the support surface. This influences the generation of APAs due to the fact that APAs are strongly dependent on the afferent input from the initial biomechanical conditions (Aruin et al 2003).
- His lack of stability during sit to stand leads to perturbation expressed by increased flexor activity in his left arm, which he uses as a postural fixation strategy.
- The asymmetrical weight bearing through the lower limbs in the last phase of sit to stand in which HS mostly loads his right leg, which leaves him with no alternative to initiate walking with his left leg.

■ Human Gait

Depending on the relationship between the foot and the support surface, the human gait is usually divided into two phases: stance and swing. The period of time when the foot is in contact with the surface is termed stance, and in the swing phase the foot is in the air for limb advancement. The human gait cycle consists of 60% stance and 40% swing phase. The gait cycle for one leg can be described in terms of initial contact, loading response, midstance, terminal stance, preswing, initial swing; midswing; and terminal swing (Raine et al 2009). Preswing is the transitional phase between a single-leg stance on one limb and limb advancement of the other.

The fundamental requirements of human walking include balance, stability, and progression (Shumway-Cook 2011). *Stable gait* refers to step-to-step repeatable walking (IJmker et al 2014); a gait flexible with regard to external and internal perturbations (Terrier & Dériaz 2011); or to the ability to maintain an upright stance during walking (Menz et al 2003).

Energy is required to generate muscle force for walking. Stroke patients expend up to twice as much energy as compared with healthy subjects walking at the same speed (Stoquart et al 2012; Platts et al 2006). The nature of this increase in energy cost is not fully understood. It may be due to increased muscle work because of stroke-related impairments, such as increased muscle tone, and/or the use of compensatory strategies. The latter is supported by Stoquart and colleagues (2012), who found that the increased energy cost in walking after a stroke was mainly due to mechanical work done by the healthy limb, mainly to lift the CoM.

Generation of the appropriate anteroposterior (AP) ground reaction forces by which the body CoM is advanced is essential for progression (Turns et al 2007). During normal walking, the propulsive ground reaction force (GRF) occurs in the second half of the stance phase (McGowan et al 2008).

The AP GRF of normal subjects is bilaterally symmetrical; however, subjects with hemiparesis often demonstrate significant asymmetries between the two legs. Consequently, to maintain a given walking speed, the nonparetic leg must compensate and generate a greater propulsive impulse (Bowden et al 2006).

Introduction to Initial Contact (Heel Strike)

The stance phase is the basis for generating and building up kinetic energy for the next swing: the stronger and longer the stance phase, the better the swing (Raine et al 2009). Proper foot motion, specifically subtalar pronation and supination, is critical to achieving stability and propulsion in this phase (Cote et al 2005). In healthy subjects a stance begins with the heel making contact with the floor in a slightly supinated position. Early in the loading response phase, the subtalar joint moves into pronation and achieves maximum pronation in midstance (Cote et al 2005). Subtalar pronation influences joints proximal as well as distal to it and reduces rotational stresses that would otherwise be transferred proximally. Adequate initial heel contact with the ground creates

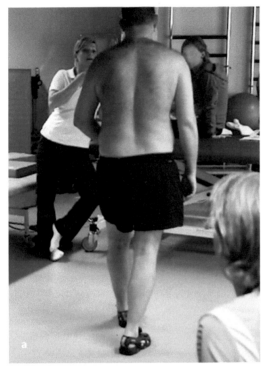

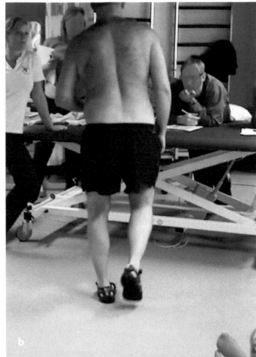

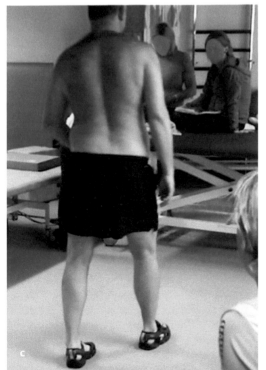

a basis for the role of the foot during stance, and a stable heel contact with the ground is essential for selective knee and hip movement in midstance (Raine et al 2009).

Following heel contact the trunk tends to rotate forward and over the stance leg causing rapid stride-to-stride horizontal accelerations of the trunk (Winter 1995). In the plane of progression, erector spinae activity and almost equal and opposite hip extensor moments are generated to prevent unbalancing of the trunk early in the stance phase (Anders et al 2007).

Initial Heel Contact for HS

HS demonstrates a supinated rather than pronated subtalar joint, with excessive torsion on the tibia; consequently he is not obtaining stable contact with the floor (**Fig. 4.3a**). At this moment in the gait cycle HS is at the end stance on the right leg. He demonstrates a suboptimal stance phase with right knee flexion, right lateral pelvic tilt, and forward rotation of the right shoulder girdle, and there is a lack of axial extension through the whole right side of the body.

Fig. 4.3 **(a)** Initial heel contact. **(b)** Initial midstance phase on the left (loading response to midstance). **(c)** Initial double-stance phase (preswing phase on the left).

Midstance Phase on the Left (Loading Response to Midstance)

When moving from heel strike to loading response, the subtalar joint should immediately pronate (Bolgla & Malone 2004), and maximum pronation is achieved in midstance (Cote et al 2005). This unlocks the subtalar joint and gives a flexible foot, allowing for adaptation to the ground, weight bearing, and stability of the body over the foot (Qaquish & McLean 2010). An important determinant of gait stability is the ability to maintain single-limb support.

Midstance for HS

During this phase, HS shows excessive supination and external rotation of the leg; hence the weight is carried on the lateral aspect of the foot (**Fig. 4.3b**). The adaptation of the foot to the ground is reduced and gives him a biomechanical disadvantage with regard to loading the leg and using the triceps surae for propulsion. Furthermore, his supinated foot gives a smaller contact area between the foot and the ground and consequently less sensory feedback to the central nervous system (CNS) to support the demand for stability during this phase (Cote et al 2005) .Thus, to maintain balance in walking, the demand on other parts of the body increase as compensation. HS demonstrates poor acquisition of midstance due to factors already mentioned; in addition he demonstrates weakness of hip and pelvic extension and abduction and thereby poor alignment of the hip/pelvis on the stance side.

The Role of the Trunk in Midstance

The trunk plays an important role in human locomotion. During walking, translation and orientation of the trunk serve the roles of navigation and upright stability, respectively (Anson et al 2013). The main muscle activity to maintain the posture against gravity and to facilitate propulsion is *extension.*

The trunk is a central key area of the body, and trunk control is a prerequisite for strength and control of the distal limb. Trunk control during gait involves keeping the body upright, adjusting weight shift, and performing selective movements to maintain the CoM within the base of support (BOS) (Karthikbabu et al 2011). The APAs in the trunk during walking prepare the trunk against the destabilizing forces imposed by the movement of the limbs and orient the trunk in space so that the desired motor output can be achieved via the focal movement. During the single-leg stance, trunk muscles need to stabilize against the moment caused by gravity. Furthermore, in the transverse plane, trunk muscle activity controls stride-related rotations around the longitudinal axis (Hu et al 2012). Activity in the erector spinae and hip extensor muscles is generated to prevent unbalancing of the trunk early in the stance phase (Kavanagh 2009). The hip abductor apparatus provides pelvic stabilization, and the gluteus maximus acts as a principle stabilizer of the trunk, controlling trunk extension at heel strike during the single-leg stance. The gluteus maximus makes a large contribution to gait, and ineffective muscle function can compromise many aspects of the gait cycle. The muscle contributes most significantly to support the lower limb via the vertical GRF during the early stance phase from foot flat to just after contralateral toe-off (Arnold et al 2005).

During walking, excessive trunk motion has been related to instability in older individuals and individuals with balance disorders (Allum et al 2002).

Trunk Control Midstance for HS

HS demonstrates trunk rotation to the left and lateral flexion to the left in this phase of the gait cycle (**Fig. 4.3b**); there is a lack of segmental selective extension bilaterally and therefore reduced postural control on both right and left sides. Reduced stability causes HS to compensate, which elicits significant associated reactions in the left upper limb.

Double Stance Phase

Walking speed after a stroke depends largely on the person's ability to control the paretic leg during preswing (Peterson et al 2010). Therefore, this phase in the gait cycle is important for both forward acceleration and generating knee flexion during swing. From midstance to toe-off the subtalar joint supinates and the foot is transformed into the rigid lever arm needed for propulsion (Qaquish & McLean 2010). In healthy walkers the gastrocnemius and soleus are important for generating plantar flexion moments about the ankle from midstance through the beginning of preswing (Francis et al 2013; Liu et al 2006). The ankle plantar flexor group and the hip extensors are important for creating propulsion of walking; therefore, the combination of increasing ankle and hip power generation has been proposed as an important mechanism in increasing walking speed. In addition to creating propulsion, the gastrocnemius muscle produces knee flexor activity during midstance by which knee hyperextension is prevented.

Double Stance Phase for HS (Preswing Phase on the Left)

During this phase of walking, the alignment of HS's left ankle joint is still dominated by excessive calcaneal supination and inversion (**Fig. 4.3c**); the plantar flexors are therefore unable to generate appropriate plantar flexion moments about the ankle, thereby reducing the propulsion force from this leg and consequently affecting his walking speed.

Efficient locomotion depends on the coordination of movement of the two hips (Hyngstrom et al 2010). HS demonstrates reduced right hip extension and an orientation of this hip toward internal rotation. Given the importance of hip sensory afferents for the regulation of locomotion, it is plausible that this alignment of the hip may interrupt the ability of accessing central pattern generator (CPG) activity with respect to limb loading and hip stability. Internal rotation of the hip combined with forward rotation of the right pelvic half makes it difficult to generate the abduction/extension and lateral tilt necessary for an optimal stance phase and propulsion of the right leg.

In this phase, HS's right upper trunk and shoulder girdle move anteriorly, causing a reduction of scapular setting, which increases the anterior displacement of the shoulder and contributes to the difficulty of appropriately activating the upper body over the lower trunk.

▨ Clinical Reasoning and the Formation of Hypotheses

Through clinical reasoning, the physiotherapist deduces the main problem that needs resolution and develops a hypothesis as to possible causes.

▨ Main Problem

The physiotherapist concludes that HS's main problem consists of reduced antigravity activity in the ipsilateral (right) trunk and weakness of the left hip and pelvis. Initially, there might have been a lesion to the ipsilateral pontine reticular pathway causing loss of preparatory postural adjustments (pAPAs) on the right side. In addition, the coma might induce the problems in the postural system.

▨ Hypotheses

The Main Problem Causes

The physiotherapist hypothesizes that HS's main problem leads to the following difficulties:

- Inefficient postural alignment for obtaining a stable stance phase and for head and neck alignment, which may further influence the function of the vestibular system and contribute to HS's balance problems.
- Too much lateral displacement of the pelvis and a poor acquisition of midstance on his left side during walking, which interfere with gaining appropriate alignment and stability of the left scapula on the thorax.
- Reduced gait speed, which may be related to weakness of hip extensors and ankle plantar flexors not working optimally due to the malalignment in the ankle joint. Weak plantar flexors can also contribute to hyperextension of the knee and loss of propulsive force (Moseley et al 1993). HS has problems with knee hyperextension in the stance phase, but he compensates for this by walking with a flexed knee.
- Loss of scapular setting increases displacement of the shoulder complex and contributes to the difficulty of activating the upper body over the lower trunk.

Compensatory Strategies

Reduced antigravity activity in the ipsilateral (right) trunk leads to an inability to support his trunk against gravity and causes a need to compensate with the following strategies:

- Excessive activity of the right shoulder, which, combined with weakness in the left lower limb, creates a biomechanical disadvantage and prevents HS from regaining optimal alignment and activation of the trunk.
- Excessive activity of the right upper limb and right lower limb hip flexors, hip adductors, and hip internal rotators results in asymmetrical weight bearing and reduced activation of APAs on the left side.

- Excessive activity of the left upper limb, associated reactions, and leads to postural fixation.

Compensatory Strategies Causes
- Retraction of the left side of the pelvis.
- Malalignment in the left foot: excessive supination and plantar flexion compromise the initial heel contact.
- Shortening of the plantar flexors and limited range of dorsiflexion impair movement of the tibia over the foot during the loading response and midstance (Cooper & Alghamdi 2002).
- Left leg becomes too short to reach the floor. The triceps surae and tibialis anterior fire premature during limb loading. As a consequence, the stance phase is shortened during walking, and the buildup of kinetic energy for the next swing is further compromised. The malalignment in the foot may cause the loss of an important source of information to the balance control system, which may further compromise balance in all standing activities.
- Reduced forward motion of the body over the left leg in stance phase leads to a posterior displacement of the center of gravity.

Additional Problems
- Limited awareness and integration of the left side of the body into his body schema leads to an insufficient anticipatory control to create a more appropriate postural set in sit to stand and for walking.

▨ Intervention

The following is an account of twice-daily physiotherapy over a 3-week period (3 × 5 days). The aim of the interventions was to identify if treatment based on the Bobath Concept would have a positive effect on the efficiency of sit to stand and gait in a patient with chronic stroke.

■ Intervention Overview

Both sides of the body play their respective roles for harmonizing balance and function (Pandian et al 2014) and are therefore important for organizing dynamic balance. Thus the first main goal of therapy was to increase the ipsilateral postural stability in the trunk and thereby reduce the need to compensate (**Fig. 4.4**). Furthermore, the weakness in his left side as well as the retraction of the pelvis and malalignment of the ankle had to be addressed. By improving the alignment of the foot to the ground his ankle strategy could work better and consequently improve his postural control in sit to stand and all standing activities, as well as further reduce his need for compensatory fixation. Due to the foregoing factors the alignment and activity of the left foot and ankle were important to address (**Fig. 4.5**). Plantar intrinsic muscles originate and insert within the foot itself and function to enhance the alignment in the foot, control the position of the arch, and stimulate proprioceptors on the sole of the foot to aid in standing balance. Impaired function of the intrinsic foot muscles leads to disadvantageous alterations in foot posture (Fiolkowski et al 2003). whereas training the intrinsic foot muscles may lead to improvement in foot posture (Headlee et al 2008). Research has demonstrated that the intrinsic foot muscles play an important role in supporting the medial longitudinal arch (Fiolkowski et al 2003; Headlee et al 2008) and contribute to balance control (Moon et al 2014; Mulligan & Cook 2013). In addition, the weakness in the left side was addressed both in pat and whole task practice, where specific muscle activation patterns combined with task specific sensory input were used for successful achievement of the task (Graham et al 2009) (**Fig. 4.6, Fig. 4.7, Fig. 4.8, Fig. 4.9, Fig. 4.10, Fig. 4.11, Fig. 4.12, Fig. 4.13, Fig. 4.14**).

The shoulder complex does not function in isolation. It is a part of the kinetic chain, including the lower limb and trunk (Kaur et al 2014). The scapula provides a link between the arm and trunk. Therefore, the scapula and the scapula–thoracic junction on the left side also had to be addressed (**Fig. 4.10**). Enhanced thoracic mobility and activity may facilitate scapular setting and improve trunk postural control and single-leg stance on the left. Scapular stability allows the upper arm to be laterally positioned on the trunk and in the appropriate alignment for swing during the gait. Improved scapular stability may facilitate better trajectory of the left upper limb and improve the alignment of the hand/arm.

The hand is represented in a vast cortical area, and sensory information from the hand is a potent source for enhancing body orientation and axial tone (Baccini et al 2007); therefore, it was important to include HS's left hand in treatment. This was done by facilitating contractual hand orientation response (CHOR) of the left hand during different interventions. The CHOR is a frictional contact of the hand to a surface that allows for the hand to begin its functional roles (Porter & Lemon 1995; Raine et al 2009) and can be used in treatment to facilitate the following (Raine et al 2009):

- Midline orientation.
- "Light touch contact" for increasing axial tone.
- Limb support and limb loading.

Treatment in Sitting and Kneeling

To reduce the fixation pattern of right shoulder flexion, purposeful and oriented distal movement demands the ability to recruit proximal stability and activation of both the ipsilateral and the contralateral trunk APAs (Raine et al 2009) (**Fig. 4.4a, b**). The left hand is kept in CHOR to improve interaction between both sides

Mobilization and Activation of Trunk and Hip Muscles in Various Postural Sets to Improve Integration between the Two Sides for Reciprocal Activity

The intervention aims to achieve linear extension of the trunk and letting go of this activity, reinforcing graded trunk extension and encouraging selective activity of trunk muscles (**Fig. 4.6a–c**). On this basis, the following functional activities may be facilitated: anterior pelvic tilt with upper trunk extension; forward reach; initiation of the transition between sitting to standing; and lateral weight shifts with trunk rotation for the transition from sitting to supine. Specific and selective activation of trunk muscles may lead to selective trunk activity and improved timing of APAs, and reduce the need for compensatory activity. Reciprocal activation of lower limbs may thereby be facilitated, as well as the possibility of training selective activity of the left upper limb. Improvement of core stability for more efficient forward movement of the trunk over the left foot provides a better basis for efficient weight bearing during sit to stand, which may result in reduced associated reactions in the left upper limb.

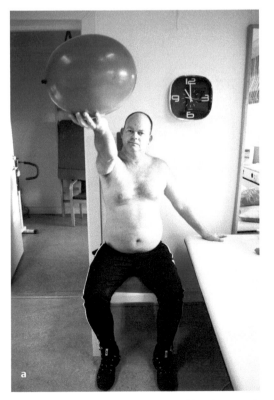
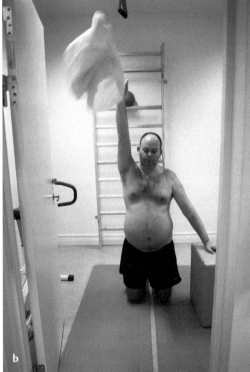

Fig. 4.4   (a, b) Intervention in sitting and kneeling to reduce right upper limb fixation and to enhance postural control.

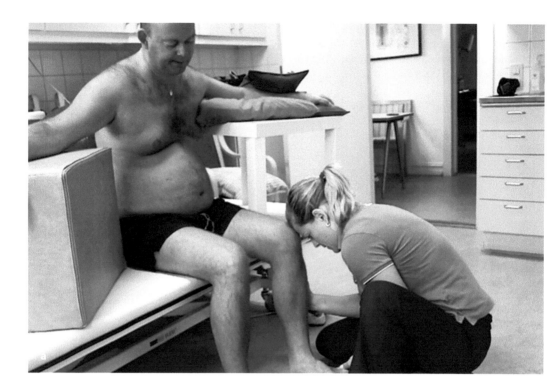

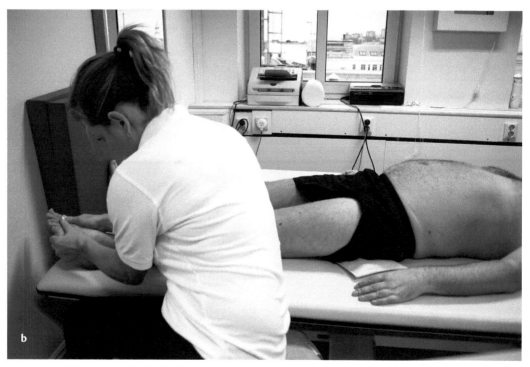

Fig. 4.5   (a) Activation of triceps surae for foot/floor interaction with gastrocnemius coactivating with eccentric soleus for heel down. **(b)** Using sensory stimulation to activate the intrinsic muscles of the foot.

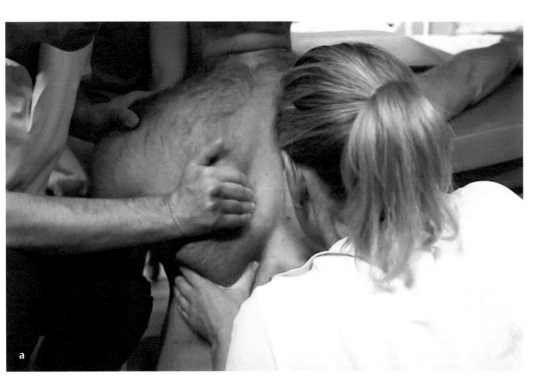

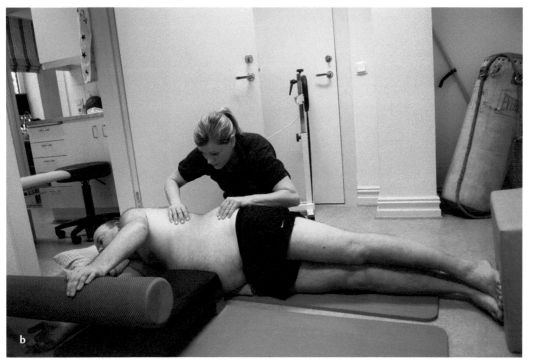

Fig. 4.6 (a) Intervention to mobilize and activate trunk musculature in sitting. One therapist facilitates scapular setting and the other trunk mobility. (b) Patient in side lying for activation of selective activity of pelvic and hip musculature. (*Continued*)

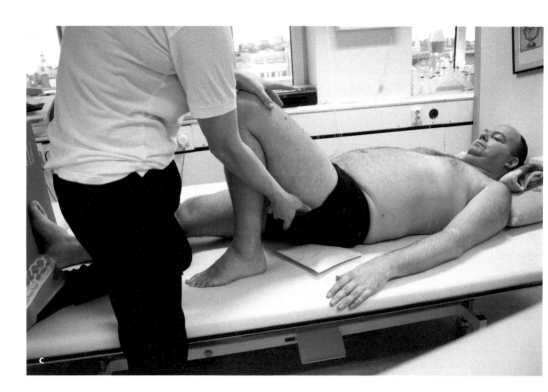

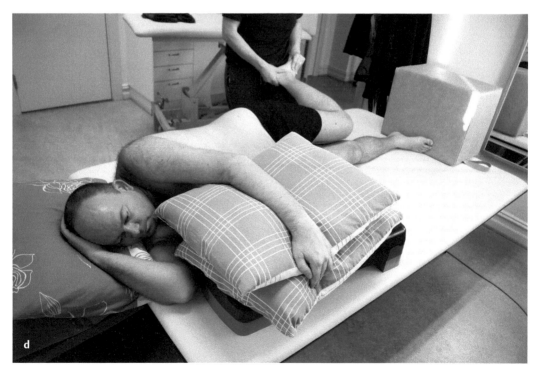

Fig. 4.6 (*continued*) **(c)** Selective activation of right hip extensors combined with facilitation of forward weight transfer over the foot as a basis for selective pelvic tilt. **(d)** Hip extension in side lying to improve sensory-motor integration.

In Right Side Lying, Stabilizing the Ipsilateral Side (Right) for Postural Stability for Contralateral Lower Limb Activity

A side-lying postural set may create the perception of a relationship between a stance leg and a moving leg that is context based to locomotion. HS's right leg was placed in an extended position to simulate a stance phase of walking (**Fig. 4.6b**). This might ensure that the cerebellum receives contextual proprioceptive information to increase the APAs in the right trunk. The left upper limb is kept in CHOR. The intervention aims to improve reciprocal activity of the trunk and pelvis with the purpose of preventing the retraction pattern in the pelvis and improving the alignment of the left lower limb, as well as achieving selective activity of pelvic and core musculature.

Selective Activation of Left Hip Extensors, Combined with Facilitation of Forward Weight Transfer over the Foot as a Basis for Selective Pelvic Tilt

This involves creation of active crook lying through activation of the foot as a basis for selective hip extension and pelvic tilt to strengthen the reciprocal activity in the hip and core muscles and facilitate forward weight transfer over the left foot (**Fig. 4.6c**). The hip and pelvic floor musculature serve as the base of support for the core. The hip musculature is involved with stabilization of the trunk as well as force and power generation during lower extremity movements (Sharrock et al 2011). An increase in hip extension, especially for the latter part of the stance phase, is important because hip extension strength is associated with moving the trunk forward over the stance foot. Thus the hip flexors are given an improved mechanical advantage for the generation of a swinging leg, resulting in a larger step length and an increased speed (Teixeira-Salmela et al 2001).

Hip Extension in Side Lying to Improve Sensory Motor Integration

The therapist facilitates hip extension from the heel of the left foot in side lying (**Fig. 4.6d**). Overuse of vision to check the foot position on the ground is a commonly used compensation for reduced body schema of the lower limb. Thus working in side lying allows emphasis on sensory-guided muscle activation of the leg without vision.

Part Task Practice: Facilitate Stop Standing with Bilateral CHOR

Facilitation of selective activity in core and hip musculature may be achieved through the task of stand to sit (stop standing) (**Fig. 4.7**). The transition from standing to sitting demands the ability to lower the body mass using eccentric muscle activity while sustaining postural stability (Raine et al 2009).

The intervention starts in standing with bilateral CHOR, and the therapist facilitates pelvic and hip movement in different stages of the stand-to-sit activity. In the Bobath Concept, facilitation is about building the patient's body schema. The facilitation given is always related to the task; the therapist aims to provide the patient with appropriate sensory information, which would be experienced during the specific voluntary movement in a healthy person. Therefore, in this example, the therapist uses hands-on to hip extensors and lower abdominals to facilitate activity in the main muscle groups involved in this task.

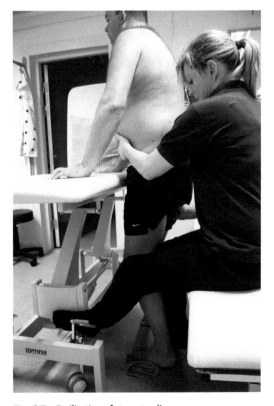

Fig. 4.7   Facilitation of stop standing.

Activation and Mobilization of the Left Foot/ Ankle

The following interventions aim to enhance the foot–floor contact by improving alignment and muscle activity in the foot and ankle joint (**Fig. 4.5a, b**). This may increase the afferent information from the left side; improve the orientation to the left side; improve the possibility to load the left leg in different activities; and further increase the extensor activity of this leg.

Facilitation of Selective Knee Extension with Dorsiflexion of the Ankle

Knee and ankle extensors are both antigravity muscles; an abnormal coactivation could contribute to hemiparetic gait disabilities (Dyer et al 2011). Impaired coordination may be manifested by the inability to activate muscles selectively. This intervention aims for strength training across multiple joints, by which movement of the entire lower limb is produced, and may result in improved coactivation, a greater increase in motor unit activity, and muscle reeducation, compared with training of muscle strength across single joints of the lower limbs (Son et al 2014). The patient sits with the arms out of compensatory patterns to prevent pushing down from the head, arms, and upper trunk (**Fig. 4.8**). Distal facilitation of the left foot is used to realign the foot and ankle and gain recruitment of knee extension, postural activity at the left hip, and contralateral core stability.

Task Practice: Training Sitting to Standing

As the patient achieved improved core stability in the trunk and a better alignment in the ankle, he achieved a more efficient forward movement of the trunk over the left foot during sit to stand. With the left hand in CHOR the intervention aims for activating the left ankle in a good alignment (**Fig. 4.9**). The patient lifts a balloon with the right arm to initiate the sit to stand without using the right arm for compensation. The use of the left hand in CHOR emphasizes the role of the hands

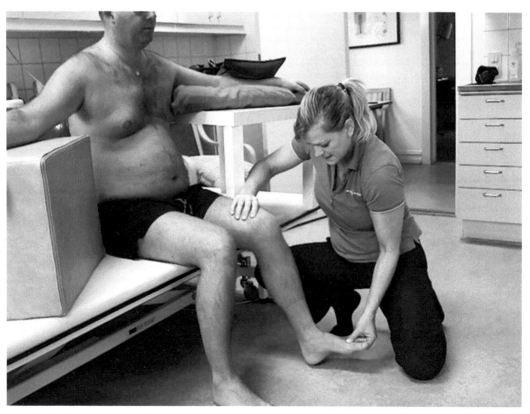

Fig. 4.8 Facilitation of selective knee extension with dorsiflexion of the ankle.

for interaction with the environment and disengages it from a role of fixator resulting from a lack of stability. With the hand in CHOR the CNS receives information about postural sway and enables feedforward motor adjustments, thereby facilitating the patient to more efficiently stand up from sitting.

Scapular Setting in Prone Lying

The treatment goal is to improve the interaction between the left shoulder girdle and the trunk, and selective strengthening of the muscles that facilitate scapular posterior tilting (SPT), which refers to movement of the coracoid process in a posterior and cranial direction while the inferior or angle of the scapula moves in an anterior and caudal direction (Clarkson 2005) (**Fig. 4.10**). The scapular stability is dependent on the activity and mobility of the thoracic spine, which serves as the base for its movements (Stewart et al 1995).

Strengthening the Plantar Flexors of the Foot

The intervention aims to improve the strength and reciprocal activity of the plantar flexors to increase the propulsion and thus walking speed (**Fig. 4.11**). Activation of the gastrocnemius facilitates eccentric control of the soleus. The soleus and gastrocnemius play key roles in forward progression and swing initiation, respectively, primarily during the double support phase of gait (Neptune et al 2004).

Exploring Upper Limb Movements with the Left Arm in CHOR for Increasing Postural Control in Standing

Fig. 4.12a demonstrates an intervention to integrate postural control and task performance (Graham et al 2009). The practice of a dynamic task in standing is a functional challenge to postural stability and allows the exploration of stability limits. However, free standing caused too much freedom of movement and thus compensatory fixation, therefore the standing position

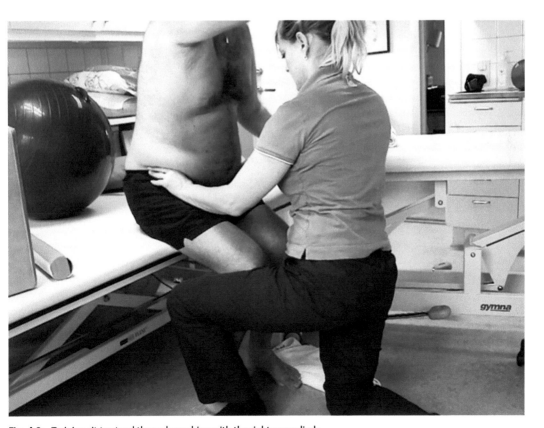

Fig. 4.9   Training sit to stand through reaching with the right upper limb.

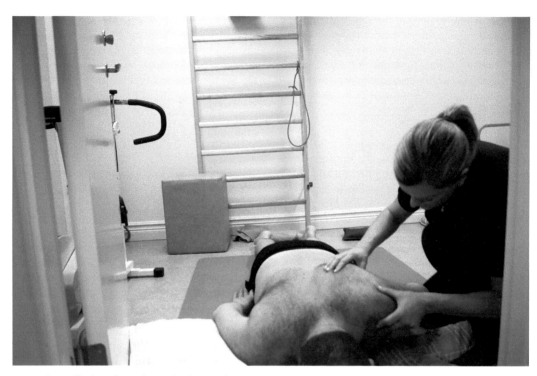

Fig. 4.10 Facilitation of scapular setting in prone lying.

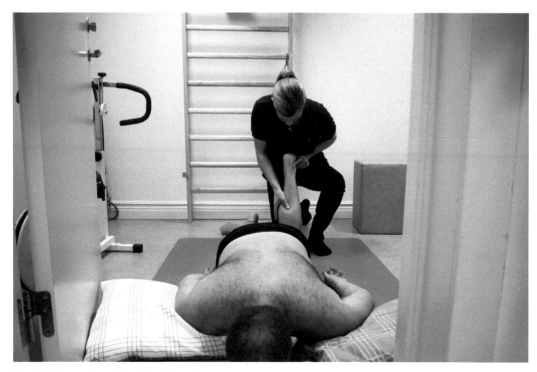

Fig. 4.11 Strength training of the plantar flexors.

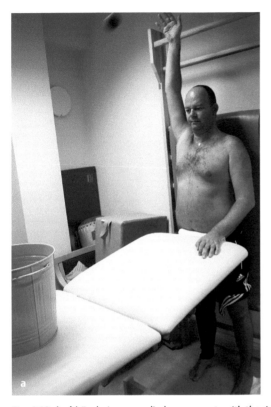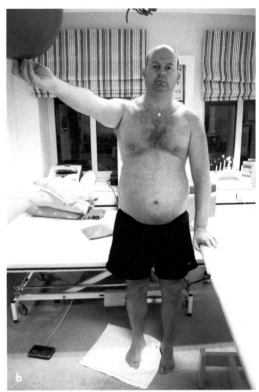

Fig. 4.12 (a, b) Exploring upper limb movements with the right arm in contractual hand orientation response (CHOR).

needed to be adapted. Changing the environment and providing an appropriate external support enabled the patient to perform complex motor tasks that, in turn, can improve postural control and selective movement (Graham et al 2009). With the use of CHOR and the wall as a support behind the patient, the degrees of freedom were limited, and the sensory input was maximized. In this way, standing postural control was optimized. A CHOR of the left hand was created; light touch on a stable surface appears to decrease postural sway during stance because of an associated increase in hip axial muscle tone (Franzén et al 2011). The task was to throw balls of different weight into a bucket using only the wrist and hand (distal selective movement). The throwing movement will demand APAs, and, due to the different weights of the objects to be thrown, compensatory balance strategies. Training that involves a functional activity, such as throwing a ball, may affect the generation of APAs prior to a predictable perturbation as well as the effect of the enhanced APAs on subsequent balance control (Aruin et al ok).

HS's standing stability improved to the point where he could increase the degrees of freedom and

still maintain balance without compensatory fixation (**Fig. 4.12b**), and he could start to explore right upper limb activity in a straight-line pattern while still keeping the left arm in CHOR.

Training Single Leg Stance on the Left with Left Hand in CHOR

This intervention aims to explore left leg stance control facilitating interaction of the left hand with the environment, thereby disengaging it from the fixator role (**Fig. 4.13**). Improved core control and enhanced alignment of the left foot to the floor allowed treatment to progress to the left stance phase to further improve postural activity.

Task Practice: Treadmill Training with Facilitation of Hip Extension of Leg and Lower Abdominal Activity to Promote CPG Activity and Gait Speed

Decreased paretic propulsion in gait may be due to decreased paretic leg extension in late stance (Peterson et al 2010). Activation of lower limb

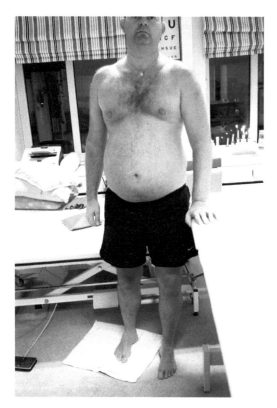

Fig. 4.13 Sliding a towel forward/backward with the right leg while standing on the left leg and maintaining contractual hand orientation response (CHOR) with the left arm.

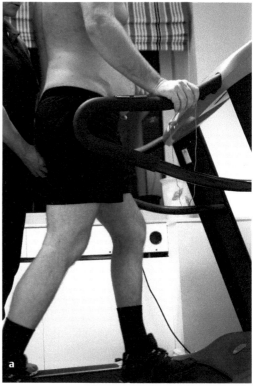

Fig. 4.14 **(a)** Treadmill training with facilitation of hip extension to promote reciprocal patterns of leg movements and gait speed. *(Continued)*

extensors for weight bearing during gait is known to be partly dependent on sensory input (Beres-Jones & Harkema 2004), and may be enhanced by treadmill training (**Fig. 4.14a**). The aim of the intervention was activation of CPGs for walking, which may potentially be achieved by facilitating appropriate loading and unloading of the limb, and hip alignment in the stance phase (Rossignol et al 2006).

Facilitation of Backward Walking
We walk backward daily, such as when stepping away from the sink, when opening a door, or when stepping back as a car passes by. It has been suggested that backward walking demands more balance and motor control (Hao & Chen 2011), as well as more stability than forward walking (Hoogkamer et al 2014). Without visual cues, backward walking relies more heavily on proprioception than forward walking and consequently can be used to update the body schema of the lower limbs. Backward walking puts focus on posi-

tioning the foot behind the body and thus facilitates hip extension (**Fig. 4.14b**). Using a step backward to initiate forward movement can increase force and power at pushoff and improve the temporal characteristics of the first step (Frost et al 2015).

Evaluation

Outcome Measures

5-Meter Walking Test
Self-paced walking speed is the most common outcome measure for gait-training strategies and reflects the ability to transport the body from one place to another in a timely manner (**Fig. 4.15**). The most used test is 10 m walking, but, for practical reasons, shorter walking tests can also be used. Here, a 5 m test was used; time was measured for the intermediate 5 m to allow for acceleration and deceleration; altogether a 7 m distance was used.

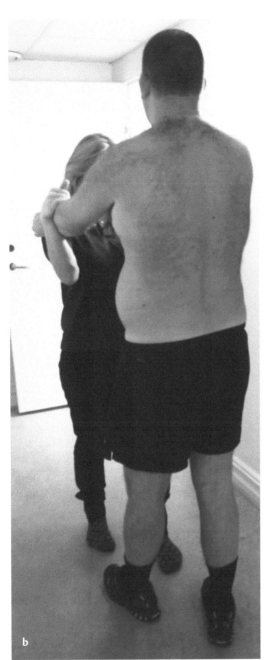

Fig. 4.14   (*continued*) **(b)** Facilitating backward walking.

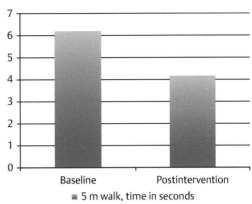

Fig. 4.15   The 5-meter walking test results pre- and postintervention.

(**Fig. 4.16**). A prerequisite for scoring is the ability to sit upright without support for 10 seconds. The scale consists of six items, giving a total sum of 0 to 16 points (16 highest).

Maximum Step Length (MSL)

Maximum step length (MSL) is the maximum distance that a person can step forward and successfully return to the original position without losing balance. The MSL test is as good a predictor of mobility performance and balance confidence as standard clinical balance tests (Goldberg et al 2010). The MSL test is a complex activity requiring coordinated activity of the proximal and distal lower extremity, as well as trunk musculature (Goldberg et al 2010).

HS's walking speed was 0.8 m/s in the preintervention period, and 1.2 m/s postintervention, which is an improvement in walking speed of 0.4 m/s (**Fig. 4.17**).

In a recent study, 0.05 m/s change in walking speed was calculated as the change needed for a meaningful improvement (Perera et al 2006). For patients who have a slower walking speed than normal, an improvement in walking speed of at least 0.1 m/s is a useful predictor of well-being (Purser et al 2005).

■ Sitting Posture

Comparison of HS's sitting posture preintervention (**Fig. 4.18**) and postintervention (**Fig. 4.19**) shows marked improvement in the following areas:

- More symmetrical head position.
- Improved axial extension

The Trunk Impairment Scale—Modified Norwegian Version (TIS-modNV)

The Trunk Impairment Scale–Modified Norwegian Version (TIS-modNV) (Gjelsvik et al 2012) was used to evaluate the quality of trunk control in sitting

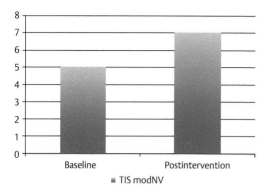

Fig. 4.16 Trunk Impairment Scale–Modified Norwegian Version (TIS-modNV) pre- and postintervention.

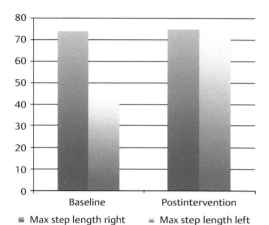

Max step length right centimeters   Max step length left centimeters

Fig. 4.17 Maximum step length pre- and postintervention.

- Thoracic spine in more extension.
- Pelvic component in better alignment.
- More symmetrical resting position of the scapulae and the upper limbs.

■ Observational Movement Analysis

HS's observational movement analysis covered sit to stand and several phases of gait.

Sit to Stand
HS showed improvement in a comparison of preintervention (**Fig. 4.20a–c**) and postintervention (**Fig. 4.21a–c**) sit to stand:
- Initiation of sit to stand using less compensatory strategies through the right side enables transfers from sit to stand with better symmetry.

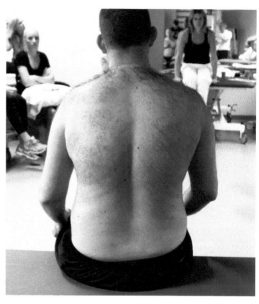

Fig. 4.18 Initial sitting posture.

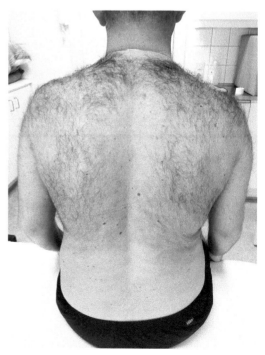

Fig. 4.19 Sitting posture postintervention.

- Improved core control and ability to coordinate forward displacement of the trunk and head. This improved timing and feed-forward control and reduced unwanted compensatory strategies.
- Improved lower limb strategies and alignment of the foot to the floor allow improved left leg involvement in the task and improved rise into extension.
- Loading of both legs gives HS the choice of initiating walking with either leg.

Gait

HS also showed improvement in pre- and postintervention comparisons of several phases of gait.

- Initial contact (heel strike) (**Fig. 4.22a, Fig. 4.23a**).
  - Longer step with left leg.
  - Improved heel contact with the floor with better alignment of the subtalar joint, providing a better contact with the floor.
  - Better stance phase with improved knee and hip extension on the contralateral leg.
- Midstance phase on the left (single-leg support) (**Fig. 4.22b, Fig. 4.23b**).
  - Some improvement of knee extension on the left side and improved alignment of the hip and pelvis on the left side.
  - Improved alignment of the trunk with less rotation and better extension, and, consequently, a better alignment of the head.
  - Less flexion of the right leg (hypothesis: HS demonstrates a less cortically driven flexion pattern and consequently a more automatic and CPG-driven walking pattern).
- Double-stance phase (**Fig. 4.22c, Fig. 4.23c**).
  - Improved step length of the right leg.

  - Improved extension of the left hip with better alignment of the hip/pelvis.
  - Improved stability of upper trunk and shoulder girdle over the lower trunk, with more trunk extension and better scapular setting.

■ Discussion

The aim of this case was to identify if intervention based on the Bobath Concept would have a positive effect on the efficiency of two activities: sit to stand and gait, in a patient with chronic stroke. Five main impairment areas were found in the assessment: (1) reduced antigravity activity in the trunk, (2) malalignment of the left ankle/foot component, (3) reduced strength in the left pelvis, (4) hip and knee and malalignment, and (5) weakness in the left upper limb. It was hypothesized that specific and selective activation of trunk muscles and improved alignment in the left ankle would improve trunk control, lower limb weight bearing, and whole body postural control as well as reduce compensatory fixations, and consequently improve the patient's ability to sit to stand and to walk.

■ Conclusion

Outcomes of this case study suggest that a patient with chronic stroke undergoing an intense, individually designed, 2-week intervention based on the Bobath Concept can improve walking and sit-to-stand function.

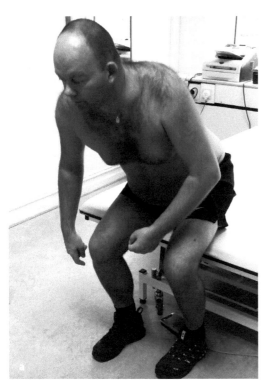
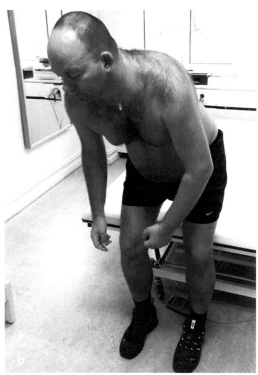

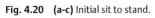
Fig. 4.20   (a-c) Initial sit to stand.

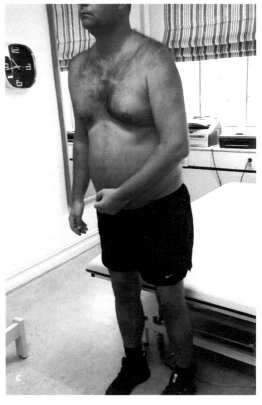

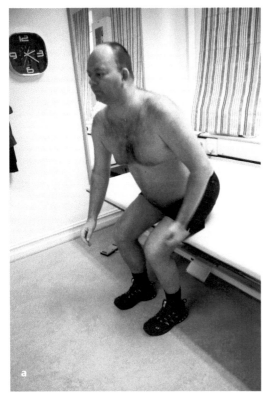
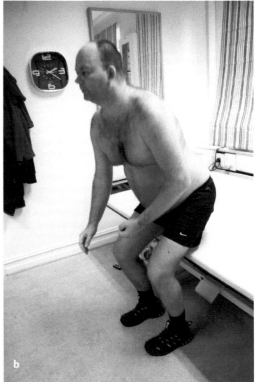
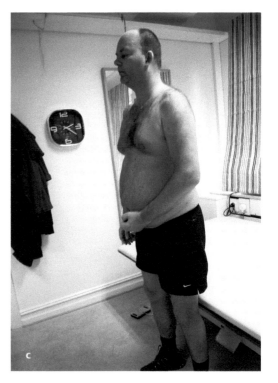

Figs. 4.21 (a–c) Sit-to-stand postintervention.

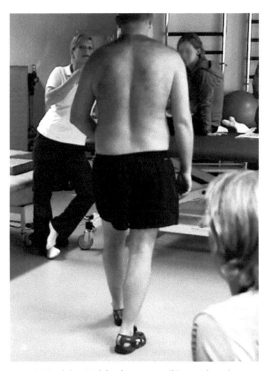

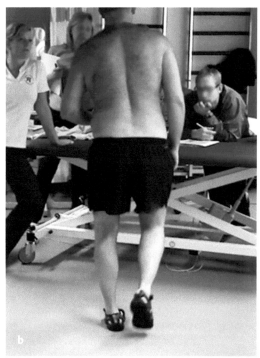

Fig. 4.22 (a) Initial heel contact. **(b)** Initial midstance phase on the left (loading response to midstance). **(c)** Initial double-stance phase (preswing phase on the left).

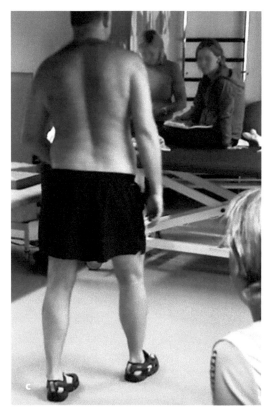

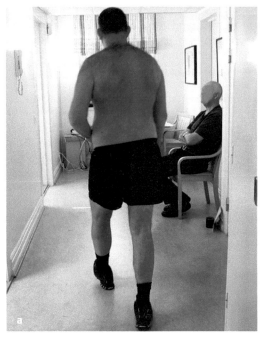

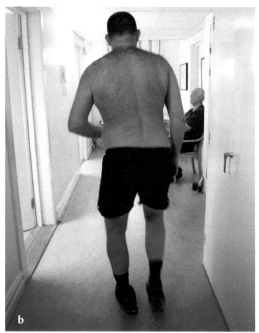

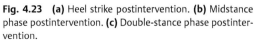

Fig. 4.23 **(a)** Heel strike postintervention. **(b)** Midstance phase postintervention. **(c)** Double-stance phase postintervention.

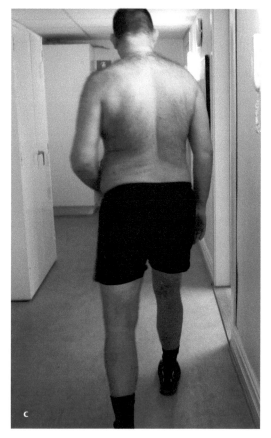

4.2   Cerebellar Ataxia: Assessment, Treatment, and Evaluation

▮▮ Social History and Activities

Avelino is 57 years old, and a baker in his own bakery-pastry shop. He is married and has three children. He lives with his wife and daughter. His hobbies were cycling and hiking.

▮▮ Medical History

He has a history of hypertension. He fractured his left leg at the age of 12 in a motorcycle accident (the proximal third of the femur and the distal third of the tibia and fibula). In April 2012 he suffered a hemorrhagic stroke in the cerebellum. A week later, his condition deteriorated, and he became unconscious. Repeated brain tomography showed a left hemispheric cerebellar hematoma and obstructive hydrocephalus. He underwent evacuation of the left hemispheric hematoma and received a ventricular shunt. Thereafter, he showed clinically and radiographically favorable development. At that time he had no balance in standing with marked incoordination of the left body side. He was an inpatient for almost 1 month for rehabilitation. After discharge he attended the rehabilitation outpatient unit three times per week.

▮▮ Initial Assessment

Table 4.2 summarizes the problem list for Avelino according to the ICF.

▮▮ Clinical Reasoning

Avelino shows decreased postural control; observed through the reduction of postural orientation and postural stability in standing. The malalignment in this position is caused by the difficulty in integrating the left leg in his body geometry (Fig. 4.24). The left foot orientation influences the entire lower limb alignment, contributing to the decrease of hip APAs, thereby favoring a pattern of left hip external rotation. The

patient uses a wide base of support and overuses the contralateral hip adductors in a fixation strategy (instead of the abductors and extensors) in an attempt to find stability against gravity. The reduced stability limits lead to a reduction in anticipatory postural control. The wide base of support is a safety strategy that impairs the creation of a single-leg stance on the left. The creation of a left single-leg stance is not possible because of difficulties in controlling the ankle strategy and thereby moving the pelvis to neutral/posterior with adequate hip activity as a basis for core stability. The difficulty in creating the left lateral extensor component influences the ability for selective movement on the right side. The lack of adaptation and orientation of the left foot to the ground further accentuates the weakness of the left pelvic girdle, thereby negatively influencing the role of the hip/pelvis as a base for core stability muscles and trunk stability. The patient has a kyphosis of his thoracic spine (Fig. 4.24), causing a malalignment of both scapulae on the ribcage; decreased activity of the dynamic stabilizers of the left scapula is most evident (Fig. 4.24). Loss of scapular setting increases the anterior displacement of the shoulder and contributes to the difficulty of activating the upper body over the lower trunk. All this contributes to forward head displacement and right head rotation interfering with interpretation of vestibular information from cervical afferents (Fig. 4.24). *Hypothesis: the foregoing findings may be the basis for the projection of the center of mass forward, which negatively influences postural control in standing.*

The patient shows difficulty in combining the appropriate anticipatory activity across several muscles and modifying that muscle activity in response to changing demands, leading to compensatory proximal fixing strategies for the performance of distal movements. Loss of APAs of the left scapula also increases the left-hand dysmetria and affects the capacity for multijoint movements like sit to stand and stand to sit.

Fear of falling, as reported by the patient, influences the APAs, causing a stiffening strategy that limits the movement choices. Automatic balance strategies in response to external perturbations are affected, and the patient is unable to scale the size of his postural responses to stance perturbations and tends to overrespond. The patient's first pattern of choice for controlling upright sway is the hip strategy (instead of ankle strategy, which would

Table 4.2 The problem list for Avelino according to the International Classification of Function, Disability, and Health (ICF)

Health condition	Cerebellar ataxia after surgery for evacuation left hemisphere cerebellar hematoma obstructive hydrocephalus
Body functions and structures Domain	Poor core control Weakness (L) shoulder and (L) pelvis girdle Decomposition of movement (L) Dysmetria (L) Head fixation (R) Shoulder and (R) pelvis girdle fixation ↓ Multijoint movements Difficulty in dual-task ↓ Adaptation to the environment ↓ Postural control in standing • Malalignment in standing • ↓ Anticipatory postural adjustments • Modified stability limits • Difficulty in creating a (L) single-leg stance • ↓ Ankle strategy • Overresponds with hip strategy • ↑ Postural sway Gait • Wide base of support (BOS) • Visual dependence • Prolonged double support period • ↓ Interlimb coupling • Compensatory activity in upper limb
Activity Dimension	Mobility activities • Inability to get up from the floor • Inability to carry objects with both hands • Inability to stand up from a low chair • Inability to walk at fast speed and in uneven terrain Daily activities • Inability to dress and undress in standing position • Difficulties in using the left arm during feeding activities and fine dexterity, such as pushing buttons
Participation Dimension	Participation restrictions • Get out of home alone • Provide own meals • Take care of own health • Go out to public places alone • Cannot develop his profession

Contextual Factors

Environment Factors		Personal Factors
Facilitators	**Barriers**	• Collaboration
• Family support • Friends support • Spacious house with garden	• Stairs at home	• Motivation • Fear of falling • Hypertension • At age 12 fractured left leg in two places (proximal third of femur and the distal third of tibia and fibula)

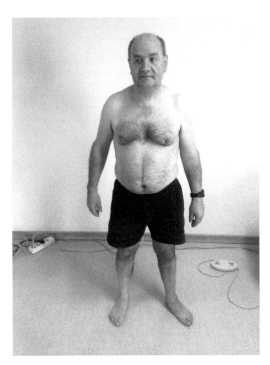

Fig. 4.24 Initial standing posture.

be used normally), which further increases the postural instability.

Initial Standing Posture

Impaired balance in standing increases the cortical regulation of gait, making it more cognitive instead of an automatic gait, thereby hindering dual-task ability. Variability of foot placement and stride length increases postural instability and leads to excessive use of vision. The wide base of support affects the activation of hip abductors for selective lateral extension and selective weight transfer through propulsion, increasing compensatory use of the right arm that attempts to guide the left leg and thereby limits the interlimb coupling between arms and legs (**Fig. 4.25a, b**). Double support time is increased, further reducing gait rhythm and speed.

Hypotheses

- Improving selective activation of core muscle control promotes efficiency of feedforward and

feedback postural control strategies and the ability to control the center of mass (CoM) over the base of support (BoS) and thereby improve stability limits.

- Improving alignment of the head and neck as the head fixation strategy negatively impacts the interpretation of vestibular information from cervical afferents.
- Improving ankle strategy leads to improved stability in standing.
- Creation of the left single-leg stance facilitates internal representation of stability limits and a reciprocal gait pattern.

Outcome Measures

Balance Evaluation Systems Test (BESTest)

The BESTest consists of 36 items, grouped into six systems: Biomechanical Constraints, Stability Limits/Verticality, Anticipatory Postural Adjustments, Postural Responses, Sensory Orientation, and Stability in Gait.

The BESTest is easy to administer, with excellent reliability and very good validity. It is unique in allowing clinicians to determine the type of balance problems to direct specific treatments for their patients and is the most comprehensive clinical balance tool available (Horak et al 2009).

International Cooperative Ataxia Rating Scale (ICARS)

The International Cooperative Ataxia Rating Scale (ICARS) is a commonly used evaluation tool and is composed of four clinical subscores: posture and gait, limb coordination, speech, and oculomotor function.

The ICARS has demonstrated high interrater reliability, even without prior observer standardization, and is sensitive to a range of ataxia severities, from very mild to severe (Storey et al 2004).

Falls Efficacy Scale

This 10-item scale measures confidence in performing a range of specific activities of daily living without falling. The Falls Efficacy Scale-International (FES-I) has acceptable reliability and validity in different samples in different countries. This tool measures the level of concern about falling

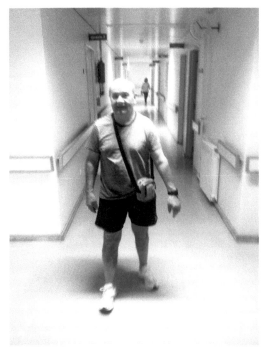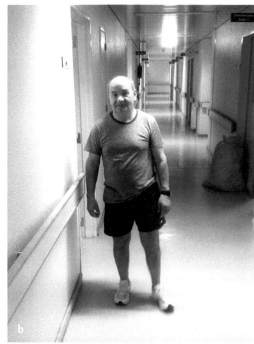

Fig. 4.25   (a, b) Initial gait pattern.

during social and physical activities inside and outside the home whether or not the person actually does the activity. The level of concern is measured on a four point Likert scale (1=not at all concerned to 4=very concerned) (Yardley et al., 2005).

Intervention

The patient received treatment three times per week (1 hour of treatment per session) for 10 weeks. During this period, the patient was assessed at three time points. The intervention was based on the Bobath Concept and included detailed assessment, clinical reasoning, and intervention processes related to assessment findings. This intervention was based on the type of interventions described in Raine et al (2009). The treatment intervention was developed according to the patient's goals—to walk outdoors independently without fear of falling and return to work—as well as the main goal of therapy, which was to increase postural stability to reduce fixation strategies and thereby improve postural control in standing.

Initially, alignment/orientation of the left foot was provided as a reference for appropriate activation of the left leg (**Fig. 4.26**), allowing a reduction

of the wide base of support and the potential for improving extensor activity of the left hip and activation of core stability (**Fig. 4.27**).

At the same time, creation of a right CHOR assists the recruitment of postural control. During stance, postural tone and postural sway may be influenced through light touch because touching a stable contact with the hand provides an additional reference system for trunk postural control that may strongly influence perception of self- and world-motion (Gurfinkel & Levik 1993; Lackner et al 1999; Franzén et al 2011). Improved alignment in the midline enabled facilitation of selective standing to sitting (stop standing) through the pelvis (**Fig. 4.28**).

In sitting, the stability of the right side of the trunk was maintained by using a plinth on the patient's right side to prevent compensatory strategies, limit the degrees of freedom in the trunk, and better isolate movements of the left hip. This postural set was essential for the specific mobilization of the left hip in relation to a stable trunk (**Fig. 4.29**).

Improved postural control in sitting allows for selective facilitation from sitting to supine to specifically activate core stability muscles. Training of core muscles improves the expression of APAs and thereby stabilizes the body axis to free the limbs.

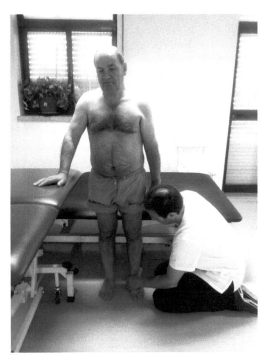

Fig. 4.26   Left foot alignment/orientation with a contractual hand orientating response (CHOR) to facilitate postural control in standing.

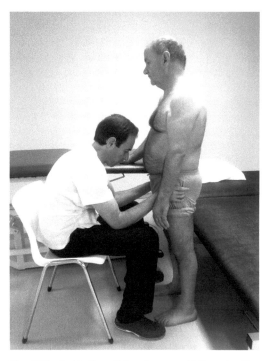

Fig. 4.27   Facilitation of hip extensors activity and activation of core stability.

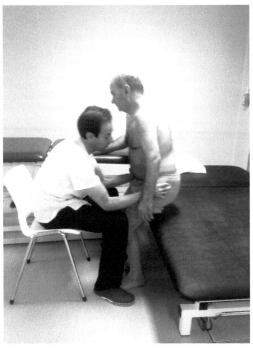

Fig. 4.28   Facilitation of stop standing.

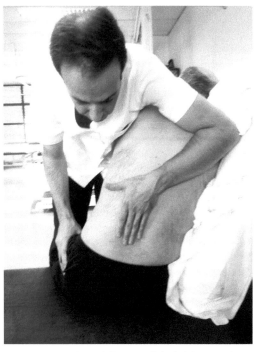

Fig. 4.29   Specific mobilization of the left hip in relation to a stable trunk.

Core stability involves dynamically controlling and transferring large forces from the upper and lower extremities through the core to maximize performance and promote efficient biomechanics. A weak core results in less force production and inefficient movement patterns (Sharrock et al 2011). Sitting on a ball with the patient's legs resting on the legs of the therapist facilitated posterior tilt of the pelvis for selective activation of abdominals using the movement of the ball together with the therapist's trunk extension; this activated the patient's core muscles combined with hip extension (**Fig. 4.30**).

The combination of core muscle recruitment depends on the demands of the task (Behm et al 2010). Different core exercises that challenge the core musculature at different intensities of muscle activation are required to result in stability or strength enhancements (Hibbs et al 2008). Core exercises were performed to strengthen these muscles, initially with the assistance of a second therapist to facilitate head control to improve a better relationship of the head to the trunk to stop the patient using head hyperextension to activate core muscles (**Fig. 4.31, Fig. 4.32**).

Two patterns of APAs in neck muscles are used in anticipation of perturbation acting directly on the head: a time-shifted (reciprocal) pattern is more likely to be used in anticipation of a perturbation acting directly on the head, and a simultaneous activation (coactivation) pattern is used when direction of head perturbation cannot be predicted with certainty (Danna-Dos-Santos et al 2007). Giving a strong reference to the right foot in stable crook lying, facilitated from left foot dorsiflexion as a basis for selective hip extension activation, the patient increases extension through his right side (**Fig. 4.33**).

The gluteal muscles stabilize the trunk over a planted leg to supply power for forward leg motion (Sharrock et al 2011). Improved pelvic stability allowed for better organization of the lower trunk to achieve stable side lying. This postural set creates the perception of the relationship between a stance leg and a moving leg, which is context based to locomotion. Activation and strengthening of hip abductors are a prerequisite for creating a single-leg stance to the left (**Fig. 4.34**). There is a close association between hip abductor function and segmental alignment of the femur, pelvis, and trunk (Grimaldi 2011).

With better pelvis and lower trunk activation it was possible to achieve a more active sitting posture to explore scapular–thoracic alignment. Scapular setting is a prerequisite to achieve ankle strategy,

head-placing response, and reaching. Forward trunk flexion reduces head overactivity through head stabilization and allows facilitation of scapular setting (**Fig. 4.35**). The key scapular muscles for scapular stability and mobility are the upper and lower trapezius and serratus anterior (Kibler et al 2013). These stabilizing muscles need to be recruited before movement of the upper limb (Mottram 1997). Improvement of scapular setting decreases shoulder anterior displacement and allows a better relationship of the head with the upper trunk, which facilitates APAs in the trunk for the creation of selective extension in sitting.

Single-leg stance involves greater postural control and APAs and is a bilateral movement with different demands to each side of the body. A single-leg stance requires the postural control system to reorganize the total body CoM over a narrow BOS (Riemann & Schmitz 2012). Facilitation from high sitting will allow the creation of a single-leg stance over the left leg (**Fig. 4.36**). Using concentric dorsiflexion to achieve ground contact, hip and knee extension are facilitated.

Improving single-leg stance facilitates a reciprocal gait pattern. Similar ankle–hip coordination patterns in walking and single-limb standing might imply a unique biomechanical configuration in the lower extremity (Liu et al 2012). Subsequently, the patient was given a strong reference for hip abductors in the direction of the heel to control the displacement, and the patient was able to explore upper limb movements in single-leg stance (**Fig. 4.37**).

The patient's head fixation strategy limits his oculomotor responses to visual stimuli. The postural relationship of the head with the trunk is a major factor determining the integration of sensory feedback and can be interfered with by varying head orientation (Johnson & Van Emmerik R 2012). Head orientation was facilitated in sitting (**Fig. 4.38**), and later in standing with bilateral hand contractual orientating responses (**Fig. 4.39**). Light touch on a stable surface appears to decrease postural sway during stance because of an associated increase in hip axial muscle tone (Franzén et al 2011). Consistent changes in the orientation of the head require flexible coordination of lower extremity and lower trunk segments with motion of the cervical spine (Park et al 2012).

In standing, with bilateral CHOR, active plantar flexion was facilitated, followed by selective eccentric activation of this muscle group (**Fig. 4.40**).

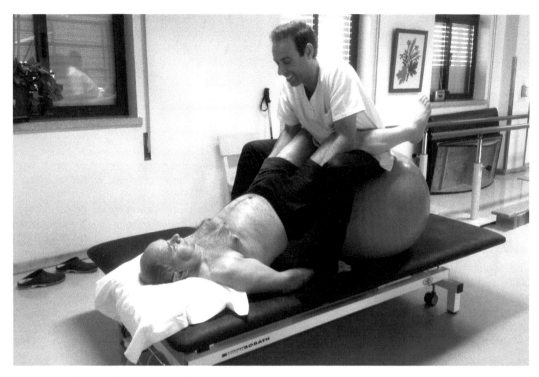

Fig. 4.30   Facilitation of core control with hip extension.

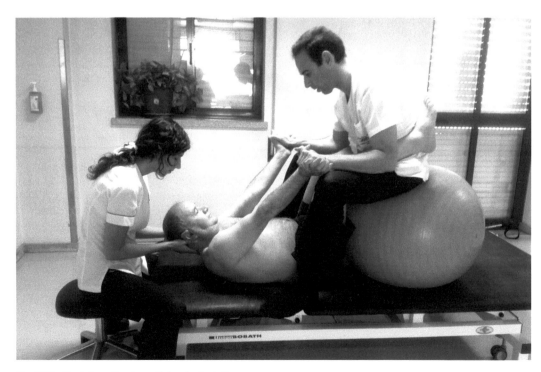

Fig. 4.31   Core strengthening with head orientation.

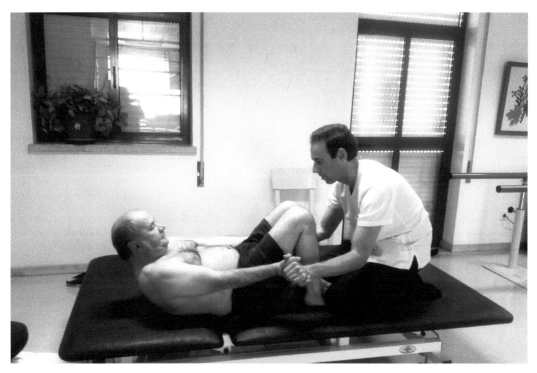

Fig. 4.32   Core strengthening through reach of the arms.

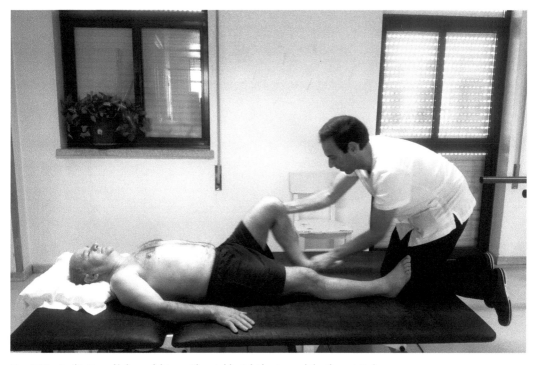

Fig. 4.33   Facilitation of left crook lying with a stable right leg toward the therapist's knee.

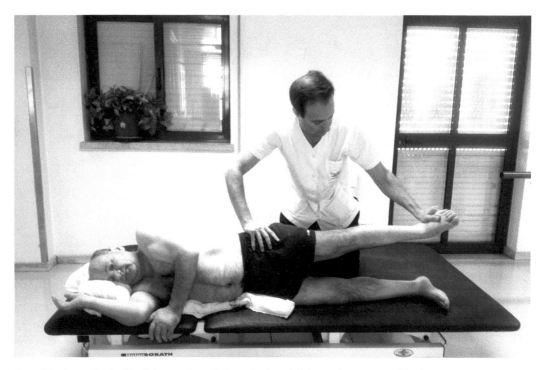

Fig. 4.34   Strengthening hip abductors through the activation of abductor digiti minimi of the foot.

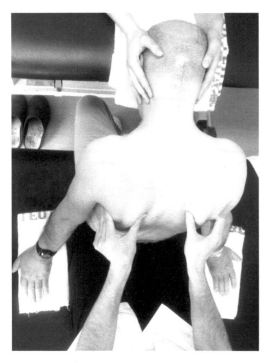

Fig. 4.35   Facilitation of scapular setting with head stabilization to reduce head overactivity.

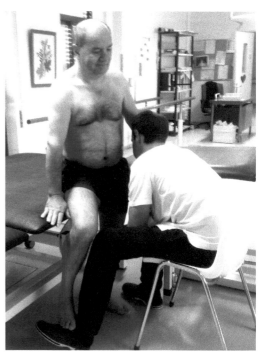

Fig. 4.36   Facilitation of single-leg stance from higher plinth.

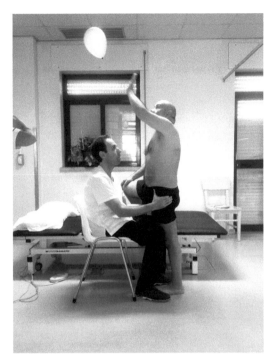

Fig. 4.37 Exploring upper limb movements in single-leg stance.

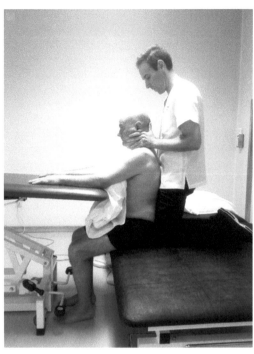

Fig. 4.38 Head orientation to midline in sitting with a stable trunk.

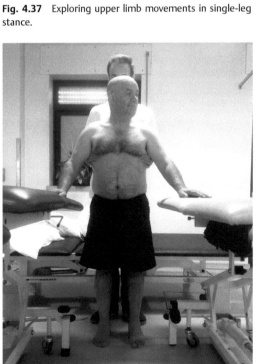

Fig. 4.39 Standing with light touch to explore free head movements.

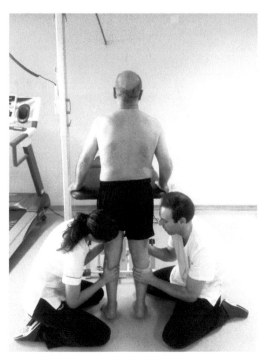

Fig. 4.40 Facilitation of active plantar flexion in standing with bilateral light touch.

Strength training (steadiness practice) to the plantar flexor muscles improves postural stability during quiet standing, even though the practice is low frequency and low intensity (Oshita & Yano 2011).

Ankle strategy was then facilitated through displacement of a big roll to increase the patient's capacity to control postural sway in standing (**Fig. 4.41**). In upright standing the ankle strategy is usually sufficient to correct small deviations in the CoM position and is primarily adopted during less demanding balance tasks when the sway frequency is low (Clifford & Holder-Powell 2010). Ankle strategy is a prerequisite for independent sit to stand and stand to sit, and it has components similar to those of propulsion and heel strike during locomotion.

Creating a stable upright posture allows the patient to explore a backward step. With the arms placed at 90° combined with pelvis restriction, one therapist facilitates hip and knee extension and another a step backward through the foot (**Fig. 4.42**). The development of a backward step reduces the overuse of vision, improves trunk and hip extension, and improves step length. Using a step backward to initiate forward movement can

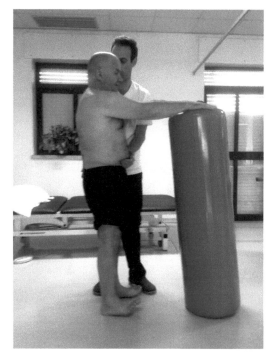

Fig. 4.41 Facilitation of ankle strategy.

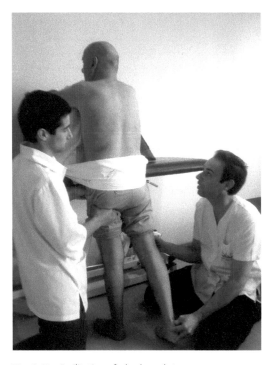

Fig. 4.42 Facilitation of a backward step.

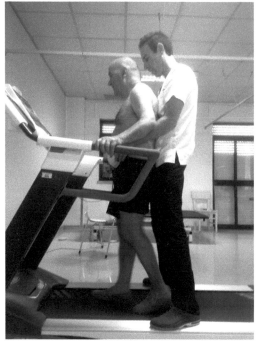

Fig. 4.43 Treadmill training (gradual modulation of velocity) with abdominal activation.

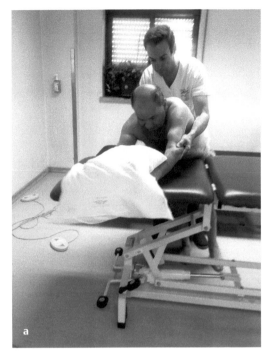

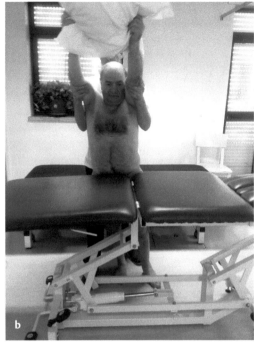

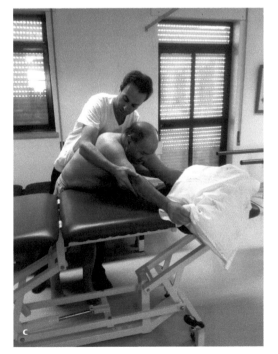

Fig. 4.44   (a–c) Facilitation of multijoint movements.

increase force and power at pushoff and improve the temporal characteristics of the first step (Frost & Cronin 2011).

The achievement of hip extension enables the practice of locomotion on a treadmill to promote reciprocal patterns of leg movements and gait speed. Gait variability, and therefore walking stability, is critically dependent on walking speed in patients with cerebellar ataxia. At the preferred walking speed, however, variability is minimal and similar to that in healthy subjects (Wuehr et al 2013). Treadmill training may have a positive effect on mobility, balance, and quality of gait in ataxic subjects (Vaz et al 2008). The velocity was modified gradually in acceleration and deceleration to reduce the size error in locomotion (**Fig. 4.43**). Cerebellar patients can adapt to a perturbation when it is introduced gradually rather than abruptly (Criscimagna-Hemminger et al 2010).

Patients with cerebellar ataxia benefit from using whole body movements to train trunk–limb coordination (Ilg et al 2009). Breaking complex movements into a series of simpler movements can be viewed as an adaptive strategy to deal with the lack of coordinated sensory data (**Fig. 4.44a–c**).

This training had a positive effect in reducing decomposition of movement and established fixation strategies.

The Bobath Concept emphasizes integrating postural control and task performance, and views this as integral to the choice of intervention strategies (Graham et al 2009). The practice of a dynamic task in standing was a challenge to postural stability and allowed the exploration of stability limits. At the same time, upper-limb weight bearing was reduced, which is important to improve gait and balance (**Fig. 4.45**). Postural control improved following task-oriented arm training in standing without explicit postural control goals, instruction, or feedback. Current training paradigms of isolated postural control training with conscious attention directed to center of pressure location and movement were thereby challenged.

There is evidence to suggest that motor skills learned prior to a cerebellar lesion may still be accessible to a patient (Petrosini et al 2003), whereas learning new skills, especially in a foreign environment, may be much more difficult. The use of previously enjoyed activities and important functional goals will increase the engagement in the task and the likelihood of success (Saywell & Taylor 2008).

Considering the patient's job and his previous daily living activities, several dynamic whole task practice were included in the rehabilitation process (**Fig. 4.46a, b**). The Bobath Concept views training in different real-life situations as appropriate, and not only in the therapy department (Graham et al 2009).

▐ Evaluation

By the end of the intervention, the patient had improved his postural control in standing, which caused a more automatic gait pattern as demonstrated by the figures of standing posture (**Fig. 4.47a-d**) and gait pattern (**Fig. 4.48a–d**). These changes were also demonstrated in the outcome measures.

Comparing the initial to the posttreatment posture in standing, it is possible to observe the following: a more active posture in standing with more extension in the gravity line; better ankle/foot alignment and more appropriate contact with the support surface to allow a narrower base of support; improved pelvic stability that increased core stability activation and decreased forward trunk displacement; more activation of hip abductors and extensors leading to a better integration of the left leg in

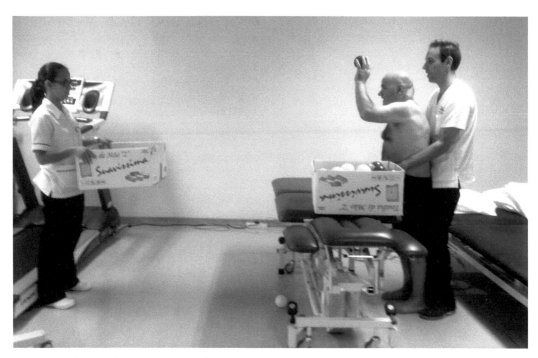

Fig. 4.45 Task-oriented arm training in standing.

the body geometry; and improvement in scapular setting leading to a decreased fixation on the right arm, which allowed head orientation in midline.

The improvements in balance and postural orientation reduced the postural instability and the need for visual dependency, and allowed dual task during walking. The variability of foot placement decreased. Improvements in propulsion enabled a better lateral extension on the left, which decreased the need to compensate with the right arm. The head was free to explore the environment, and more efficient interlimb coupling improved the walking rhythm.

Outcome Measures

At first assessment, the ICARS score was 50 points and in the last assessment 14 points (**Fig. 4.49a**). The patient improved in all ICARS subscales (**Fig. 4.49b**), especially in posture and gait disturbance (23 points in first assessment and 6 points in third assessment).

The initial score in the BESTest was 24.4% compared with 77.8% at the last assessment (**Fig. 4.50a**). The patient improved in all BESTest sections (**Fig. 4.50b**), especially in the APAs section, which had the poorest result at the initial assessment (from 9.5 to 77.8%).

From baseline to the final assessment the scores on the FES were lower (80 points in the first assessment and 45 points in the third assessment) (**Fig. 4.51**).

Discussion

The outcomes from this case study suggest that a patient with cerebellar ataxia learned to improve his postural control in standing while reporting improvements in postural stability and, as a result, decreased his fixation strategies and fear of falling following a 10-week individually designed intervention based on the Bobath Concept.

Recent evidence indicates that motor learning is possible in the presence of cerebellar damage (Boyd et al 2004; Crowdy et al 2002; Carr & Shepherd 1998; Criscimagna-Hemminger et al 2010) suggesting that physiotherapy intervention, including functional motor retraining aimed at promoting neural plasticity, may be appropriate for people with cerebellar dysfunction (Martin et al 2009). Specifically, the Bobath Concept considers that neuromuscular plasticity is a key element of functional recovery (Graham et al 2009). The Bobath practice involves active learning

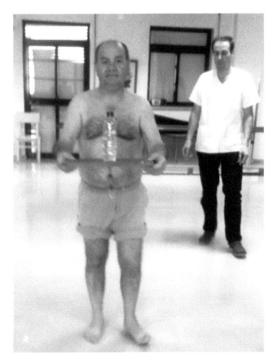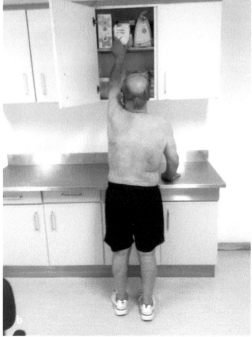

Fig. 4.46   (a, b) Dynamic task practice that challenges stability and explores stability limits.

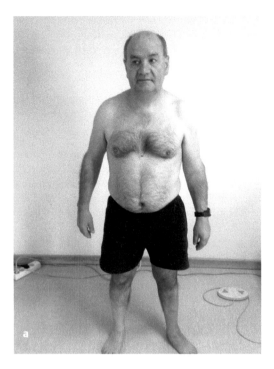
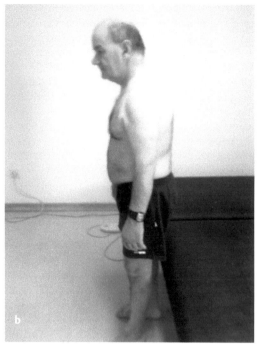
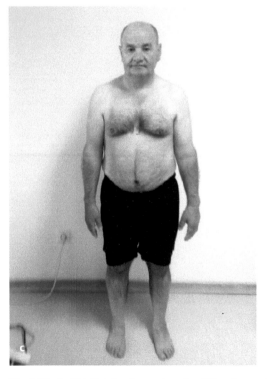
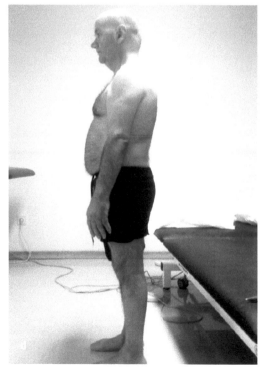

Fig. 4.47   **(a, b)** Initial standing posture. **(c, d)** Standing posture postintervention period.

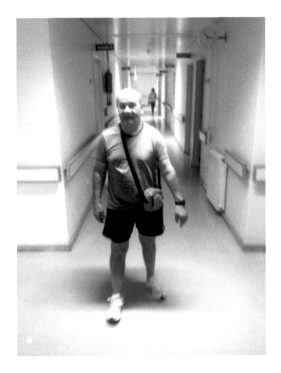
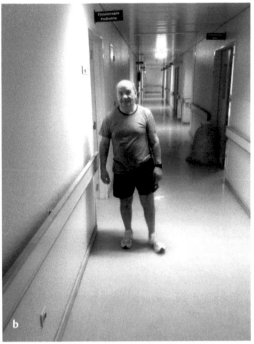
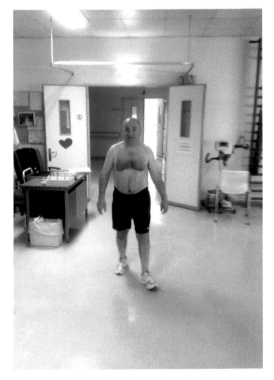
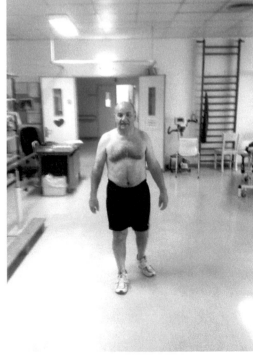

Fig. 4.48   Gait pattern changes. **(a, b)** Initial gait. **(c, d)** Gait postintervention.

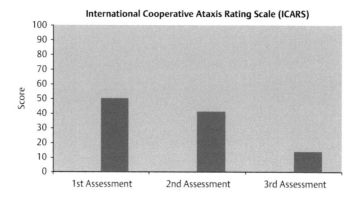

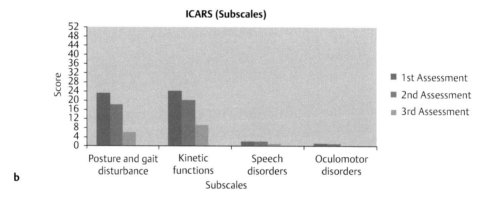

Fig. 4.49   (a) International Cooperative Ataxia Rating Scale (ICARS) results. (b) ICARS subscales.

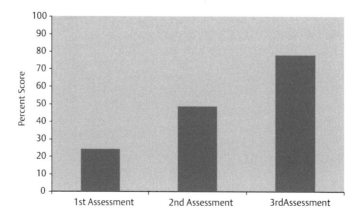

Fig. 4.50   (a) The Balance Evaluation Systems Test (BESTest) results. (Continued)

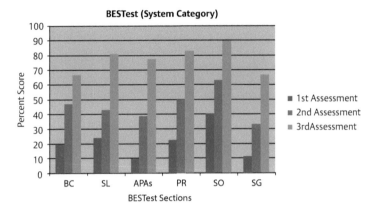

b

Fig. 4.50   *(continued)* **(b)** BESTest sections results. APA, anticipatory postural adjustment; BC, biochemical constraints; SG, stability in gait; PR, postural responses; SL, stability limits; SO, sensory orientation.

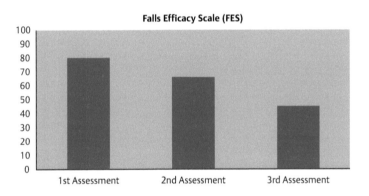

Fig. 4.51   Falls efficacy scale results.

processes in environments that enable the individual to learn to perform self-initiated actions within naturally occurring constraints (Levin & Panturin 2011; Graham et al 2009).

At the end of study, the patient had a lower score on ICARS. According to Saute et al (2012) and Trouillas et al (1997), a high ICARS score means worsening of a patient's impairments The assessment of postural control requires considering the many physiological systems underlying a person's ability to stand, walk and interact with the environment in a safe and efficient manner. A disorder in any one or a combination of these systems leads to postural instability (Horak 2009; Horak 2006). The results in BESTest show an improvement in all system categories, representing an improvement in functional

performance of postural stability, which is necessary for optimal postural control in standing.

The worst result in BESTest sections was found in gait stability, as well as in the posture and gait disturbance ICARS subscale, followed by the kinetic functions subscale. Consistent with Ilg et al (2007), ataxic gait is influenced by both balance-related impairments and deficits related to limb control and intralimb coordination. This implies that increased temporal variability of intralimb coordination is a specific characteristic of cerebellar dysfunction, which causes balance deficits and increased gait variability.

Postural stability depends on the capacity to develop efficient APAs (Yiou et al 2012). According to Horak & Diener (1994), cerebellar subjects are unable to learn how to use predictive feedforward control to scale their postural responses to expected perturbation amplitudes. However, in the beginning of the study, the APAs BESTest section had the lowest percentage score (9.5%), and at the end of the study the percentage score was 77%, indicating that the patient could learn to adjust for predictable postural perturbations. The fixation strategies decreased during the study as a result of recovery of postural stability and consequent reduction in fear of falling. Patients with cerebellar lesions may be able to learn to improve their postural stability (Gill-Body et al 1997). Human subjects tune in to task stability when stability is high, but they use more active compensation when stability is reduced (Wei et al 2008). Specific deficits in balance control occur in subjects with fear of falling (Uemura et al 2012). There is a direct relationship between fear of falling and the strategies used for human postural control (Davis et al 2009). Thus improvements in specific balance strategies are effective in reducing fear of falling (Nitz & Choy 2004; Gusi et al 2012).

Conclusion

The results suggest that patients with cerebellar ataxia may be able to learn to improve their postural control in standing as a result of a reduction of fixation strategies due to improved postural stability by the use of an intervention based on the Bobath Concept. Additional research on the effects of the Bobath Concept as an intervention for postural control in ataxic patients may contribute to clinical decision making in the context of evidence-based practice.

Bibliography

Chapter 1
Applied Neurophysiology

Chapter 1.1
The Organization of the Central Nervous System: An Overview

Academy of Medical Sciences. Restoring Neurological Function: Putting the Neurosciences to Work in Neurorehabilitation. London: Academy of Medical Sciences; 2004

Blitz DM, Nusbaum MP. Neural circuit flexibility in a small sensorimotor system. Curr Opin Neurobiol 2011;21(4):544–552

Brodal P. The Central Nervous System: Structure and Function. 4th ed. New York, NY: Oxford University Press Inc; 2010

Brownstone RM, Bui TV. Spinal interneurons providing input to the final common path during locomotion. Prog Brain Res 2010;187(902):81–95

Cornall C. Self-propelling wheelchairs: The effects on spasticity in hemiplegic patients. Physiother Theory Pract 1991;7(1):13–21

Crone C, Johnsen LL, Biering-Sørensen F, Nielsen JB. Appearance of reciprocal facilitation of ankle extensors from ankle flexors in patients with stroke or spinal cord injury. Brain 2003;126(Pt 2):495–507

D'Amico JM, Condliffe EG, Martins KJ, Bennett DJ, Gorassini MA. Recovery of neuronal and network excitability after spinal cord injury and implications for spasticity. Front Integr Neurosci 2014;8:36

Faist M, Blahak C, Duysens J, Berger W. Modulation of the biceps femoris tendon jerk reflex during human locomotion. Exp Brain Res 1999;125(3):265–270

Goulding M, Bourane S, Garcia-Campmany L, Dalet A, Koch S. Inhibition downunder: an update from the spinal cord. Curr Opin Neurobiol 2014;26:161–166

Hayes HB, Chang Y-H, Hochman S. Stance-phase force on the opposite limb dictates swing-phase afferent presynaptic inhibition during locomotion. J Neurophysiol 2012;107(11):3168–3180

Kandel E, Schwartz J, Jessell T, Siegelbaum S, Hudspeth AJ. Principles of Neural Science. 5th ed. New York, NY: McGraw-Hill Professional; 2013

Knikou M. Plasticity of corticospinal neural control after locomotor training in human spinal cord injury. Neural Plast 2012;2012:254948

Molnár Z, Brown RE. Insights into the life and work of Sir Charles Sherrington. Nat Rev Neurosci 2010;11(6):429–436

Mukherjee A, Chakravarty A. Spasticity mechanisms - for the clinician. Front Neurol 2010;1:149

Nielsen JB, Crone C, Hultborn H. The spinal pathophysiology of spasticity—from a basic science point of view. Acta Physiol (Oxf) 2007;189(2):171–180

Rothwell J. Control of Human Voluntary Movement. 2nd ed. London: Chapman and Hall; 1994

Ward NS, Cohen LG. Mechanisms underlying recovery of motor function after stroke. Arch Neurol 2004;61(12):1844–1848

Zeilhofer HU, Wildner H, Yévenes GE. Fast synaptic inhibition in spinal sensory processing and pain control. Physiol Rev 2012;92(1):193–235

Chapter 1.2
Systems Control: Systems and Structures Concerned with Movement and Sensorimotor Integration

Ab Aziz CB, Ahmad AH. The role of the thalamus in modulating pain. Malays J Med Sci 2006;13(2):11–18

Ada L, Canning CG. Anticipating and avoiding muscle shortening. In: Ada L, Canning CG, eds. Key Issues in Neurological Physiotherapy. Series: Physiotherapy: Foundations for Practice. New York, NY: Oxford University Press; 1990:219–236

af Klint R, Mazzaro N, Nielsen JB, Sinkjaer T, Grey MJ. Load rather than length sensitive feedback contributes to soleus muscle activity during human treadmill walking. J Neurophysiol 2010;103(5):2747–2756

Aimonetti J-M, Hospod V, Roll JP, Ribot-Ciscar E. Cutaneous afferents provide a neuronal population vector that encodes the orientation of human ankle movements. J Physiol 2007;580(Pt. 2):649–658

Allum JHJ, Carpenter MG, Honegger F, Adkin AL, Bloem BR. Age-dependent variations in the directional sensitivity of balance corrections and compensatory arm movements in man. J Physiol 2002;542(Pt 2):643–663

Alvarez FJ, Benito-Gonzalez A, Siembab VC. Principles of interneuron development learned from Renshaw cells and the motoneuron recurrent inhibitory circuit. Ann N Y Acad Sci 2013;1279:22–31

Angelaki DE, Cullen KE. Vestibular system: the many facets of a multimodal sense. Annu Rev Neurosci 2008;31:125–150

Asaka T, Wang Y. Feedforward postural muscle modes and multi-mode coordination in mild cerebellar ataxia. Exp Brain Res 2011;210(1):153–163

Ausim Azizi S. … And the olive said to the cerebellum: organization and functional significance of the olivo-cerebellar system. Neuroscientist 2007;13(6):616–625

Baker SN. The primate reticulospinal tract, hand function and functional recovery. J Physiol 2011;589(Pt 23):5603–5612

Bakker M, Allum JH, Visser JE, et al. Postural responses to multidirectional stance perturbations in cerebellar ataxia. Exp Neurol 2006;202(1):21–35

Bard C, Paillard J, Lajoie Y, et al. Role of afferent information in the timing of motor commands: a comparative study with a deafferented patient. Neuropsychologia 1992;30(2):201–206

Bard C, Turrell Y, Fleury M, Teasdale N, Lamarre Y, Martin O. Deafferentation and pointing with visual double-step perturbations. Exp Brain Res 1999;125(4):410–416

Bares M, Lungu OV, Liu T, Waechter T, Gomez CM, Ashe J. The neural substrate of predictive motor timing in spinocerebellar ataxia. Cerebellum 2011;10(2):233–244

Bastian AJ. Understanding sensorimotor adaptation and learning for rehabilitation. Curr Opin Neurol 2008;21(6):628–633

Bastian AJ. Moving, sensing and learning with cerebellar damage. Curr Opin Neurobiol 2011;21(4):596–601

Bastian AJ, Martin TA, Keating JG, Thach WT. Cerebellar ataxia: abnormal control of interaction torques across multiple joints. J Neurophysiol 1996;76(1):492–509

Berlucchi G, Aglioti SM. The body in the brain revisited. Exp Brain Res 2010;200(1):25–35

Beudel M, Zijlstra S, Mulder T, Zijdewind I, de Jong BM. Secondary sensory area SII is crucially involved in the preparation of familiar movements compared to movements never made before. Hum Brain Mapp 2011;32(4):564–579

Bloem BR, Hausdorff JM, Visser JE, Giladi N. Falls and freezing of gait in Parkinson's disease: a review of two interconnected, episodic phenomena. Mov Disord 2004;19(8):871–884

Blood AJ. New hypotheses about postural control support the notion that all dystonias are manifestations of excessive brain postural function. Biosci Hypotheses 2008;1(1):14–25

Blood AJ. Imaging studies in focal dystonias: a systems level approach to studying a systems level disorder. Curr Neuropharmacol 2013;11(1):3–15

Borgmann R. Behandling av spastisk torticollis med butolinumtoxin. Tidsskriftet Norske legeforening 1997;13:1889–1891

Bostan AC, Strick PL. The cerebellum and basal ganglia are interconnected. Neuropsychol Rev 2010;20(3):261–270

Bostan AC, Dum RP, Strick PL. The basal ganglia communicate with the cerebellum. Proc Natl Acad Sci U S A 2010;107(18):8452–8456

Bottini G, Karnath HO, Vallar G, et al. Cerebral representations for egocentric space: functional–anatomical evidence from caloric vestibular stimulation and neck vibration. Brain 2001;124(Pt 6):1182–1196

Brodal P. The Central Nervous System: Structure and Function. 4th ed. New York, NY: Oxford University Press; 2010

Brown LE, Halpert BA, Goodale MA. Peripheral vision for perception and action. Exp Brain Res 2005;165(1):97–106

Bruttini C, Esposti R, Bolzoni F, Vanotti A, Mariotti C, Cavallari P. Temporal disruption of upper-limb anticipatory postural adjustments in cerebellar ataxic patients. Exp Brain Res 2015;233(1):197–203

Buneo CA, Andersen RA. The posterior parietal cortex: sensorimotor interface for the planning and online control of visually guided movements. Neuropsychologia 2006;44(13):2594–2606

Burbeck CA, Yap YL. Two mechanisms for localization? Evidence for separation-dependent and separation-independent processing of position information. Vision Res 1990;30(5):739–750

Bussel B, Roby-Brami A, Néris OR, Yakovleff A. Evidence for a spinal stepping generator in man. Electrophysiological study. Acta Neurobiol Exp (Warsz) 1996;56(1):465–468

Capaday C, Ethier C, Van Vreeswijk C, Darling WG. On the functional organization and operational principles of the motor cortex. Front Neural Circuits 2013;7:66

Cappe C, Rouiller EM, Barone P. Multisensory anatomical pathways. Hear Res 2009;258(1-2):28–36

Cardini F, Longo MR, Haggard P. Vision of the body modulates somatosensory intracortical inhibition. Cereb Cortex 2011;21(9):2014–2022

Coffman KA, Dum RP, Strick PL. Cerebellar vermis is a target of projections from the motor areas in the cerebral cortex. Proc Natl Acad Sci U S A 2011;108(38):16068–16073

Collins DF, Refshauge KM, Todd G, Gandevia SC. Cutaneous receptors contribute to kinesthesia at the index finger, elbow, and knee. J Neurophysiol 2005;94(3):1699–1706

Cordo PJ, Horn JL, Künster D, Cherry A, Bratt A, Gurfinkel V. Contributions of skin and muscle afferent input to movement sense in the human hand. J Neurophysiol 2011;105(4):1879–1888

Criscimagna-Hemminger SE, Bastian AJ, Shadmehr R. Size of error affects cerebellar contributions to motor learning. J Neurophysiol 2010;103(4):2275–2284

Cullen KE. The vestibular system: multimodal integration and encoding of self-motion for motor control. Trends Neurosci 2012;35(3):185–196

Cullen KE. The neural encoding of self-generated and externally applied movement: implications for the perception of self-motion and spatial memory. Front Integr Neurosci 2014;7:108

Dakin CJ, Inglis JT, Chua R, Blouin JS. Muscle-specific modulation of vestibular reflexes with increased locomotor velocity and cadence. J Neurophysiol 2013;110(1):86–94

Davidoff RA. The pyramidal tract. Neurology 1990;40(2):332–339

de Lau LML, Breteler MMB. Epidemiology of Parkinson's disease. Lancet Neurol 2006;5(6):525–535

de Lima-Pardini AC, Papegaaij S, Cohen RG, Teixeira LA, Smith BA, Horak FB. The interaction of postural and voluntary strategies for stability in Parkinson's disease. J Neurophysiol 2012;108(5):1244–1252

de Oliveira-Souza R. The human extrapyramidal system. Med Hypotheses 2012;79(6):843–852

Dietz V. Human neuronal control of automatic functional movements: interaction between central programs and afferent input. Physiol Rev 1992;72(1):33–69

Dietz V. Spinal cord pattern generators for locomotion. Clin Neurophysiol 2003;114(8):1379–1389

Dietz V. Neuroplasticity after a spinal cord injury: effects of functional training and neurorehabilitation. 2010:2196–2205

Dietz V, Duysens J. Significance of load receptor input during locomotion: a review. Gait Posture 2000;11(2):102–110

Dietz V, Zijlstra W, Duysens J. Human neuronal interlimb coordination during split-belt locomotion. Exp Brain Res 1994;101(3):513–520

Dietz V, Grillner S, Trepp A, Hubli M, Bolliger M. Changes in spinal reflex and locomotor activity after a complete spinal cord injury: a common mechanism? Brain 2009;132(Pt 8):2196–2205

Dijkerman HC, de Haan EHF. Somatosensory processes subserving perception and action. Behav Brain Sci 2007;30(2):189–201, discussion 201–239

Doucet BM, Lam A, Griffin L. Neuromuscular electrical stimulation for skeletal muscle function. Yale J Biol Med 2012;85(2):201–215

Duysens J, Clarac F, Cruse H. Load-regulating mechanisms in gait and posture: comparative aspects. Physiol Rev 2000;80(1):83–133

Duysens J, Van de Crommert HW. Neural control of locomotion; The central pattern generator from cats to humans. Gait Posture 1998;7(2):131–141

Flavell SW, Greenberg ME. Signaling mechanisms linking neuronal activity to gene expression and plasticity of the nervous system. Annu Rev Neurosci 2008;31:563–590

Floeter M. Structure and function of muscle fibers and motor units. In: Karpati G, Hilton-Jones D, eds. Disorders of Voluntary Muscle. New York, NY: Cambridge University Press; 2010:1–10

Flynn JR, Graham BA, Galea MP, Callister RJ. The role of propriospinal interneurons in recovery from spinal cord injury. Neuropharmacology 2011;60(5):809–822

Forbes PA, Siegmund GP, Schouten AC, Blouin JS. Task, muscle and frequency dependent vestibular control of posture. Front Integr Nuerosci 2015;8:94

Forget R, Lamarre Y. Postural adjustments associated with different unloadings of the forearm: effects of proprioceptive and cutaneous afferent deprivation. Can J Physiol Pharmacol 1995;73(2):285–294

Franceschini M, Agosti M, Cantagallo A, Sale P, Mancuso M, Buccino G. Mirror neurons: action observation treatment as a tool in stroke rehabilitation. Eur J Phys Rehabil Med 2010;46(4):517–523

Frey SH, Fogassi L, Grafton S, et al. Neurological principles and rehabilitation of action disorders: computation, anatomy, and physiology (CAP) model. Neurorehabil Neural Repair 2011; 25(5, Suppl)6S–20S

Gallager S. How the Body Shapes the Mind. New York, NY: Oxford University Press; 2005

Genewein T, Braun DA. A sensorimotor paradigm for Bayesian model selection. Front Hum Neurosci 2012;6(October):1–16

Gilbert SJ, Burgess PW. Executive function. Curr Biol 2008;18(3):R110–R114

Gjerstad L, Kerty E, Nyberg Hansen R. Behandling av fokale dystonier med botulinumtoksin. Tidsskrift Norske legeforening 1991;111:2637–2639

Goldspink G, Williams P. Muscle fibre and connective tissue changes associated with use and disuse. In: Ada L, Canning C, eds. Key Issues in Neurological Physiotherapy. Boston, MA: Butterworth-Heinemann; 1991:197–218

Grabli D, Karachi C, Welter ML, et al. Normal and pathological gait: what we learn from Parkinson's disease. J Neurol Neurosurg Psychiatry 2012;83(10):979–985

Graham JV, Eustace C, Brock K, Swain E, Irwin-Carruthers S. The Bobath concept in contemporary clinical practice. Top Stroke Rehabil 2009;16(1):57–68

Gray V, Rice CL, Garland SJ. Factors that influence muscle weakness following stroke and their clinical implications: a critical review. Physiother Can 2012;64(4):415–426

Grillner S. Biological pattern generation: the cellular and computational logic of networks in motion. Neuron 2006;52(5):751–766

Grillner S, Wallén P, Saitoh K, Kozlov A, Robertson B. Neural bases of goal-directed locomotion in vertebrates—an overview. Brain Res Brain Res Rev 2008;57(1):2–12

Grol, MJ Madjandzić J, Stephan KE, et al. Parieto-frontal connectivity during visually guided grasping. J Neurosci 2007;27(44):11877–11887

Guertin PA. Central pattern generator for locomotion: anatomical, physiological, and pathophysiological considerations. Front Neurol 2012;3:183

Guertin PA. The spinal cord: functional organization, diseases, and dysfunctions. In: Aldskogius H, ed. Animal Models of Spinal Cord Repair: Neuromethods. Totowa, NJ: Humana Press; 2013

Haber SN, Calzavara R. The cortico-basal ganglia integrative network: the role of the thalamus. Brain Res Bull 2009;78(2-3):69–74

Harris P, Nagy S, Vardaxis N. Mosby's Dictionary of Medicine, Nursing and Health Professions. 9th ed. Atlanta, GA: Elsevier; 2010

Henneman E. The size-principle: a deterministic output emerges from a set of probabilistic connections. J Exp Biol 1985;115:105–112

Holmes NP, Spence C. The body schema and the multisensory representation(s) of peripersonal space. Cogn Process 2004;5(2):94–105

Honeycutt CF, Kharouta M, Perreault EJ. Evidence for reticulospinal contributions to coordinated finger movements in humans. J Neurophysiol 2013;110(7):1476–1483

Horak FB, Diener HC, Nashner LM. Influence of central set on human postural responses. J Neurophysiol 1989;62(4):841–853

Hubli M, Dietz V. The physiological basis of neurorehabilitation—locomotor training after spinal cord injury. J Neuroeng Rehabil 2013;10:5

Hufschmidt A, Mauritz KH. Chronic transformation of muscle in spasticity: a peripheral contribution to increased tone. J Neurol Neurosurg Psychiatry 1985;48(7):676–685

Imamizu H, Kawato M. Cerebellar internal models: implications for the dexterous use of tools. Cerebellum 2012;11(2):325–335

Ioffe ME, Chernikova LA, Ustinova KI. Role of cerebellum in learning postural tasks. Cerebellum 2007;6(1):87–94

Ivry R. Exploring the role of the cerebellum in sensory anticipation and timing: commentary on Tesche and Karhu. Hum Brain Mapp 2000;9(3):115–118

Ivry RB, Spencer RMC. The neural representation of time. Curr Opin Neurobiol 2004;14(2):225–232

Jacobs JV, Horak FB. Cortical control of postural responses. J Neural Transm 2007;114(10):1339–1348

Jacobs JVJ. Why we need to better understand the cortical neurophysiology of impaired postural responses with age, disease, or injury. Front Integr Neurosci 2014;8:69

Jang SH. The corticospinal tract from the viewpoint of brain rehabilitation. J Rehabil Med 2014;46(3):193–199

Jankowska E, Hammar I, Slawinska U, Maleszak K, Edgley SA. Neuronal basis of crossed actions from the reticular formation on feline hindlimb motoneurons. J Neurosci 2003;23(5):1867–1878

Jankowska E, Edgley SA. How can corticospinal tract neurons contribute to ipsilateral movements? A question with implications for recovery of motor functions. Neuroscientist 2006;12(1):67–79

Jeannerod M, Arbib MA, Rizzolatti G, Sakata H. Grasping objects: the cortical mechanisms of visuomotor transformation. Trends Neurosci 1995;18(7):314–320

Jimenez-Shahed J. A new treatment for focal dystonias: incobotulinumtoxinA (Xeomin®), a botulinum neurotoxin type A free from complexing proteins. Neuropsychiatr Dis Treat 2012;8:13–25

Jobst EE, Melnick ME, Byl NN, Dowling GA, Aminoff MJ. Sensory perception in Parkinson disease. Arch Neurol 1997;54(4):450–454

Johansson RS, Flanagan JR. Coding and use of tactile signals from the fingertips in object manipulation tasks. Nat Rev Neurosci 2009;10(5):345–359

Juvin L, Le Gal JP, Simmers J, Morin D. Cervicolumbar coordination in mammalian quadrupedal locomotion: role of spinal thoracic circuitry and limb sensory inputs. J Neurosci 2012;32(3):953–965

Kaji R, Urushihara R, Murase N, Shimazu H, Goto S. Abnormal sensory gating in basal ganglia disorders. J Neurol 2005;252(Suppl 4):IV13–IV16

Kammers MPM, Kootker JA, Hogendoorn H, Dijkerman HC. How many motoric body representations can we grasp? Exp Brain Res 2010;202(1):203–212

Kandel E, Jessell T, Siegelbaum S, Schwartz J, Hudspeth AJ. Principles of Neural Science. 5th ed. New York, NY: McGraw-Hill Professional; 2013

Kanning KC, Kaplan A, Henderson CE. Motor neuron diversity in development and disease. Annu Rev Neurosci 2010;33:409–440

Karl JM, Whishaw IQ. Different evolutionary origins for the reach and the grasp: an explanation for dual visuomotor channels in primate parietofrontal cortex. Front Neurol 2013;4:208

Kars HJ, Hijmans JM, Geertzen JH, Zijlstra W. The effect of reduced somatosensation on standing balance: a systematic review. J Diabetes Sci Tech 2009;3(4):931–943

Kavounoudias A, Roll R, Roll JP. The plantar sole is a 'dynamometric map' for human balance control. Neuroreport 1998;9(14):3247–3252

Kern DS, Kumar R. Deep brain stimulation. Neurologist 2007;13(5):237–252

Kerty E. Vision rehabilitation after brain injury. Tidsskrift Norske legeforening. 2005:125–146

Khan AZ, Crawford JD, Blohm G, Urquizar C, Rossetti Y, Pisella L. Influence of initial hand and target position on reach errors in optic ataxic and normal subjects. J Vis 2007;7(5):1–16

Kidd G. The myotatic reflex. In: Downie P, ed. Cash's Textbook of Neurology for Physiotherapists. London: Faber & Faber; 1986:85–103

Kidd G, Lawes N, Musa I. Understanding Neuromuscular Plasticity: A Basis for Clinical Rehabilitation. London: Edward Arnold; 1992

Kishore A, Meunier S, Popa T. Cerebellar influence on motor cortex plasticity: behavioral implications for Parkinson's disease. Front Neurol 2014;5:68–69

Kitago T, Krakauer JW. Motor learning principles for neurorehabilitation. Handb Clin Neurol 2013;110:93–103

Klatzky RL, Lederman SJ, Metzger VA. Identifying objects by touch: an "expert system". Percept Psychophys 1985;37(4):299–302

Knapp HD, Taub E, Berman AJ. Movements in monkeys with deafferented forelimbs. Exp Neurol 1963;7:305–315

Koziol LF, Budding D, Andreasen N, et al. Consensus paper: the cerebellum's role in movement and cognition. Cerebellum 2014;13(1):151–177

Koziol LF, Budding DE, Chidekel D. Adaptation, expertise, and giftedness: towards an understanding of cortical, subcortical, and cerebellar network contributions. Cerebellum 2010;9(4):499–529

Koziol LF, Budding DE, Chidekel D. Sensory integration, sensory processing, and sensory modulation disorders: putative functional neuroanatomic underpinnings. Cerebellum 2011;10(4):770–792

Kravitz DJ, Saleem KS, Baker CI, Mishkin M. A new neural framework for visuospatial processing. Nat Rev Neurosci 2011;12(4):217–230

Kreitzer AC, Malenka RC. Striatal plasticity and basal ganglia circuit function. Neuron 2008;60(4):543–554

Lacquaniti F, Ivanenko YP, Zago M. Patterned control of human locomotion. J Physiol 2012;590(Pt 10):2189–2199

Lamontagne A, Paquette C, Fung J. Stroke affects the coordination of gaze and posture during preplanned turns while walking. Neurorehabil Neural Repair 2007;21(1):62–67

Lan N, He X. Fusimotor control of spindle sensitivity regulates central and peripheral coding of joint angles. Front Comput Neurosci 2012;6(August):66

Lang CE, Schieber MH. Reduced muscle selectivity during individuated finger movements in humans after damage to the motor cortex or corticospinal tract. J Neurophysiol 2004;91(4):1722–1733

Laube R, Govender S, Colebatch JG. Vestibular-dependent spinal reflexes evoked by brief lateral accelerations of the heads of standing subjects. J Appl Physiol (1985) 2012;112(11):1906–1914

Lavoie BA, Cody FWJ, Capaday C. Cortical control of human soleus muscle during volitional and postural activities studied using focal magnetic stimulation. Exp Brain Res 1995;103(1):97–107

Lederman SJ, Klatzky RL. Extracting object properties through haptic exploration. Acta Psychol (Amst) 1993;84(1):29–40

Lederman SJ, Klatzky RL. Haptic perception: a tutorial. Atten Percept Psychophys 2009;71(7):1439–1459

Lemon RN. Descending pathways in motor control. Annu Rev Neurosci 2008;31:195–218

Lemon RN. What drives corticospinal output? F1000 Biol Rep 2010;2:51

Lemon RN, Griffiths J. Comparing the function of the corticospinal system in different species: organizational differences for motor specialization? Muscle Nerve 2005;32(3):261–279

Levi DM, Klein SA. Limitations on position coding imposed by undersampling and univariance. Vision Res 1996;36(14):2111–2120

Longo MR, Cardozo S, Haggard P. Visual enhancement of touch and the bodily self. Conscious Cogn 2008;17(4):1181–1191

Lopez C, Blanke O. The thalamocortical vestibular system in animals and humans. Brain Res Brain Res Rev 2011;67(1-2):119–146

Lopez C, Schreyer HM, Preuss N, Mast FW. Vestibular stimulation modifies the body schema. Neuropsychologia 2012;50(8):1830–1837

Lumpkin EA, Marshall KL, Nelson AM. The cell biology of touch. J Cell Biol 2010;191(2):237–248

Lundy-Ekman. Neuroscience, Fundamentals for Rehabilitation. 3rd ed. Elsevier Health Sciences; 2007

Mackay-Lyons M. Central pattern generation of locomotion: a review of the evidence. Phys Ther 2002;82(1):69–83

Maki BE, McIlroy WE. The r ole of limb movements in maintaining upright stance: the "change-in-support" strategy. Phys Ther 1997;77(5):488–507

Mani S, Mutha PK, Przybyla A, Haaland KY, Good DC, Sainburg RL. Contralesional motor deficits after unilateral stroke reflect hemisphere-specific control mechanisms. Brain 2013;136(Pt 4):1288–1303

Manto M. Mechanisms of human cerebellar dysmetria: experimental evidence and current conceptual bases. J Neuroeng Rehabil 2009;6:10

Manto M, Haines D. Cerebellar research: two centuries of discoveries. Cerebellum 2012;11(2):446

Manto M, Bower JM, Conforto AB, et al. Consensus paper: roles of the cerebellum in motor control—the diversity of ideas on cerebellar involvement in movement. Cerebellum 2012;11(2):457–487

Manuel M, Zytnicki D. Alpha, beta and gamma motoneurons: functional diversity in the motor system's final pathway. J Integr Neurosci 2011;10(3): 243–276

Marchand-Pauvert V, Iglesias C. Properties of human spinal interneurones: normal and dystonic control. J Physiol 2008;586(5):1247–1256

Markham CH. Vestibular control of muscular tone and posture. Can J Neurol Sci 1987;14(3, Suppl):493–496

Marsden CD, Quinn NP. The dystonias. BMJ 1990;300(6718):139–144

Massion J. Movement, posture and equilibrium: interaction and coordination. Prog Neurobiol 1992;38(1):35–56

Massion J, Alexandrov A, Frolov A. Why and how are posture and movement coordinated? Prog Brain Res 2004;143:13–27

Matsakas A, Patel K. Skeletal muscle fibre plasticity in response to selected environmental and physiological stimuli. Histol Histopathol 2009;24(5):611–629

Mendell LM. The size principle: a rule describing the recruitment of motoneurons. J Neurophysiol 2005;93(6):3024–3026

Milner AD, Goodale MA. Two visual systems re-viewed. Neuropsychologia 2008;46(3):774–785

Mishkin M, Ungerleider LG, Macko KA. Object vision and spatial vision: two cortical pathways. Trends Neurosci 1983;6:414–417

Molinari M. Plasticity properties of CPG circuits in humans: impact on gait recovery. Brain Res Bull 2009;78(1):22–25

Molinari M, Chiricozzi FR, Clausi S, Tedesco AM, De Lisa M, Leggio MG. Cerebellum and detection of sequences, from perception to cognition. Cerebellum 2008;7(4):611–615

Morton SM, Bastian AJ. Cerebellar control of balance and locomotion. Neuroscientist 2004;10(3):247–259

Morton SM, Bastian AJ. Cerebellar contributions to locomotor adaptations during splitbelt treadmill walking. J Neurosci 2006;26(36):9107–9116

Mottolese C, Richard N, Harquel S, Szathmari A, Sirigu A, Desmurget M. Mapping motor representations in the human cerebellum. Brain 2013;136(Pt 1):330–342

Mudge S, Rochester L. Neurophysiological rationale of treadmill training: evaluating evidence for practice. New Zealand Journal of Physiotherapy 2001;29(2):7–18

Mulder T, Nienhuis B, Pauwels J. The assessment of motor recovery: A new look at an old problem. J Electromyogr Kinesiol 1996;6(2):137–145

Nachev P, Kennard C, Husain M. Functional role of the supplementary and pre-supplementary motor areas. Nat Rev Neurosci 2008;9(11):856–869

Nagai K, Yamada M, Mori S, et al. Effect of the muscle coactivation during quiet standing on dynamic postural control in older adults. Arch Gerontol Geriatr 2013;56(1):129–133

Nielsen JB. Sensorimotor integration at spinal level as a basis for muscle coordination during voluntary movement in humans. J Appl Physiol (1985) 2004;96(5):1961–1967

Nowak DA, Glasauer S, Hermsdorfer J. How predictive is grip force control in the complete absence of somatosensory feedback? Brain 2004;127(Pt 1):182–192

Petersen NT, Pyndt HS, Nielsen JB. Investigating human motor control by transcranial magnetic stimulation. Exp Brain Res 2003;152(1):1–16

Pettorossi VE, Schieppati M. Neck proprioception shapes body orientation and perception of motion. Front Hum Neurosci 2014;8:895

Porter R, Lemon RN. Corticospinal Function and Voluntary Movement. New York, NY: Oxford University Press; 1995

Riddle CN, Edgley SA, Baker SN. Direct and indirect connections with upper limb motoneurons from the primate reticulospinal tract. J Neurosci 2009;29(15):4993–4999

Rizzolatti G, Cattaneo L, Fabbri-Destro M, Rozzi S. Cortical mechanisms underlying the organization of goal-directed actions and mirror neuron-based action understanding. Physiol Rev 2014;94(2):655–706

Rizzolatti G, Craighero L. The mirror-neuron system. Annu Rev Neurosci 2004;27:169–192

Rizzolatti G, Sinigaglia C. The functional role of the parieto-frontal mirror circuit: interpretations and misinterpretations. Nat Rev Neurosci 2010;11(4):264–274

Robertson JV, Roche N, Roby-Brami A. Influence of the side of brain damage on postural upper-limb control including the scapula in stroke patients. Exp Brain Res 2012;218(1):141–155

Rondi-Reig L, Paradis AL, Lefort JM, Babayan BM, Tobin C. How the cerebellum may monitor sensory information for spatial representation. Front Syst Neurosci 2014;8:205

Rosenkranz K, Rothwell JC. Modulation of proprioceptive integration in the motor cortex shapes human motor learning. J Neurosci 2012;32(26):9000–9006

Rossignol S, Dubuc R, Gossard JP. Dynamic sensorimotor interactions in locomotion. Physiol Rev 2006;86(1):89–154

Rossignol S, Barrière G, Frigon A, et al. Plasticity of locomotor sensorimotor interactions after peripheral and/or spinal lesions. Brain Res Rev 2008;57(1):228–240

Rothgangel AS, Braun SM, Beurskens AJ, Seitz RJ, Wade DT. The clinical aspects of mirror therapy in rehabilitation: a systematic review of the literature. Int J Rehabil Res 2011;34(1):1–13

Rothwell J, Lennon S. Control of Human Voluntary Movement. 2nd ed. London, UK: Chapman and Hall; 1994

Rowe FJ, Wright D, Brand D, et al. Profile of Gaze Dysfunction following Cerebrovascular Accident. ISRN Ophthalmol 2013;2013:264604

Rubinstein NA, Kelly AM. Development of muscle fiber specialization in the rat hindlimb. J Cell Biol 1981;90(1):128–144

Ryczko D, Dubuc R. The multifunctional mesencephalic locomotor region. Curr Pharm Des 2013;19(2 4):4448–4470

Sahrmann S. Posture and muscle imbalance. Physiotherapy 1992;78(1):1–19

Sahrmann SA. Diagnosis and Treatment of Movement Impairment Syndromes. White K, ed. St. Louis, MO: Mosby; 2002

Sand KM, Midelfart A, Thomassen L, Melms A, Wilhelm H, Hoff JM. Visual impairment in stroke patients—a review. Acta Neurol Scand Suppl 2013;127(196):52–56

Santos MJMMJ, Kanekar N, Aruin AS. The role of anticipatory postural adjustments in compensatory control of posture: 2. Biomechanical analysis. J Electromyogr Kinesiol 2010;20(3):398–405

Sarlegna FR, Mutha PK. The influence of visual target information on the online control of movements. Vision Research. 2014:1–11

Saunders JA, Knill DC. Visual feedback control of hand movements. J Neurosci 2004;24(13):3223–3234

Schepens B, Drew T. Independent and convergent signals from the pontomedullary reticular formation contribute to the control of posture and movement during reaching in the cat. J Neurophysiol 2004;92(4):2217–2238

Schepens B, Drew T. Descending signals from the pontomedullary reticular formation are bilateral, asymmetric, and gated during reaching movements in the cat. J Neurophysiol 2006;96(5):2229–2252

Schepens B, Stapley P, Drew T. Neurons in the pontomedullary reticular formation signal posture and movement both as an integrated behavior and independently. J Neurophysiol 2008;100(4):2235–2253

Schiaffino S, Reggiani C. Fiber types in mammalian skeletal muscles. Physiol Rev 2011;91(4):1447–1531

Schieber MH, Lang CE, Reilly KT, McNulty P, Sirigu A. Selective activation of human finger muscles after stroke or amputation. Adv Exp Med Biol 2009;629:559–575

Schlerf J, Ivry RB, Diedrichsen J. Encoding of sensory prediction errors in the human cerebellum. J Neurosci 2012;32(14):4913–4922

Schmahmann JD. Vascular syndromes of the thalamus. Stroke 2003;34(9):2264–2278

Scott W, Stevens J, Binder-Macleod SA. Human skeletal muscle fiber type classifications. Phys Ther 2001;81(11):1810–1816

Seger CA. The basal ganglia in human learning. Neuroscientist 2006;12(4):285–290

Shumway-Cook AWM. Motor Control: Translating Research into Clinical Practice. 4th ed. Philadelphia, PA: Lippincott Williams & Wilkins; 2011

Shumway-Cook A, Woollacott MH. Motor Control: Translating Research into Clinical Practice. 3rd ed. Philadelphia, PA: Lippincott Williams & Wilkins; 2006

Sieck GC. Highlighted Topics series: Plasticity in Skeletal, Cardiac, and Smooth Muscle. J Appl Physiol 2001;90:1158–1164

Silva CC, Silva A, Sousa A, et al. Co-activation of upper limb muscles during reaching in post-stroke subjects: an analysis of the contralesional and ipsilesional limbs. J Electromyogr Kinesiol 2014;24(5):731–738

Simons DG, Mense S. Understanding and measurement of muscle tone as related to clinical muscle pain. Pain 1998;75(1):1–17

Stenneken P, Prinz W, Cole J, Paillard J, Aschersleben G. The effect of sensory feedback on the timing of movements: evidence from deafferented patients. Brain Res 2006;1084(1):123–131

Stokes M. Neurological Physiotherapy, London, UK: Mosby; 1998

Stoodley CJ, Schmahmann JD. Evidence for topographic organization in the cerebellum of motor control versus cognitive and affective processing. Cortex 2010;46(7):831–844

Sullivan JE, Hedman LD. Sensory dysfunction following stroke: incidence, significance, examination, and intervention. Top Stroke Rehabil 2008;15(3):200–217

Suzuki M, Omori Y, Sugimura S, et al. Predicting recovery of bilateral upper extremity muscle strength after stroke. J Rehabil Med 2011;43(10):935–943

Takakusaki K. Neurophysiology of gait: from the spinal cord to the frontal lobe. Mov Disord 2013;28(11):1483–1491

Takakusaki K, Saitoh K, Harada H, Kashiwayanagi M. Role of basal ganglia-brainstem pathways in the control of motor behaviors. Neurosci Res 2004;50(2):137–151

Takakusaki K, Obara K, Okumura T. Possible Contribution of the Basal Ganglia Brainstem System to the Pathogenesis of Parkinson's Disease. INTECH Open Access Publisher. 2010. http://www.intechopen.com/source/pdfs/21584/InTech-Possible_contribution_of_the_basal_ganglia_brainstem_system_to_the_pathogenesis_of_parkinson_s_disease.pdf. Accessed March 24, 2013

Takakusaki K, Tomita N, Yano M. Substrates for normal gait and pathophysiology of gait disturbances with respect to the basal ganglia dysfunction. J Neurol 2008;255(Suppl 4):19–29

Thach WT, Bastian AJ. Role of the cerebellum in the control and adaptation of gait in health and disease. Prog Brain Res 2004;143:353–366

Thomas CL. ed. Taber's Cyclopedic Medical Dictionary. 18th ed. Philadelphia, PA: F.A. Davis; 1997

Torres-Oviedo G, Bastian AJ. Natural error patterns enable transfer of motor learning to novel contexts. J Neurophysiol 2012;107(1):346–356

Trew M, Everett T. Human Movement: An Introductory Text. 3rd ed. Philadelphia, PA: Churchill Livingstone; 1998

Tyldesley B, Grieve J. Muscles, Nerves and Movement: Kinesiology in Daily Living. 2nd ed. Hoboken, NJ: Blackwell Sciences; 1996

Van Ingen Schenau GJ, Bobbert MF, Rozendal RH. The unique action of bi-articular muscles in leg extensions. In: Winters JM, Woo SL-Y, eds. Multiple Muscle Systems: Biomechanics and Movement Organization I. New York, NY: Springer-Verlag; 1990:1–5

Vesia M, Crawford JD. Specialization of reach function in human posterior parietal cortex. Exp Brain Res 2012;221(1):1–18 PubMed

de Vignemont F. Body schema and body image—pros and cons. Neuropsychologia 2010a;48(3):669–680

de Vignemont F. Widening the body to rubber hands and tools: what's the difference? Neurosciences Cognitives 2010b;2:203–211

Visser JE, Bloem BR. Role of the basal ganglia in balance control. Neural Plast 2005;12(2-3):161–174, discussion 263–272

Wall PD, Lidierth M. Five sources of a dorsal root potential: their interactions and origins in the superficial dorsal horn. J Neurophysiol 1997;78(2):860–871

Ward N. Assessment of cortical reorganisation for hand function after stroke. J Physiol 2011;589(Pt 23):5625–5632

Wichmann T, DeLong MR. Basal ganglia discharge abnormalities in Parkinson's disease. J Neural Transm Suppl 2006;70(70):21–25

Wolpaw JR. The complex structure of a simple memory. Trends Neurosci 1997;20(12):588–594

Wolpert DM, Miall RC, Kawato M. Internal models in the cerebellum. Trends Cogn Sci 1998;2(9):338–347

Wright WG, Ivanenko YP, Gurfinkel VS. Foot anatomy specialization for postural sensation and control. J Neurophysiol 2012;107(5):1513–1521

Yakovenko S, Drew T. A motor cortical contribution to the anticipatory postural adjustments that precede reaching in the cat. J Neurophysiol 2009;102(2):853–874

Yeo SS, Chang PH, Jang SH. The ascending reticular activating system from pontine reticular formation to the thalamus in the human brain. Front Hum Neurosci 2013;7:416

Zackowski KM, Dromerick AW, Sahrmann SA, Thach WT, Bastian AJ. How do strength, sensation, spasticity and joint individuation relate to the reaching deficits of people with chronic hemiparesis? Brain 2004;127(Pt 5):1035–1046

Zehr EP, Duysens J. Regulation of arm and leg movement during human locomotion. Neuroscientist 2004;10(4):347–361

Zehr EP, Hundza SR, Vasudevan EV. The quadrupedal nature of human bipedal locomotion. Exerc Sport Sci Rev 2009;37(2):102–108

Chapter 1.3
Motor Learning and Plasticity

Aboderin I, Venables G. Stroke management in Europe. Pan European Consensus Meeting on Stroke Management. J Intern Med 1996;240(4):173–180

Academy of Medical Sciences. Restoring Neurological Function: Putting the Neurosciences to Work in Neurorehabilitation. London, UK: Academy of Medical Sciences; 2004

Ada L, Canning C. Anticipating and avoiding muscle shortening. In: Ada L, Canning C, eds. Key Issues in Neurological Physiotherapy. Oxford, UK: Butterworth-Heinemann; 1991:219–236. Physiotherapy: Foundations for Practice

Adkins DL, Boychuk J, Remple MS, Kleim JA. Motor training induces experience-specific patterns of plasticity across motor cortex and spinal cord. J Appl Physiol (1985) 2006;101(6):1776–1782

Agnati LF, Zoli M, Biagini G, Fuxe K. Neuronal plasticity and ageing processes in the frame of the 'Red Queen Theory'. Acta Physiol Scand 1992;145(4):301–309

Allred RP, Jones TA. Experience—a double edged sword for restorative neural plasticity after brain damage. Future Neurol 2008;3(2):189–198

Allred RP, Cappellini CH, Jones TA. The "good" limb makes the "bad" limb worse: experience-dependent interhemispheric disruption of functional outcome after cortical infarcts in rats. Behav Neurosci 2010;124(1):124–132

Allred RP, Kim SY, Jones TA. Use it and/or lose it-experience effects on brain remodeling across time after stroke. Front Hum Neurosci 2014;8(June):379

Ashburn A. Physical recovery following stroke. Physiotherapy 1997;83:480–490

Avanzino L, Bassolino M, Pozzo T, Bove M. Use-dependent hemispheric balance. J Neurosci 2011;31(9):3423–3428

Bailey CH, Kandel ER. Structural changes accompanying memory storage. Annu Rev Physiol 1993;55:397–426

Bastian AJ. Understanding sensorimotor adaptation and learning for rehabilitation. Curr Opin Neurol 2008;21(6):628–633

Benowitz LI, Routtenberg A. GAP-43: an intrinsic determinant of neuronal development and plasticity. Trends Neurosci 1997;20(2):84–91

Bernhardt J, Thuy MN, Collier JM, Legg LA. Very early versus delayed mobilisation after stroke. Cochrane Database Syst Rev 2009;(1):CD006187

Bobath B. Adult Hemiplegia Evaluation and Treatment. 3rd ed. Oxford, UK: Butterworth-Heinemann; 1990

Bose PK, Hou J, Parmer R, Reier PJ, Thompson FJ. Altered patterns of reflex excitability, balance, and locomotion following spinal cord injury and locomotor training. Front Phys 2012;3:258

Boulenguez P, Vinay L. Strategies to restore motor functions after spinal cord injury. Curr Opin Neurobiol 2009;19(6):587–600

Brodal P. The Central Nervous System: Structure and Function. 4th ed. New York, NY: Oxford University Press; 2010

Bütefisch CM, Kleiser R, Seitz RJ. Post-lesional cerebral reorganisation: evidence from functional neuroimaging and transcranial magnetic stimulation. J Physiol Paris 2006;99(4-6):437–454

Butz M, Wörgötter F, van Ooyen A. Activity-dependent structural plasticity. Brain Res Brain Res Rev 2009;60(2):287–305

Cai L, Chan JS, Yan JH, Peng K. Brain plasticity and motor practice in cognitive aging. Front Aging Neurosci 2014;6:31

Calautti C, Jones PS, Naccarato M, et al. The relationship between motor deficit and primary motor cortex hemispheric activation balance after stroke: longitudinal fMRI study. J Neurol Neurosurg Psychiatry 2010;81(7):788–792

Calayan LMS, Dizon J. A systematic review on the effectiveness of mental practice with motor imagery in the neurologic rehabilitation of stroke patients. The Internet J Allied Health Sci Pract 2009;7(2)

Carmichael ST. Translating the frontiers of brain repair to treatments: starting not to break the rules. Neurobiol Dis 2010;37(2):237–242

Cayre M, Canoll P, Goldman JE. Cell migration in the normal and pathological postnatal mammalian brain. Prog Neurobiol 2009;88(1):41–63

Chen H, Epstein J, Stern E. Neural plasticity after acquired brain injury: evidence from functional neuroimaging. PM R 2010; 2(12, Suppl 2)S306–S312

Cotman CW, Berchtold NC, Christie L-A. Exercise builds brain health: key roles of growth factor cascades and inflammation. Trends Neurosci 2007;30(9):464–472

Craik R. Recovery processes: maximizing function. In: Contemporary Management of Motor Control Problems: Proceedings of the II STEP Conference. Foundation for Physical Therapy; 1991:165–173

Cramer SC, Sur M, Dobkin BH, et al. Harnessing neuroplasticity for clinical applications. Brain 2011;134(Pt 6):1591–1609

Criscimagna-Hemminger SE, Bastian AJ, Shadmehr R. Size of error affects cerebellar contributions to motor learning. J Neurophysiol 2010;103(4):2275–2284

Dancause N, Nudo RJ. Shaping plasticity to enhance recovery after injury. Prog Brain Res 2011;192(192):273–295

Darian-Smith C. Synaptic plasticity, neurogenesis, and functional recovery after spinal cord injury. Neuroscientist 2009;15(2):149–165

Demain S, Wiles R, Roberts L, McPherson K. Recovery plateau following stroke: fact or fiction? Disabil Rehabil 2006;28(13-14):815–821

Dietz V. Proprioception and locomotor disorders. Nat Rev Neurosci 2002;3(10):781–790

Diniz LP, Matias IC, Garcia MN, Gomes FC. Astrocytic control of neural circuit formation: highlights on TGF-beta signaling. Neurochem Int 2014;78(August):18–27

Doyon J, Benali H. Reorganization and plasticity in the adult brain during learning of motor skills. Curr Opin Neurobiol 2005;15(2):161–167

Eccles J. Evolution of the Brain: Creation of the Self. New York, NY: Routledge; 1990

Elbert T, Rockstroh B. Reorganization of human cerebral cortex: the range of changes following use and injury. Neuroscientist 2004;10(2):129–141

Ergul A, Alhusban A, Fagan SC. Angiogenesis: a harmonized target for recovery after stroke. Stroke 2012;43(8):2270–2274

Eriksson PS, Perfilieva E, Björk-Eriksson T, et al. Neurogenesis in the adult human hippocampus. Nat Med 1998;4(11):1313–1317

Fantini P, Aggarwal P. Monitoring brain activity using near-infrared light. American Laboratory. 2001:15–17. http://www.nmr.mgh.harvard.edu/DOT/people/mari/papers/Fantini_AmLab_2001.pdf

Faralli A, Bigoni M, Mauro A, Rossi F, Carulli D. Noninvasive strategies to promote functional recovery after stroke. Neural Plast 2013;2013:854597

Ferguson AR, Huie JR, Crown ED, et al. Maladaptive spinal plasticity opposes spinal learning and recovery in spinal cord injury. Front Phys 2012;3(October):399

Feuerstein R, Falik LH, Feuerstein RS. The cognitive elements of neural plasticity. 2013. http://www.neuropsychotherapist.com/cognitive-elements-neural-plasticity. Accessed Sept 11, 2015

Feys H, De Weerdt W, Verbeke G, et al. Early and repetitive stimulation of the arm can substantially improve the long-term outcome after stroke: a 5-year follow-up study of a randomized trial. Stroke 2004;35(4):924–929

Gorgoni M, D'Atri A, Lauri G, Rossini PM, Ferlazzo F, De Gennaro L. Is sleep essential for neural plasticity in humans, and how does it affect motor and cognitive recovery? Neural Plast 2013;2013:103949

Graham JV, Eustace C, Brock K, Swain E, Irwin-Carruthers S. The Bobath Concept in contemporary clinical practice. Top Stroke Rehabil 2009;16(1):57–68

Greenberg DA. Neurogenesis and stroke. CNS Neurol Disord Drug Targets 2007;6(5):321–325

Hallett M. The plastic brain. Ann Neurol 1995;38(1):4–5

Hori J, Ng TF, Shatos M, Klassen H, Streilein JW, Young MJ. Neural progenitor cells lack immunogenicity and resist destruction as allografts. Stem Cells 2003;21(4):405–416

Huber R, Ghilardi MF, Massimini M, et al. Arm immobilization causes cortical plastic changes and local-

ly decreases sleep slow wave activity. Nat Neurosci 2006;9(9):1169–1176

Hubli M. Plasticity of Human Spinal Locomotor Circuitry. ETH Zurich; 2011

Hubli M, Dietz V. The physiological basis of neurorehabilitation—locomotor training after spinal cord injury. J Neuroeng Rehabil 2013;10:5

Jellinger KA, Attems J. Neuropathological approaches to cerebral aging and neuroplasticity. Dialogues Clin Neurosci 2013;15(1):29–43

Johansson BB. Brain plasticity in health and disease. Keio J Med 2004;53(4):231–246

Johansson BB. Current trends in stroke rehabilitation. A review with focus on brain plasticity. Acta Neurol Scand 2011;123(3):147–159

Jones TA, Allred RP, Adkins DL, Hsu JE, O'Bryant A, Maldonado MA. Remodeling the brain with behavioral experience after stroke. Stroke 2009;40(3, Suppl):S136–S138

Kandel E, Schwartz J, Jessell T, Siegelbaum S, Hudspeth AJ. Principles of Neural Science. 5th ed., New York, NY: McGraw-Hill Professional; 2013

Karger AG. Guidelines for management of ischaemic stroke and transient ischaemic attack 2008. Cerebrovasc Dis 2008;25:457–507

Kempermann G, Kuhn HG, Winkler J, Gage FH. New nerve cells for the adult brain. Adult neurogenesis and stem cell concepts in neurologic research [in German]. Nervenarzt 1998;69(10):851–857

Khedr EM, Abdel-Fadeil MR, Farghali A, Qaid M. Role of 1 and 3 Hz repetitive transcranial magnetic stimulation on motor function recovery after acute ischaemic stroke. Eur J Neurol 2009;16(12):1323–1330

Kidd G, Lawes N, Musa I. Understanding Neuromuscular Plasticity: A Basis for Clinical Rehabilitation. London: Edward Arnold; 1992

Kitago T, Krakauer JW. Motor learning principles for neurorehabilitation. Handb Clin Neurol 2013;110:93–103

Kleim JA. Neural plasticity and neurorehabilitation: teaching the new brain old tricks. J Commun Disord 2011;44(5):521–528

Kleim JA, Jones TA, Schallert T. Motor enrichment and the induction of plasticity before or after brain injury. Neurochem Res 2003;28(11):1757–1769

Kleim JA, Jones TA. Principles of experience-dependent neural plasticity: implications for rehabilitation after brain damage. J Speech Lang Hear Res 2008;51(1):S225–S239

Komitova M, Johansson BB, Eriksson PS. On neural plasticity, new neurons and the postischemic milieu: an integrated view on experimental rehabilitation. Exp Neurol 2006;199(1):42–55

Krakauer JW. Motor learning: its relevance to stroke recovery and neurorehabilitation. Curr Opin Neurol 2006;19(1):84–90

Kwakkel G, Kollen B, Lindeman E. Understanding the pattern of functional recovery after stroke: facts and theories. Restor Neurol Neurosci 2004;22(3-5):281–299

Kwakkel G, Kollen B, Twisk J. Impact of time on improvement of outcome after stroke. Stroke 2006;37(9):2348–2353

Lam T, Noonan VK, Eng JJ; SCIRE Research Team. A systematic review of functional ambulation outcome measures in spinal cord injury. Spinal Cord 2008;46(4):246–254

Lamprecht R, LeDoux J. Structural plasticity and memory. Nat Rev Neurosci 2004;5(1):45–54

Langhorne P, Bernhardt J, Kwakkel G. Stroke rehabilitation. Lancet 2011;377(9778):1693–1702

Lee RG, van Donkelaar P. Mechanisms underlying functional recovery following stroke. Can J Neurol Sci 1995;22(4):257–263

Lee TD, Schmidt RA. Motor Learning and Memory. In J. Byrne, ed. Cognitive Psychology of Memory. 2008:645–662

Levin MF, Kleim JA, Wolf SL. What do motor "recovery" and "compensation" mean in patients following stroke? Neurorehabil Neural Repair 2009;23(4):313–319

Luo C, Tu S, Peng Y, et al. Long-term effects of musical training and functional plasticity in salience system. Neural Plast;2014:18013

Lynskey JV, Belanger A, Jung R. Activity-dependent plasticity in spinal cord injury. J Rehabil Res Dev 2008;45(2):229–240

Mally J. Non-invasive brain stimulation and its supposed site of action in the rehabilitation of Parkinson's disease and stroke. NeuroRehabilitation 2014;1:e103

Makin TR, Cramer AO, Scholz J, Hahamy A, Henderson Slater D, Tracey I, Johansen-Berg H. Deprivation-related and use-dependent plasticity go hand in hand. Elife 2013;12(2):e01273

Martin JL, Magistretti PJ. Regulation of gene expression by neurotransmitters in the central nervous system. Eur Neurol 1998;39(3):129–134

Molinari M. Plasticity properties of CPG circuits in humans: impact on gait recovery. Brain Res Bull 2009;78(1):22–25

Muir GD, Steeves JD. Sensorimotor stimulation to improve locomotor recovery after spinal cord injury. Trends Neurosci 1997;20(2):72–77

Nakamura T, Hillary FG, Biswal BB. Resting network plasticity following brain injury. PLoS ONE 2009;4(12):e8220

Nielsen JB, Willerslev-Olsen M, Christiansen L, Lundbye-Jensen J, Lorentzen J. Science-based neurorehabilitation: recommendations for neurorehabilitation from basic science. J Mot Behav 2015;47(1):7–17

Nudo RJ. Adaptive plasticity in motor cortex: implications for rehabilitation after brain injury. J Rehabil Med 2003; 35(41, Suppl)7–10

Nudo RJ. Neural bases of recovery after brain injury. J Commun Disord 2011;44(5):515–520

Nudo RJ, Milliken GW, Jenkins WM, Merzenich MM. Use-dependent alterations of movement representations in primary motor cortex of adult squirrel monkeys. J Neurosci 1996a;16(2):785–807

Nudo RJ, Wise BM, SiFuentes F, Milliken GW. Neural substrates for the effects of rehabilitative training on motor recovery after ischemic infarct. Science 1996b;272(5269):1791–1794

Olson L. Neurotrophic factors in the CNS: increasing numbers of proteins with clinical potential [in Swedish]. Nord Med 1996;111(1):3–6

Onifer SM, Smith GM, Fouad K. Plasticity after spinal cord injury: relevance to recovery and approaches to facilitate it. Neurotherapeutics 2011;8(2):283–293

Orban de Xivry JJ, Criscimagna-Hemminger SE, Shadmehr R. Contributions of the motor cortex to adaptive control of reaching depend on the perturbation schedule. Cereb Cortex 2011;21(7):1475–1484

Oudega M, Perez MA. Corticospinal reorganization after spinal cord injury. J Physiol 2012;590(Pt 16):3647–3663

Pekna M, Pekny M, Nilsson M. Modulation of neural plasticity as a basis for stroke rehabilitation. Stroke 2012;43(10):2819–2828

Raffin E, Siebner HR. Transcranial brain stimulation to promote functional recovery after stroke. Curr Opin Neurol 2014;27(1):54–60

Raine S, Meadows L, Lynch-Ellerington M. Bobath Concept: Theory and Clinical Practice in Neurological Rehabilitation. Hoboken, NJ: Wiley-Blackwell; 2009

Rank MM, Flynn JR, Battistuzzo CR, Galea MP, Callister R, Callister RJ. Functional changes in deep dorsal horn interneurons following spinal cord injury are enhanced with different durations of exercise training. J Physiol 2015;593(1):331–345

Reisman DS, Wityk R, Silver K, Bastian AJ. Locomotor adaptation on a split-belt treadmill can improve walking symmetry post-stroke. Brain 2007;130(Pt 7):1861–1872

Reisman DS, Bastian AJ, Morton SM. Neurophysiologic and rehabilitation insights from the split-belt and other locomotor adaptation paradigms. Phys Ther 2010;90(2):187–195

Richards L, Hanson C, Wellborn M, Sethi A. Driving motor recovery after stroke. Top Stroke Rehabil 2008;15(5):397–411

Rossignol S, Frigon A. Recovery of locomotion after spinal cord injury: some facts and mechanisms. Annu Rev Neurosci 2011;34:413–440

Seil FJ. Recovery and repair issues after stroke from the scientific perspective. Curr Opin Neurol 1997;10(1):49–51

Shadmehr R, Smith MA, Krakauer JW. Error correction, sensory prediction, and adaptation in motor control. Annu Rev Neurosci 2010;33:89–108

Shmuelof L, Krakauer JW, Mazzoni P. How is a motor skill learned? Change and invariance at the levels of task success and trajectory control. J Neurophysiol 2012;108(2):578–594

Siengsukon CF, Boyd LA. Does sleep promote motor learning? Implications for physical rehabilitation. Phys Ther 2009;89(4):370–383

Small SL, Hlustik P, Noll DC, Genovese C, Solodkin A. Cerebellar hemispheric activation ipsilateral to the paretic hand correlates with functional recovery after stroke. Brain 2002;125(Pt 7):1544–1557

Stein DG, Brailowsky P, Will B. Brain Repair. New York, NY: Oxford University Press; 1997

Stephenson R. A Review of Neuroplasticity: Some Implications for Physiotherapy in the Treatment of Lesions of the Brain. Physiotherapy 1993;79:699–704

Takeuchi N, Izumi S. Maladaptive plasticity for motor recovery after stroke: mechanisms and approaches. Neural Plast 2012;2012:359728

Takeuchi N, Izumi S. Rehabilitation with poststroke motor recovery: a review with a focus on neural plasticity. Stroke Res Treat 2013;2013:128641

Troen H, Edgar H. The regulation of neuronal gene expression. Trends Neurosci 1982;7:311–313

Ullian EM, Christopherson KS, Barres BA. Role for glia in synaptogenesis. Glia 2004;47(3):209–216

van Praag H. Exercise and the brain: something to chew on. Trends Neurosci 2009;32(5):283–290

Ward NS, Cohen LG. Mechanisms underlying recovery of motor function after stroke. Arch Neurol 2004;61(12):1844–1848

Winstein C, Stewart J. Conditions of task practice for individuals with neurologic impairments. In: Selzer ME, Clarke S, Cohen LG, et al, eds. Textbook of Neural Repair and Rehabilitation. Cambridge, UK: Cambridge University Press; 2006:89–102

Woldag H, Stupka K, Hummelsheim H. Repetitive training of complex hand and arm movements with shaping is beneficial for motor improvement in patients after stroke. J Rehabil Med 2010;42(6):582–587

Wolpert DM, Ghahramani Z, Jordan MI. An internal model for sensorimotor integration. Science 1995;269(5232):1880–1882

Chapter 1.4
Consequences of and Reorganization after CNS Lesions

Ashburn A, Lynch-Ellerington M. Disadvantages of the early use of wheelchairs in the treatment of hemiplegia. Clin Rehabil 1988;2:327–331

Barnes M, Johnson G. An overview of the clinical management of spasticity. In: Barnes MR, Johnson GR, eds. Upper Motor Neurone Syndrome and Spasticity: Clinical Management and Neurophysiology. Cambridge, UK: Cambridge University Press; 2008:931

Bobath B. Adult Hemiplegia Evaluation and Treatment. 2nd ed. London, UK: William Heinemann; 1978

Bobath B. Adult Hemiplegia Evaluation and Treatment. 3rd ed. Oxford, UK: Butterworth-Heinemann; 1990

Bohannon R, Andrews A. Limb muscle strength is impaired bilaterally after stroke. J Phys Ther Sci 1995;7:1–7

Bohannon RW. Muscle strength and muscle training after stroke. J Rehabil Med 2007;39(1):14–20

Brodal P. The Central Nervous System: Structure and Function. 4th ed. New York, NY: Oxford University Press; 2010

Brown P. Pathophysiology of spasticity. J Neurol Neurosurg Psychiatry 1994;57(7):773–777

Burke D. Spasticity as an adaptation to pyramidal tract injury. Adv Neurol 1988;47:401–423

Burke D, Wissel J, Donnan GA. Pathophysiology of spasticity in stroke. Neurology 2013;80(3, Suppl 2):S20–S26

Burridge JH, Wood DE, Hermens HJ, et al. Theoretical and methodological considerations in the measurement of spasticity. Disabil Rehabil 2005;27(1-2):69–80

Canning CG, Ada L, Adams R, O'Dwyer NJ. Loss of strength contributes more to physical disability after stroke than loss of dexterity. Clin Rehabil 2004;18(3):300–308

Carr J, Shepherd R. A Motor Relearning Programme for Stroke. Aspen Systems Corporation; 1983

Carr JH, Shepherd RB, Ada L. Spasticity: research findings and implications for intervention. Physiotherapy 1995;81:421–427

Cornall C. Self-propelling wheelchairs: The effects on spasticity in hemiplegic patients. Physiother Theory Pract 1991;7(1):13–21

Cramer SC, Bastings EP. Mapping clinically relevant plasticity after stroke. Neuropharmacology 2000;39(5):842–851

Cramer SC, Nelles G, Benson RR, et al. A functional MRI study of subjects recovered from hemiparetic stroke. Stroke 1997;28(12):2518–2527

Dietz V, Sinkjaer T. Spastic movement disorder: impaired reflex function and altered muscle mechanics. Lancet Neurol 2007;6(8):725–733

Dvir Z, Panturin E. Measurement of spasticity and associated reactions in stroke patients before and after physiotherapeutic intervention. Clin Rehabil 1993;7(1):15–21

Edwards S. Neurological Physiotherapy: A Problem-Solving Approach. Philadelphia, PA: Churchill Livingstone; 1996

Fujiwara T, Sonoda S, Okajima Y, Chino N. The relationships between trunk function and the findings of transcranial magnetic stimulation among patients with stroke. J Rehabil Med 2001;33(6):249–255

Giovannoni G. Multiple sclerosis related fatigue. J Neurol Neurosurg Psychiatry 2006;77(1):2–3

Goldspink G, Williams P. 1991. Muscle fibre and connective tissue changes associated with use and disuse. In: Ada L, Canning C, eds. Key Issues in Neurological Physiotherapy. Oxford, UK: Butterworth-Heinemann; 1996:197–218

Gracies J-M. Pathophysiology of spastic paresis, I: Paresis and soft tissue changes. Muscle Nerve 2005;31(5):535–551

Gray V, Rice CL, Garland SJ. Factors that influence muscle weakness following stroke and their clinical implications: a critical review. Physiother Can 2012;64(4):415–426

Haaland KY, Delaney HD. Motor deficits after left or right hemisphere damage due to stroke or tumor. Neuropsychologia 1981;19(1):17–27

Hufschmidt A, Mauritz KH. Chronic transformation of muscle in spasticity: a peripheral contribution to increased tone. J Neurol Neurosurg Psychiatry 1985;48(7):676–685

Kitsos GH, Hubbard IJ, Kitsos AR, Parsons MW. The ipsilesional upper limb can be affected following stroke. ScientificWorldJournal 2013;2013:684860

Kline TL, Schmit BD, Kamper DG. Exaggerated interlimb neural coupling following stroke. Brain 2007;130 (Pt 1):159–169

Lerdal A, Bakken LN, Kouwenhoven SE, et al. Post-stroke fatigue—a review. J Pain Symptom Manage 2009;38(6):928–949

Maas MB, Safdieh JE. Ischemic stroke: pathophysiology and principles of localization. Neurology 2009; 30(1):1-16

Malhotra S, Pandyan AD, Day CR, Jones PW, Hermens H. Spasticity, an impairment that is poorly defined and poorly measured. Clin Rehabil 2009;23(7):651–658

Mani S, Mutha PK, Przybyla A, Haaland KY, Good DC, Sainburg RL. Contralesional motor deficits after unilateral stroke reflect hemisphere-specific control mechanisms. Brain 2013;136(Pt 4):1288–1303

Pandyan AD, Gregoric M, Barnes MP, et al. Spasticity: clinical perceptions, neurological realities and meaningful measurement. Disabil Rehabil 2005;27(1-2):2–6

Patten C, Lexell J, Brown HE. Weakness and strength training in persons with poststroke hemiplegia: rationale, method, and efficacy. J Rehabil Res Dev 2004;41(3A):293–312

Platz T, Eickhof C, Nuyens G, Vuadens P. Clinical scales for the assessment of spasticity, associated phenomena, and function: a systematic review of the literature. Disabil Rehabil 2005;27(1-2):7–18

Rothwell J, Lennon S. Control of Human Voluntary Movement. 2nd ed. London, UK: Chapman and Hall; 1994

Shumway-Cook A, Woollacott MH. Motor Control: Translating Research into Clinical Practice. 3rd ed. Philadelphia, PA: Lippincott Williams & Wilkins; 2006

Soderlund A, Malterud K. Why did I get chronic fatigue syndrome? A qualitative interview study of causal attributions in women patients. Scand J Prim Health Care 2005;23(4):242–247

Stokes M. Neurological Physiotherapy. London, UK: Mosby; 1998

Thibaut A, Chatelle C, Ziegler E, Bruno MA, Laureys S, Gosseries O. Spasticity after stroke: physiology, assessment and treatment. Brain Inj 2013;27(10):1093–1105

Toft E. Mechanical and electromyographic stretch responses in spastic and healthy subjects. Acta Neurol Scand Suppl 1995;163:1–24

Turton A, Pomeroy V. When should upper limb function be trained after stroke? Evidence for and against early intervention. NeuroRehabilitation 2002;17(3):215–224

Tyldesley B, Grieve J. Muscles, Nerves and Movement: Kinesiology in Daily Living. 2nd ed. Oxford, UK: Blackwell Sciences; 1996

Vattanasilp W, Ada L, Crosbie J. Contribution of thixotropy, spasticity, and contracture to ankle stiffness after stroke. J Neurol Neurosurg Psychiatry 2000;69(1):34–39

Voerman GE, Gregoric M, Hermens HJ. Neurophysiological methods for the assessment of spasticity: the Hoffmann reflex, the tendon reflex, and the stretch reflex. Disabil Rehabil 2005;27(1-2):33–68

Walshe FMR. The decerebrate rigidity of Sherrington in man: its recognition and differentiation from other forms of tonic muscular contraction. Arch Neur Psych 1923;10(1):1–28

Ward NS, Brown MM, Thompson AJ, Frackowiak RS. Neural correlates of motor recovery after stroke: a longitudinal fMRI study. Brain 2003;126(Pt 11):2476–2496

Ward NS, Cohen LG. Mechanisms underlying recovery of motor function after stroke. Arch Neurol 2004;61(12):1844–1848

Wood DE, Burridge JH, van Wijck FM, et al. Biomechanical approaches applied to the lower and upper limb for the measurement of spasticity: a systematic review of the literature. Disabil Rehabil 2005;27(1-2):19–32

Yarkony GM, Sahgal V. Contractures. A major complication of craniocerebral trauma. Clin Orthop Relat Res 1987; (219):93–96

Yelnik AP, Simon O, Parratte B, Gracies JM. How to clinically assess and treat muscle overactivity in spastic paresis. J Rehabil Med 2010;42(9):801–807

Young RR. Spasticity: a review. Neurology 1994; 44(11, Suppl 9) S12–S20

Chapter 2
Human Movement

Aaslund MK, Moe-Nilssen R. Treadmill walking with body weight support effect of treadmill, harness and body weight support systems. Gait Posture. 2008;28:303–308

Abe H, Kondo T, Oouchida Y, Suzukamo Y, Fujiwara S, Izumi S. Prevalence and length of recovery of pusher syndrome based on cerebral hemispheric lesion side in patients with acute stroke. Stroke 2012;43(6):1654–1656

Ada L, Canning CG. Anticipating and avoiding muscle shortening. In: Ada L, Canning CG, eds. Key Issues in Neurological Physiotherapy. New York, NY: Oxford University Press; 1990:219–236. Physiotherapy: Foundations for Practice

Ada L, Dorsch S, Canning CG. Strengthening interventions increase strength and improve activity after stroke: a systematic review. Aust J Physiother 2006;52(4):241–248

Ada L, Foongchomcheay A, Canning C. Supportive devices for preventing and treating subluxation of the shoulder after stroke. Cochrane Database Syst Rev 2005;(1):CD003863

Alexandrov AV, Frolov AA, Horak FB, Carlson-Kuhta P, Park S. Feedback equilibrium control during human standing. Biol Cybern 2005;93(5):309–322

Alfieri FM, Riberto M, Gatz LS, Ribeiro CP, Lopes JA, Battistella LR. Functional mobility and balance in community-dwelling elderly submitted to multisensory versus strength exercises [published correction appears in Clin Interv Aging 2010;5:363. Santarém, José Maria removed]. Clin Interv Aging 2010;5:181–185

Aruin A, Almeida G. A coactivation strategy in anticipatory postural adjustments in persons with Down syndrome. Motor Control 1997;1:178–191

Aruin AS. The effect of asymmetry of posture on anticipatory postural adjustments. Neurosci Lett 2006;401(1-2e):150–153

Aruin AS, Latash ML. Anticipatory postural adjustments during self-initiated perturbations of different magnitude triggered by a standard motor action. Electroencephalogr Clin Neurophysiol 1996;101(6):497–503

Asberg KH. Orthostatic tolerance training of stroke patients in general medical wards. An experimental study. Scand J Rehabil Med 1989;21(4):179–185

Ashburn A, Lynch-Ellerington M. Disadvantage of the early use of wheelchairs in the treatment of hemiplegia. Clin Rehabil 1988;2:327–331

Bader-Johansson C. Grundmotorik, Lund, Sweden: Studentlitteratur

Bae SH, Lee HG, Kim YE, Kim GY, Jung HW, Kim KY. Effects of trunk stabilization exercises on different support surfaces on the cross-sectional area of the trunk muscles and balance ability. J Phys Ther Sci 2013;25(6):741–745

Baldan AMS, Alouche SR, Araujo IM, Freitas SM. Effect of light touch on postural sway in individuals with balance problems: a systematic review. Gait Posture 2014;40(1):1–10

Barbieri G, Gissot AS, Fouque F, Casillas JM, Pozzo T, Pérennou D. Does proprioception contribute to the sense of verticality? Exp Brain Res 2008;185(4):545–552

Barra J, Pérennou D. Is the sense of verticality vestibular? [in French] Neurophysiol Clin 2013;43(3):197–204

Barra J, Marquer A, Joassin R, et al. Humans use internal models to construct and update a sense of verticality. Brain 2010;133(Pt 12):3552–3563

Bateni H, Maki BE. Assistive devices for balance and mobility: benefits, demands, and adverse consequences. Arch Phys Med Rehabil 2005;86(1):134–145

Bateni H, Zecevic A, McIlroy WE, Maki BE. Resolving conflicts in task demands during balance recovery: does holding an object inhibit compensatory grasping? Exp Brain Res 2004;157(1):49–58

Bayouk J-F, Boucher JP, Leroux A. Balance training following stroke: effects of task-oriented exercises with and without altered sensory input. Int J Rehabil Res 2006;29(1):51–59

Belenkiy VE, Gurfinkel VS, Paltsev EI. On elements of control of voluntary movements. Biofizika 1967;12(1):135–141

Berencsi A, Ishihara M, Imanaka K. The functional role of central and peripheral vision in the control of posture. Hum Mov Sci 2005;24(5-6):689–709

Berg W, Strang A. The Role of Electromyography (EMG) in the Study of Anticipatory Postural Adjustments. Rijeka, Croatia: InTech; 2012

Bernstein N. The Coordination and Regulation of Movements. New York, NY: Pergamon; 1967

Bharadwaj K, Sugar TG, Koeneman JB, Koeneman EJ. Design of a robotic gait trainer using spring over muscle actuators for ankle stroke rehabilitation. J Biomech Eng 2005;127(6):1009–1013

Blouin J, Bard C, Teasdale N, et al. Reference systems for coding spatial information in normal subjects and a deafferented patient. Exp Brain Res 1993;93(2):324–331

Blouin J, Saradjian AH, Lebar N, Guillaume A, Mouchnino L. Opposed optimal strategies of weighting somatosensory inputs for planning reaching movements toward visual and proprioceptive targets. J Neurophysiol 2014;112(9):2290–2301

Bobath B. Adult Hemiplegia: Evaluation and Treatment. 2nd ed. London, UK: William Heinemann; 1978

Bobath B. Adult Hemiplegia: Evaluation and Treatment. 3rd ed. Oxford, UK: Butterworth-Heinemann; 1990

Bohannon R, Andrews A. Limb Muscle Strength is Impaired Bilaterally after stroke. J Phys Ther Sci 1995;7(1):1–7

Bonan IV, Yelnik AP, Colle FM, et al. Reliance on visual information after stroke. Part II: Effectiveness of a balance rehabilitation program with visual cue deprivation after stroke: a randomized controlled trial. Arch Phys Med Rehabil 2004;85(2):274–278

Bonan IV, Guettard E, Leman MC, Colle FM, Yelnik AP. Subjective visual vertical perception relates to balance in acute stroke. Arch Phys Med Rehabil 2006;87(5):642–646

Bonan IV, Marquer A, Eskiizmirliler S, Yelnik AP, Vidal PP. Sensory reweighting in controls and stroke patients. Clin Neurophysiol 2013;124(4):713–722

Boonsinsukh R, Panichareon L, Phansuwan-Pujito P. Light touch cue through a cane improves pelvic stability during walking in stroke. Arch Phys Med Rehabil 2009;90(6):919–926

Boonsinsukh R, Panichareon L, Saengsirisuwan V, Phansuwan-Pujito P. Clinical identification for the use of light touch cues with a cane in gait rehabilitation poststroke. Top Stroke Rehabil 2011;18(1, Suppl 1):633–642

Borghuis J, Hof AL, Lemmink KA. The importance of sensory-motor control in providing core stability: implications for measurement and training. Sports Med 2008;38(11):893–916

Bouisset S, Do MC. Posture, dynamic stability, and voluntary movement. Neurophysiol Clin 2008;38(6):345–362

Bouisset S, Le Bozec S. Posturo-kinetics capacity and postural function in voluntary movement. In: Latash ML, ed. Progress in Motor Control. Champaign, IL: Human Kinetics; 2002:25–52

Bouisset S, Zattara M. A sequence of postural movements precedes voluntary movement. Neurosci Lett 1981;22:263–270

Bowden JL, Lin GG, McNulty PA. The prevalence and magnitude of impaired cutaneous sensation across the hand in the chronic period post-stroke. PLoS ONE 2014;9(8):e104153

Bowen A, Hazelton C, Pollock A, Lincoln NB. Cognitive rehabilitation for spatial neglect following stroke. Cochrane Database Syst Rev 2013;7(7):CD003586

Brady RA, Peters BT, Batson CD, Ploutz-Snyder R, Mulavara AP, Bloomberg JJ. Gait adaptability training is affected by visual dependency. Exp Brain Res 2012;220(1):1–9

Bridgewater KJ, Sharpe MH. Trunk muscle performance in early Parkinson's disease. Phys Ther 1998;78(6):566–576

Brock K, Haase G, Rothacher G, Cotton S. Does physiotherapy based on the Bobath Concept, in conjunction with a task practice, achieve greater improvement in walking ability in people with stroke compared to physiotherapy focused on structured task practice alone?: a pilot randomized controlled trial. Clin Rehabil 2011;25(10):903–912

Brodal P. Det nevrologiske grunnlaget for balanse.pdf. Fysioterapeuten 2004;(8):25–30

Brodal P. The Central Nervous System: Structure and Function. 4th ed. New York, NY: Oxford University Press; 2010

Brooks V. The Neural Basis for Motor Control. Oxford, UK: Oxford University Press; 1986

Brown LA, Shumway-Cook A, Woollacott MH. Attentional demands and postural recovery: the effects of aging. J Gerontol A Biol Sci Med Sci 1999;54(4):M165–M171

Bussel B, Roby-Brami A, Néris OR, Yakovleff A. Evidence for a spinal stepping generator in man. Electrophysiological study. Acta Neurobiol Exp (Warsz) 1996;56(1):465–468

Caillet R. The Shoulder in Hemiplegia. Philadelphia, PA: FA Davis; 1980

Caneiro JP, O'Sullivan P, Burnett A, Barach A, O'Neil D, Tveit O, Olafsdottir K. The influence of different sitting postures on head/neck posture and muscle activity. Man Ther 2010;15(1):54–60

Cambridge NA. Electrical apparatus used in medicine before 1900. Proc R Soc Med 1977;70(9):635–641

Canning CG, Ada L, Adams R, O'Dwyer NJ. Loss of strength contributes more to physical disability after stroke than loss of dexterity. Clin Rehabil 2004;18(3):300–308

Carr LJ, Harrison LM, Stephens JA. Evidence for bilateral innervation of certain homologous motoneurone pools in man. J Physiol 1994;475(2):217–227

Casadio M, Morasso P, Sanguineti V, Giannoni P. Minimally assistive robot training for proprioception enhancement. Exp Brain Res 2009;194(2):219–231

Cheng PT, Liaw MY, Wong MK, Tang FT, Lee MY, Lin PS. The sit-to-stand movement in stroke patients and its correlation with falling. Arch Phys Med Rehabil 1998;79(9):1043–1046

Cirstea MC, Levin MF. Compensatory strategies for reaching in stroke. Brain 2000;123(Pt 5):940–953

Clément G, Delière Q, Migeotte PF. Perception of verticality and cardiovascular responses during short-radius centrifugation. J Vestib Res 2014;24(1):1–8

Cornall C. Self-propelling wheelchairs: the effects on spasticity in hemiplegic patients. Physiother Theory Pract 1991;7(1):13–21

Cote KP, Brunet ME, Gansneder BM, Shultz SJ. Effects of pronated and supinated foot postures on static and dynamic postural stability. J Athl Train 2005;40(1):41–46

Cram JF, Criswell E. Introduction to Surface Electromyography. Sudbury, MA: Jones and Bartlett; 2011

Creath R, Kiemel T, Horak F, Jeka JJ. The role of vestibular and somatosensory systems in intersegmental control of upright stance. J Vestib Res 2008;18(1):39–49

Crosbie J, Kilbreath SL, Hollmann L, York S. Scapulohumeral rhythm and associated spinal motion. Clin Biomech (Bristol, Avon) 2008;23(2):184–192

Daubney ME, Culham EG. Lower-extremity muscle force and balance performance in adults aged 65 years and older. Phys Ther 1999;79(12):1177–1185

Davies P. Steps to Follow: The Comprehensive Treatment of Patients with Hemiplegia. 2nd ed. Berlin, Germany: Springer; 2003

Decety J. The neurophysiological basis of motor imagery. Behav Brain Res 1996;77(1-2):45–52

Deliagina TG, Beloozerova IN, Zelenin PV, Orlovsky GN. Spinal and supraspinal postural networks. Brain Res Brain Res Rev 2008;57(1):212–221

Dickstein R, Shefi S, Marcovitz E, Villa Y. Anticipatory postural adjustment in selected trunk muscles in post stroke hemiparetic patients. Arch Phys Med Rehabil 2004;85(2):261–267

Dietz V. Human neuronal control of automatic functional movements: interaction between central programs and afferent input. Physiol Rev 1992;72(1):33–69

Dijkerman HC, Ietswaart M, Johnston M, MacWalter RS. Does motor imagery training improve hand function in chronic stroke patients? A pilot study. Clin Rehabil 2004;18(5):538–549

Dobkin BH, Duncan PW. Should body weight-supported treadmill training and robotic-assistive steppers for locomotor training trot back to the starting gate? Neurorehabil Neural Repair 2012;26(4):308–317

Doucet BM, Lam A, Griffin L. Neuromuscular electrical stimulation for skeletal muscle function. Yale J Biol Med 2012;85(2):201–215

Ebenbichler GR, Oddsson LI, Kollmitzer J, Erim Z. Sensory-motor control of the lower back: implications for rehabilitation. Med Sci Sports Exerc 2001;33(11):1889–1898

Edwards S. Neurological Physiotherapy: A Problem-Solving Approach. 2nd ed. Philadelphia, PA: Churchill Livingstone; 1996

Eskes GA, Butler B, McDonald A, Harrison ER, Phillips SJ. Limb activation effects in hemispatial neglect. Arch Phys Med Rehabil 2003;84(3):323–328

Falla D, Jull G, Russell T, Vicenzino B, Hodges P. Effect of neck exercise on sitting posture in patients with chronic neck pain. Phys Ther 2007;87(4):408–417

Ferguson AR, Huie JR, Crown ED, et al. Maladaptive spinal plasticity opposes spinal learning and recovery in spinal cord injury. Front Phys 2012;3(October):399

Feys HM, De Weerdt WJ, Selz BE, et al. Effect of a therapeutic intervention for the hemiplegic upper limb in the acute phase after stroke: a single-blind, randomized, controlled multicenter trial. Stroke 1998;29(4):785–792

van der Fits IB, Klip AW, van Eykern LA, Hadders-Algra M. Postural adjustments accompanying fast pointing movements in standing, sitting and lying adults. Exp Brain Res 1998;120(2):202–216

Fitzpatrick R, Rogers DK, McCloskey DI. Stable human standing with lower-limb muscle afferents providing the only sensory input. J Physiol 1994;480(Pt 2):395–403

Franzén E, Gurfinkel VS, Wright WG, Cordo PJ, Horak FB. Haptic touch reduces sway by increasing axial tone. Neuroscience 2011;174(3):216–223

Gandevia SC, Refshauge KM, Collins DF. Proprioception: peripheral inputs and perceptual interactions. Adv Exp Med Biol 2002;508:61–68

Garland SJ, Gray VL, Knorr S. Muscle activation patterns and postural control following stroke. Mot Contr 2009;13(4):387–411

Garland SJ, Pollock CL, Ivanova TD. Could motor unit control strategies be partially preserved after stroke? Front Hum Neurosci 2014;8(October):864

Genthon N, Vuillerme N, Monnet JP, Petit C, Rougier P. Biomechanical assessment of the sitting posture maintenance in patients with stroke. Clin Biomech (Bristol, Avon) 2007;22(9):1024–1029

Geurts A, Mulder T, Nienhuis B, Rijken R. Influence of orthopedic footwear on postural control in patients with hereditary motor and sensory neuropathy. J Rehabil Sci 1992;5:3–9

Geurts ACH, de Haart M, van Nes IJ, Duysens J. A review of standing balance recovery from stroke. Gait Posture 2005;22(3):267–281

Graham JV, Eustace C, Brock K, Swain E, Irwin-Carruthers S. The Bobath Concept in contemporary clinical practice. Top Stroke Rehabil 2009;16(1):57–68

Gramsbergen A. Postural control in man: the phylogenetic perspective. Neural Plast 2005;12(2-3):77–88, discussion 263–272

Gribble PA, Hertel J, Plisky P. Using the Star Excursion Balance Test to assess dynamic postural-control deficits and outcomes in lower extremity injury: a literature and systematic review. J Athl Train 2012;47(3):339–357

Griffin C. Management of the hemiplegic shoulder complex. Top Stroke Rehabil 2014;21(4):316–318

Grimaldi A. Assessing lateral stability of the hip and pelvis. Man Ther 2011;16(1):26–32

Guertin PA. The spinal cord: functional organization, diseases, and dysfunctions. In: Aldskogius H, ed. Animal Models of Spinal Cord Repair. Neuromethods. Totowa, NJ: Humana Press; 2013

Gurfinkel V, Cacciatore TW, Cordo P, Horak F, Nutt J, Skoss R. Postural muscle tone in the body axis of healthy humans. J Neurophysiol 2006;96(5):2678–2687

Hacmon RR, Krasovsky T, Lamontagne A, Levin MF. Deficits in intersegmental trunk coordination during walking are related to clinical balance and gait function in chronic stroke. J Neurol Phys Ther 2012;36(4):173–181

Harvey M, Hood B, North A, Robertson IH. The effects of visuomotor feedback training on the recovery of hemispatial neglect symptoms: assessment of a 2-week and follow-up intervention. Neuropsychologia 2003;41(8):886–893

Hasan Z. The human motor control system's response to mechanical perturbation: should it, can it, and does it ensure stability? J Mot Behav 2005;37(6):484–493

Heilman KM, Valenstein E. Clinical Neuropsychology. 4th ed. New York, NY: Oxford University Press; 2003

Held J. Recovery of function after brain damage: theoretical implication for therapeutic intervention. In: Carr JH, Shepherd RB, eds. Movement Science: Foundations for Physical Therapy in Rehabilitation. Rockville, MD: Aspen Publishers; 1987:155–177

Hijmans JM, Geertzen JH, Dijkstra PU, Postema K. A systematic review of the effects of shoes and other ankle or foot appliances on balance in older people and people with peripheral nervous system disorders. Gait Posture 2007;25(2):316–323

Hilfiker R, Vaney C, Gattlen B, et al. Local dynamic stability as a responsive index for the evaluation of rehabilitation effect on fall risk in patients with multiple sclerosis: a longitudinal study. BMC Res Notes 2013;6:260

Himmelbach M, Karnath H-O. Goal-directed hand movements are not affected by the biased space representation in spatial neglect. J Cogn Neurosci 2003;15(7):972–980

Horak FB. Clinical measurement of postural control in adults. Phys Ther 1987;67(12):1881–1885

Horak FB. Clinical assessment of balance disorders. Gait Posture 1997;6:76–84

Horak FB. Postural orientation and equilibrium: what do we need to know about neural control of balance to prevent falls? Age Ageing 2006;35(Suppl 2):ii7–ii11

Horak FB, Henry SM, Shumway-Cook A. Postural perturbations: new insights for treatment of balance disorders. Phys Ther 1997;77(5):517–533

Horak FB, Nashner LM. Central programming of postural movements: adaptation to altered support-surface configurations. J Neurophysiol 1986;55(6):1369–1381

Horlings CGC, Küng UM, van Engelen BG, et al. Balance control in patients with distal versus proximal muscle weakness. Neuroscience 2009;164(4):1876–1886

Hsieh C-L, Sheu CF, Hsueh IP, Wang CH. Trunk control as an early predictor of comprehensive activities of daily living function in stroke patients. Stroke 2002;33(11):2626–2630

Hubble RP, Naughton GA, Silburn PA, Cole MH. Trunk muscle exercises as a means of improving postural stability in people with Parkinson's disease: a protocol for a randomised controlled trial. BMJ Open 2014;4(12):e006095

Hubli M, Dietz V. The physiological basis of neurorehabilitation—locomotor training after spinal cord injury. J Neuroeng Rehabil 2013;10:5

Hunter MC, Hoffman MA. Postural control: visual and cognitive manipulations. Gait Posture 2001;13(1):41–48

Ietswaart M, Johnston M, Dijkerman HC, et al. Mental practice with motor imagery in stroke recovery: randomized controlled trial of efficacy. Brain 2011;134(Pt 5):1373–1386

Inglin B, Woollacott M. Age-related changes in anticipatory postural adjustments associated with arm movements. J Gerontol 1988;43(4):M105–M113

Ivanenko YP, Cappellini G, Solopova IA, et al. Plasticity and modular control of locomotor patterns in neurological disorders with motor deficits. Front Comput Neurosci 2013;7(September):123

Jacobs JV, Horak FB. Cortical control of postural responses. J Neural Transm 2007;114(10):1339–1348

Jacobs JV, Lou JS, Kraakevik JA, Horak FB. The supplementary motor area contributes to the timing of the anticipatory postural adjustment during step initiation in participants with and without Parkinson's disease. Neuroscience 2009;164(2):877–885

Jakobs T, Miller JA, Schultz AB. Trunk position sense in the frontal plane. Exp Neurol 1985;90(1):129–138

Jeka JJ. Light touch contact as a balance aid. Phys Ther 1997;77(5):476–487

Jeka JJ, Lackner JR. Fingertip contact influences human postural control. Exp Brain Res 1994;100(3):495–502

Jeka JJ, Lackner JR. The role of haptic cues from rough and slippery surfaces in human postural control. Exp Brain Res 1995;103(2):267–276

Kamphuis JF, de Kam D, Geurts AC, Weerdesteyn V. Is weight-bearing asymmetry associated with postural instability after stroke? A systematic review. Stroke Res Treat 2013;2013:692137

Kandel ER, Schwartz JH, Jessell TM, Siegelbaum SA, Hudspeth AJ, eds. Principles of Neural Science. 5th ed. New York, NY: McGraw-Hill Professional; 2013

Kanekar N, Lee Y-J, Aruin AS. Effect of light finger touch in balance control of individuals with multiple sclerosis. Gait Posture 2013;38(4):643–647

Kang HG, Dingwell JB. Dynamic stability of superior vs. inferior segments during walking in young and older adults. Gait Posture 2009;30(2):260–263

Karatas M, Cetin N, Bayramoglu M, Dilek A. Trunk muscle strength in relation to balance and functional disability in unihemispheric stroke patients. Am J Phys Med Rehabil 2004;83(2):81–87

Karnath HO, Dieterich M. Spatial neglect—a vestibular disorder? Brain 2006;129(Pt 2):293–305

Karnath HO, Ferber S, Dichgans J. The origin of contraversive pushing: evidence for a second graviceptive system in humans. Neurology 2000;55(9):1298–1304

Kavounoudias A, Roll R, Roll JP. The plantar sole is a 'dynamometric map' for human balance control. Neuroreport 1998;9(14):3247–3252

Kavounoudias A, Roll R, Roll JP. Foot sole and ankle muscle inputs contribute jointly to human erect posture regulation. J Physiol 2001;532(Pt 3):869–878

Keijsers NLW, Admiraal MA, Cools AR, Bloem BR, Gielen CC. Differential progression of proprioceptive and visual information processing deficits in Parkinson's disease. Eur J Neurosci 2005;21(1):239–248

Kibler WB, Press J, Sciascia A. The role of core stability in athletic function. Sports Med 2006;36(3):189–198

Kidd G, Musa IM, Lawes N. Understanding Neuromuscular Plasticity: A Basis for Clinical Rehabilitation. London, UK: Edward Arnold; 1992

Kim YH, Park JW, Ko MH, Jang SH, Lee PK. Plastic changes of motor network after constraint-induced movement therapy. Yonsei Med J 2004;45(2):241–246

King AC, Wang Z, Newell KM. Asymmetry of recurrent dynamics as a function of postural stance. Exp Brain Res 2012;220(3-4):239–250

Kitsos GH, Hubbard IJ, Kitsos AR, Parsons MW. The ipsilesional upper limb can be affected following stroke. ScientificWorldJournal 2013;2013:684860

Klous M, Mikulic P, Latash ML. Early postural adjustments in preparation to whole-body voluntary sway. J Electromyogr Kinesiol 2012;22(1):110–116

Klous M, Mikulic P, Latash ML. Two aspects of feedforward postural control: anticipatory postural adjustments and anticipatory synergy adjustments. J Neurophysiol 2011;105(5):2275–2288

Krishnan V, Aruin AS, Latash ML. Two stages and three components of the postural preparation to action. Exp Brain Res 2011;212(1):47–63

Krishnan V, Kanekar N, Aruin AS. Anticipatory postural adjustments in individuals with multiple sclerosis. Neurosci Lett 2012;506(2):256–260

Kwakkel G, Van Peppen R, Wagenaar RC, et al. Effects of augmented exercise therapy time after stroke: A meta-analysis. Stroke. 2004;35:2529–2539

Lackner JR, DiZio P. Vestibular, proprioceptive, and haptic contributions to spatial orientation. Annu Rev Psychol 2005;56:115–147

Lafosse C, Kerckhofs E, Troch M, Vandenbussche E. Upper limb exteroceptive somatosensory and proprioceptive sensory afferent modulation of hemispatial neglect. J Clin Exp Neuropsychol 2003;25(3):308–323

Lakhani B, Mansfield A, Inness EL, McIlroy WE. Compensatory stepping responses in individuals with stroke: a pilot study. Physiother Theory Pract 2011;27(4):299–309

Latash ML, Aruin AS, Neyman I, Nicholas JJ. Anticipatory postural adjustments during self inflicted and predictable perturbations in Parkinson's disease. J Neurol Neurosurg Psychiatry 1995;58(3):326–334

Le Bozec S, Bouisset S. Does postural chain mobility influence muscular control in sitting ramp pushes? Exp Brain Res 2004;158(4):427–437

Lee LJ, Coppieters MW, Hodges PW. Anticipatory postural adjustments to arm movement reveal complex control of paraspinal muscles in the thorax. J Electromyogr Kinesiol 2009;19(1):46–54

Lee MY, Wong MK, Tang FT, Cheng PT, Lin PS. Comparison of balance responses and motor patterns during sit-to-stand task with functional mobility in stroke patients. Am J Phys Med Rehabil 1997;76(5):401–410

Leonard JA, Brown RH, Stapley PJ. Reaching to multiple targets when standing: the spatial organization of feedforward postural adjustments. J Neurophysiol 2009;101(4):2120–2133

Levin MF, Panturin E. Sensorimotor integration for functional recovery and the Bobath approach. Mot Contr 2011;15(2):285–301

Liepert J, Bauder H, Wolfgang HR, Miltner WH, Taub E, Weiller C. Treatment-induced cortical reorganization after stroke in humans. Stroke 2000;31(6):1210–1216

Lin KC. Right-hemispheric activation approaches to neglect rehabilitation poststroke. Am J Occup Ther 1996;50(7):504–515

Lindberg P, Schmitz C, Forssberg H, Engardt M, Borg J. Effects of passive-active movement training on upper limb motor function and cortical activation in chronic patients with stroke: a pilot study. J Rehabil Med 2004;36(3):117–123

Lockhart DB, Ting LH. Optimal sensorimotor transformations for balance. Nat Neurosci 2007;10(10):1329–1336

Logan D, Kiemel T, Dominici N, et al. The many roles of vision during walking. Exp Brain Res 2010;206(3):337–350

Logan D, Kiemel T, Jeka JJ. Asymmetric sensory reweighting in human upright stance. PLoS ONE 2014;9(6):e100418

Lopez C, Blanke O. The thalamocortical vestibular system in animals and humans. Brain Res Brain Res Rev 2011;67(1-2):119–146

Loram ID, Gollee H, Lakie M, Gawthrop PJ. Human control of an inverted pendulum: is continuous control necessary? Is intermittent control effective? Is intermittent control physiological? J Physiol 2011;589(Pt 2):307–324

Loubinoux I, Carel C, Pariente J, et al. Correlation between cerebral reorganization and motor recovery after subcortical infarcts. Neuroimage 2003;20(4):2166–2180

Ludewig PM, Reynolds JF. The association of scapular kinematics and glenohumeral joint pathologies. J Orthop Sports Phys Ther 2009;39(2):90–104

Luft CDB. Learning from feedback: the neural mechanisms of feedback processing facilitating better performance. Behav Brain Res 2014;261:356–368

Lum PS, Burgar CG, Shor PC, Majmundar M, Van der Loos M. Robot-assisted movement training compared with conventional therapy techniques for the rehabilitation of upper-limb motor function after stroke. Arch Phys Med Rehabil 2002;83(7):952–959

Lynch-Ellerington. What Are Associated Reactions? Synapse, Spring 2000;28–30

Lynskey JV, Belanger A, Jung R. Activity-dependent plasticity in spinal cord injury. J Rehabil Res Dev 2008;45(2):229–240

Macaluso A, De Vito G. Muscle strength, power and adaptations to resistance training in older people. Eur J Appl Physiol 2004;91(4):450–472

Macé MJ, Levin O, Alaerts K, Rothwell JC, Swinnen SP. Corticospinal facilitation following prolonged proprioceptive stimulation by means of passive wrist movement. J Clin Neurophysiol 2008;25(4):202–209

Mackay-Lyons M. Central pattern generation of locomotion: a review of the evidence. Phys Ther 2002;82(1):69–83

Maki BE, McIlroy WE. Control of rapid limb movements for balance recovery: age-related changes and implications for fall prevention. Age Ageing 2006;35(Suppl 2):ii12–ii18

Maki BE, McIlroy WE. The role of limb movements in maintaining upright stance: the "change-in-support" strategy. Phys Ther 1997;77(5):488–507

Maki BE, Edmondstone MA, McIlroy WE. Age-related differences in laterally directed compensatory stepping behavior. J Gerontol A Biol Sci Med Sci 2000;55(5):M270–M277

Mancini M, Horak FB. The relevance of clinical balance assessment tools to differentiate balance deficits. Eur J Phys Rehabil Med 2010;46(2):239–248

Mancini M, Zampieri C, Carlson-Kuhta P, Chiari L, Horak FB. Anticipatory postural adjustments prior to step initiation are hypometric in untreated Parkinson's disease: an accelerometer-based approach. Eur J Neurol 2009;16(9):1028–1034

Mansfield A, Inness EL, Lakhani B, McIlroy WE. Determinants of limb preference for initiating compensatory stepping poststroke. Arch Phys Med Rehabil 2012;93(7):1179–1184

Mansfield A, Inness EL, Wong JS, Fraser JE, McIlroy WE. Is impaired control of reactive stepping related to falls during inpatient stroke rehabilitation? Neurorehabil Neural Repair 2013;27(6):526–533

Marigold DS, Misiaszek JE. Whole-body responses: neural control and implications for rehabilitation and fall prevention. Neuroscientist 2009;15(1):36–46

Marigold DS, Eng JJ, Tokuno CD, Donnelly CA. Contribution of muscle strength and integration of afferent input to postural instability in persons with stroke. Neurorehabil Neural Repair 2004;18(4):222–229

Martinez KM, Mille ML, Zhang Y, Rogers MW. Stepping in persons poststroke: comparison of voluntary and perturbation-induced responses. Arch Phys Med Rehabil 2013;94(12):2425–2432

Massaad F, Levin O, Meyns P, Drijkoningen D, Swinnen SP, Duysens J. Arm sway holds sway: locomotor-like modulation of leg reflexes when arms swing in alternation. Neuroscience 2014;258:34–46

Massion J. Movement, posture and equilibrium: interaction and coordination. Prog Neurobiol 1992;38(1):35–56

Massion J. Postural control system. Curr Opin Neurobiol 1994;4(6):877–887

Massion J, Alexandrov A, Frolov A. Why and how are posture and movement coordinated? Prog Brain Res 2004;143:13–27

Massion J, Ioffe M, Schmitz C, Viallet F, Gantcheva R. Acquisition of anticipatory postural adjustments in a bimanual load-lifting task: normal and pathological aspects. Exp Brain Res 1999;128(1-2):229–235

Maurer C, Peterka RJ. A new interpretation of spontaneous sway measures based on a simple model of human postural control. J Neurophysiol 2005;93(1):189–200

Maurer C, Mergner T, Peterka RJ. Multisensory control of human upright stance. Exp Brain Res 2006;171(2):231–250

McIlroy WE, Maki BE. Age-related changes in compensatory stepping in response to unpredictable perturbations. J Gerontol A Biol Sci Med Sci 1996;51(6):M289–M296

McKenzie J. The Foot as a Half-dome. BMJ 1955;1(4921):1068–1070

McKeon PO, Hertel J, Bramble D, Davis I. The foot core system: a new paradigm for understanding intrinsic foot muscle function. Br J Sports Med 2015;49(5):290

Mehrholz J, Pohl M. Electromechanical-assisted gait training after stroke: a systematic review comparing end-effector and exoskeleton devices. J Rehabil Med 2012;44(3):193–199

Mehrholz J, Pohl M, Elsner B. Treadmill training and body weight support for walking after stroke. Cochrane Database Syst Rev 2014;1:CD002840

Melzer I, Benjuya N, Kaplanski J, Alexander N. Association between ankle muscle strength and limit of stability in older adults. Age Ageing 2009;38(1):119–123

Menz HB, Morris ME, Lord SR. Foot and ankle characteristics associated with impaired balance and functional ability in older people. J Gerontol A Biol Sci Med Sci 2005;60(12):1546–1552

Mercier C, Bertrand AM, Bourbonnais D. Comparison of strength measurements under single-joint and multi-joint conditions in hemiparetic individuals. Clin Rehabil 2005;19(5):523–530

Mergner T, Maurer C, Peterka RJ. A multisensory posture control model of human upright stance. Prog Brain Res 2003;142(1):189–201

Meyer PF, Oddsson LI, De Luca CJ. The role of plantar cutaneous sensation in unperturbed stance. Exp Brain Res 2004;156(4):505–512

Michaelsen SM, Dannenbaum R, Levin MF. Task-specific training with trunk restraint on arm recovery in stroke: randomized control trial. Stroke 2006;37(1):186–192

Michaelsen SM, Luta A, Roby-Brami A, Levin MF. Effect of trunk restraint on the recovery of reaching movements in hemiparetic patients. Stroke 2001;32(8):1875–1883

Misiaszek JE, Krauss EM. Restricting arm use enhances compensatory reactions of leg muscles during walking. Exp Brain Res 2005;161(4):474–485

Mittelstaedt H. Somatic versus vestibular gravity reception in man. Ann N Y Acad Sci 1992;656:124–139

Mittelstaedt H. Somatic graviception: biological psychology. 1996. http://www.sciencedirect.com/science/article/pii/0301051195051465. Accessed July 1, 2013

Mononen K, Konttinen N, Viitasalo J, Era P. Relationships between postural balance, rifle stability and shooting accuracy among novice rifle shooters. Scand J Med Sci Sports 2007;17(2):180–185

Morasso P, Casadio M, Mohan V, Zenzeri J. A neural mechanism of synergy formation for whole body reaching. Biol Cybern 2010;102(1):45–55

Morningstar MW, Pettibon BR, Schlappi H, Schlappi M, Ireland TV. Reflex control of the spine and posture: a review of the literature from a chiropractic perspective. Chiropr Osteopat 2005;13:16

Mulder T. A process-oriented model of human motor behavior: toward a theory-based rehabilitation approach. Phys Ther 1991;71(2):157–164

Mulder T, Nienhuis B, Pauwels J. The assessment of motor recovery: A new look at an old problem. J Electromyogr Kinesiol 1996;6(2):137–145

Mulder T, Pauwells J, Nienhuis B. Motor recovery following stroke: towards a disability oriented assesment of motor dysfunctions. In: Harrison M, ed. Physiotherapy in Stroke Management. Philadelphia, PA: Churchill Livingstone; 1995:275–282

Murnaghan C. Exploring the nature of postural sway. 2013. http://elk.library.ubc.ca/handle/2429/44079. Accessed March 23, 2014

Nashner LM. Adaptation of human movement to altered environments. Trends Neurosci 1982;5:358–361

Nawoczenski DA, Saltzman CL, Cook TM. The effect of foot structure on the three-dimensional kinematic coupling behavior of the leg and rear foot. Phys Ther 1998;78(4):404–416

Neely FG. Biomechanical risk factors for exercise-related lower limb injuries. Sports Med 1998;26(6):395–413

Nelles G. Cortical reorganization—effects of intensive therapy. Restor Neurol Neurosci 2004;22(3-5):239–244

Niedenthal PM. Embodying emotion. Science 2007;316(5827):1002–1005

Nijboer T, van de Port I, Schepers V, Post M, Visser-Meily A. Predicting functional outcome after stroke: the influence of neglect on basic activities in daily living. Front Hum Neurosci 2013;7:182

Normann B. Individualisering i nevrologisk fysioterapi. Bobathkonseptet. Hjerneslagspasienter-behandling og kunnskapsgrunnlag. University of Tromsø; 2004

Nowak DA, Glasauer S, Hermsdorfer J. How predictive is grip force control in the complete absence of somatosensory feedback? Brain 2004;127(Pt 1):182–192

Nudo RJ, Milliken GW, Jenkins WM, Merzenich MM. Use-dependent alterations of movement representations in primary motor cortex of adult squirrel monkeys. J Neurosci 1996;16(2):785–807

Nudo RJ, Wise BM, SiFuentes F, Milliken GW. Neural substrates for the effects of rehabilitative training on motor recovery after ischemic infarct. Science 1996;272(5269):1791–1794

Orr R. Contribution of muscle weakness to postural instability in the elderly. A systematic review. Eur J Phys Rehabil Med 2010;46(2):183–220

O'Sullivan PB, Grahamslaw KM, Kendell M, Lapenskie SC, Möller NE, Richards KV. The effect of different standing and sitting postures on trunk muscle activity in a pain-free population. Spine 2002;27(11):1238–1244

O'Sullivan PB, Dankaerts W, Burnett AF, et al. Effect of different upright sitting postures on spinal-pelvic curvature and trunk muscle activation in a pain-free population. Spine 2006;31(19):E707–E712

Oujamaa L, Relave I, Froger J, Mottet D, Pelissier JY. Rehabilitation of arm function after stroke. Literature review. Ann Phys Rehabil Med 2009;52(3):269–293

Paci M, Nannetti L, Rinaldi LA. Glenohumeral subluxation in hemiplegia: An overview. J Rehabil Res Dev 2005;42(4):557–568

Papegaaij S, Taube W, Baudry S, Otten E, Hortobágyi T. Aging causes a reorganization of cortical and spinal control of posture. Front Aging Neurosci 2014;6:28

Park RJ, Tsao H, Cresswell AG, Hodges PW. Anticipatory postural activity of the deep trunk muscles differs between anatomical regions based on their mechanical advantage. Neuroscience 2014;261:161–172

Pasma JH, Boonstra TA, Campfens SF, Schouten AC, Van der Kooij H. Sensory reweighting of proprioceptive information of the left and right leg during human balance control. J Neurophysiol 2012;108(4):1138–1148

Patten C, Lexell J, Brown HE. Weakness and strength training in persons with poststroke hemiplegia: rationale, method, and efficacy. J Rehabil Res Dev 2004;41(3A):293–312

Pavol MJ. Detecting and understanding differences in postural sway. Focus on "A new interpretation of spontaneous sway measures based on a simple model of human postural control". J Neurophysiol 2005;93(1):20–21

Pereira LC, Botelho AC, Martins EF. Relationships between body symmetry during weight-bearing and functional reach among chronic hemiparetic patients. Rev Bras Fisioter 2010;14(3):229–266

Pereira S, Silva CC, Ferreira S, et al. Anticipatory postural adjustments during sitting reach movement in post-stroke subjects. J Electromyogr Kinesiol 2014;24(1):165–171

Pérennou DA, Leblond C, Amblard B, Micallef JP, Rouget E, Pélissier J. The polymodal sensory cortex is crucial for controlling lateral postural stability: evidence from stroke patients. Brain Res Bull 2000;53(3):359–365

Pérennou DA, Mazibrada G, Chauvineau V, et al. Lateropulsion, pushing and verticality perception in hemisphere stroke: a causal relationship? Brain 2008;131(Pt 9):2401–2413

Perlmutter S, Lin F, Makhsous M. Quantitative analysis of static sitting posture in chronic stroke. Gait Posture 2010;32(1):53–56

Peterka RJ. Sensorimotor integration in human postural control. J Neurophysiol 2002;88(3):1097–1118

Poli P, Morone G, Rosati G, Masiero S. Robotic technologies and rehabilitation: new tools for stroke patients' therapy. Biomed Res Int 2013;2013:153872

Pollock AS, Durward BR, Rowe PJ, Paul JP. What is balance? Clin Rehabil 2000;14(4):402–406

Pontelli TE, Pontes-Neto OM, Colafêmina JF, Araújo DB, Santos AC, Leite JP. Posture control in Pusher syndrome: influence of lateral semicircular canals. Braz J Otorhinolaryngol 2005;71(4):448–452

Popovic D, Sinkjaer T. Central nervous system lesions leading to disability. J Automatic Control 2008;18(2):11–23

Porter R, Lemon RN. Corticospinal Function and Voluntary Movement. New York, NY: Oxford University Press; 1995

Pozzo T, Berthoz A, Lefort L. Head stabilization during various locomotor tasks in humans. I. Normal subjects. Exp Brain Res 1990;82(1):97–106

Pozzo T, Levik Y, Berthoz A. Head and trunk movements in the frontal plane during complex dynamic equilibrium tasks in humans. Exp Brain Res 1995;106(2):327–338

Prochazka A, Ellaway P. Sensory systems in the control of movement. Compr Physiol 2012;2(4):2615–2627

Raine S. The current theoretical assumptions of the Bobath concept as determined by the members of BBTA. Physiother Theory Pract 2007;23(3):137–152

Raine S, Meadows L, Lynch-Ellerington M. Bobath Concept Theory and Clinical Practice in Neurological Rehabilitation. Hoboken, NJ: Wiley-Blackwell; 2009

Reisman DS, Scholz JP. Workspace location influences joint coordination during reaching in post-stroke hemiparesis. Exp Brain Res 2006;170(2):265–276

Robbins SM, Houghton PE, Woodbury MG, Brown JL. The therapeutic effect of functional and transcutaneous electric stimulation on improving gait speed in stroke patients: a meta-analysis. Arch Phys Med Rehabil 2006;87(6):853–859

Robert G, Blouin J, Ruget H, Mouchnino L. Coordination between postural and movement controls: effect of changes in body mass distribution on postural and focal component characteristics. Exp Brain Res 2007;181(1):159–171

Robertson I, Hogg K, McMillan T. Rehabilitation of unilateral neglect: improving function by contralesional limb activation. Neuropsychol Rehabil 1998;8:19–29

Robertson JV, Roby-Brami A. The trunk as a part of the kinematic chain for reaching movements in healthy subjects and hemiparetic patients. Brain Res 2011;1382(25):137–146

Robertson JV, Roche N, Roby-Brami A. Influence of the side of brain damage on postural upper-limb control including the scapula in stroke patients. Exp Brain Res 2012;218(1):141–155

Robertson LC, Eglin M. Attentional search in unilateral visual neglect. In: Robertson IH, Marshall JC, eds. Unilateral Neglect: Clinical and Experimental Studies. East Sussex, UK: Lawrence Erlbaum Associates; 1993:169–191

Roby-Brami A, Feydy A, Combeaud M, Biryukova EV, Bussel B, Levin MF. Motor compensation and recovery for reaching in stroke patients. Acta Neurol Scand 2003;107(5):369–381

Ronsse R, Puttemans V, Coxon JP, et al. Motor learning with augmented feedback: modality-dependent behavioral and neural consequences. Cereb Cortex 2011;21(6):1283–1294

Rose W, Bowser B, McGrath R, Salerno J, Wallace J, Davis I. Effect of footwear on balance. American Society of Biomechanics Annual Meeting; Long Beach, CA:2011

Rossignol S, Dubuc R, Gossard JP. Dynamic sensorimotor interactions in locomotion. Physiol Rev 2006;86(1):89–154

Rothwell J, Lennon S. Control of Human Voluntary Movement. 2nd ed. London, UK: Chapman and Hall; 1994

Rousseaux M, Honoré J, Vuilleumier P, Saj A. Neuroanatomy of space, body, and posture perception in patients with right hemisphere stroke. Neurology 2013;81(15):1291–1297

Ryerson S, Byl NN, Brown DA, Wong RA, Hidler JM. Altered trunk position sense and its relation to balance functions in people post-stroke. J Neurol Phys Ther 2008;32(1):14–20

Safavynia SA, Ting LH. Task-level feedback can explain temporal recruitment of spatially fixed muscle synergies throughout postural perturbations. J Neurophysiol 2012;107(1):159–177

Sahrmann SA. Diagnosis and Treatment of Movement Impairment Syndromes. St. Louis, MO: Mosby; 2002

Sahrmann S. Posture and muscle imbalance. Physiotherapy 1992;78(1):1–19

Santello M, Flanders M, Soechting JF. Patterns of hand motion during grasping and the influence of sensory guidance. J Neurosci 2002;22(4):1426–1435

Santos MJ, Aruin AS. Effects of lateral perturbations and changing stance conditions on anticipatory postural adjustment. J Electromyogr Kinesiol 2009;19(3):532–541

Santos MJ, Aruin AS. Role of lateral muscles and body orientation in feedforward postural control. Exp Brain Res 2008;184(4):547–559

Santos MJ, Kanekar N, Aruin AS. The role of anticipatory postural adjustments in compensatory control of posture: 2. Biomechanical analysis. J Electromyogr Kinesiol 2010;20(3):398–405

Santos-Pontelli T. New insights for a better understanding of the pusher behavior: from clinical to neuroimaging features. 2011. http://cdn.intechopen.com/pdfs/24729.pdf. Accessed August 21, 2014

Schädler S, Kool J. Pushen: Syndrom oder Symptomeine Literaturubersicht. Krankengymnastik, Pflaum Verlag Publikation 2001;1:7-16

Schepens B, Drew T. Strategies for the integration of posture and movement during reaching in the cat. J Neurophysiol 2003;90(5):3066–3086

Schepens B, Drew T. Independent and convergent signals from the pontomedullary reticular formation contribute to the control of posture and movement during reaching in the cat. J Neurophysiol 2004;92(4):2217–2238

Schepens B, Drew T, Baker SN. Descending signals from the pontomedullary reticular formation are bilateral, asymmetric, and gated during reaching movements in the cat. J Neurophysiol 2006;96(5):2229–2252

Schepens B, Stapley P, Drew T. Neurons in the pontomedullary reticular formation signal posture and movement both as an integrated behavior and independently. J Neurophysiol 2008;100(4):2235–2253

Schleichkorn J. The Bobaths: A Biography of Karel and Bertha Bobath. Tuscon, Ariz: Neuro-Development Treatment Association (NDTA) and Therapy Skill Builders; 1992

Schmidt R. Motor learning principles for physical therapy. In Marilyn JL, ed. Contemporary Management of Motor Control Problems: Proceedings of the II STEP Conference. Alexandria, VA: Foundation for Physical Therapy; 1991

Shinohara J, Gribble P. Five-toed socks decrease static postural control among healthy individuals as measured with time-to-boundary analysis. Poster presentation at: American Society of Biomechanics Annual Meeting. 2009

Shmuelof L, Krakauer JW, Mazzoni P. How is a motor skill learned? Change and invariance at the levels of task success and trajectory control. J Neurophysiol 2012;108(2):578–594

Shumway-Cook, Woollacott MH. Motor Control: Translating Research into Clinical Practice. 4th ed. Philadelphia, PA: Lippincott Williams & Wilkins; 2011

Shumway-Cook A, Woollacott MH. Motor Control: Translating Research into Clinical Practice. 3rd ed.

Philadelphia, PA: Lippincott Williams & Wilkins; 2006

Slijper H, Latash ML, Mordkoff JT. Anticipatory postural adjustments under simple and choice reaction time conditions. Brain Res 2002;924(2):184–197

Smedal T, Lygren H, Myhr KM, et al. Balance and gait improved in patients with MS after physiotherapy based on the Bobath concept. Physiother Res Int 2006;11(2):104–116

Smith BA, Jacobs JV, Horak FB. Effects of magnitude and magnitude predictability of postural perturbations on preparatory cortical activity in older adults with and without Parkinson's disease. Exp Brain Res 2012;222(4):455–470

Solopova IA, Selionov VA, Sylos-Labini F, Gurfinkel VS, Lacquaniti F, Ivanenko YP. Tapping into rhythm generation circuitry in humans during simulated weightlessness conditions. Front Syst Neurosci 2015;9(February):14

Sousa AS, Santos R, Oliveira FP, Carvalho P, Tavares JM. Analysis of ground reaction force and electromyographic activity of the gastrocnemius muscle during double support. Proc Inst Mech Eng H 2012;226(5):397–405

Sousa ASP, Silva A, Santos R, Sousa F, Tavares JM. Interlimb coordination during the stance phase of gait in subjects with stroke. Arch Phys Med Rehabil 2013;94(12):2515–2522

Stapley P, Drew T, Schepens B. Neurons in the pontomedullary reticular formation signal posture and movement both as an integrated behavior and independently. J Neurophysiol. 2008;100(4):2235–2253

Stoykov MEP, Stojakovich M, Stevens JA. Beneficial effects of postural intervention on prehensile action for an individual with ataxia resulting from brainstem stroke. NeuroRehabilitation 2005;20(2):85–89

Sunderland A, Tinson DJ, Bradley EL, Fletcher D, Langton Hewer R, Wade DT. Enhanced physical therapy improves recovery of arm function after stroke. A randomised controlled trial. J Neurol Neurosurg Psychiatry 1992;55(7):530–535

Suzuki M, Omori Y, Sugimura S, et al. Predicting recovery of bilateral upper extremity muscle strength after stroke. J Rehabil Med 2011;43(10):935–943

Sylos-Labini F, Ivanenko YP, Maclellan MJ, Cappellini G, Poppele RE, Lacquaniti F. Locomotor-like leg movements evoked by rhythmic arm movements in humans. PLoS ONE 2014;9(3):e90775

Tagliabue M, Ferrigno G, Horak F. Effects of Parkinson's disease on proprioceptive control of posture and reaching while standing. Neuroscience 2009;158(4):1206–1214

Takakusaki K, Saitoh K, Harada H, Kashiwayanagi M. Role of basal ganglia-brainstem pathways in the control of motor behaviors. Neurosci Res 2004;50(2):137–151

Takeuchi N, Izumi S. Maladaptive plasticity for motor recovery after stroke: mechanisms and approaches. Neural Plast 2012;2012:359728

Taub E, Uswatt G. Constraint-induced movement therapy: answers and questions after two decades of research. NeuroRehabilitation 2006;21(2):93–95

Taub E, Uswatte G, Mark VW. The functional significance of cortical reorganization and the parallel development of CI therapy. Front Hum Neurosci 2014;8(June):396

Taub E, Uswatte G, Pidikiti R. Constraint-Induced Movement Therapy: a new family of techniques with broad application to physical rehabilitation—a clinical review. J Rehabil Res Dev 1999;36(3):237–251

Taylor B, Ellis E, Haran H. The reliability of measurement of postural alignment to assess muscle tone change. Physiotherapy 1995;81:485–490

Taylor JA, Krakauer JW, Ivry RB. Explicit and implicit contributions to learning in a sensorimotor adaptation task. J Neurosci 2014;34(8):3023–3032

Teasdale N, Simoneau M. Attentional demands for postural control: the effects of aging and sensory reintegration. Gait Posture 2001;14(3):203–210

Thach WT, Bastian AJ. Role of the cerebellum in the control and adaptation of gait in health and disease. Prog Brain Res 2004;143:353–366

Thielman G. Insights into upper limb kinematics and trunk control one year after task-related training in chronic post-stroke individuals. J Hand Ther 2013;26(2):156–160, quiz 161

Thomas CL. Taber's Cyclopedic Medical Dictionary. 18th ed. Philadelphia, PA: F.A. Davis; 1997

Thornquist E. Kroppens spennende samspill. Fysioterapeuten 1985;51:636–643

Thrasher TA, Popovic MR. Functional electrical stimulation of walking: function, exercise and rehabilitation. Ann Readapt Med Phys 2008;51(6):452–460

Ticini LF, Klose U, Nägele T, Karnath HO. Perfusion imaging in Pusher syndrome to investigate the neural substrates involved in controlling upright body position. PLoS ONE 2009;4(5):e5737

Ting LH. Dimensional reduction in sensorimotor systems: a framework for understanding muscle coordination of posture. Prog Brain Res 2007;165:299–321

Ting LH, McKay JL. Neuromechanics of muscle synergies for posture and movement. Curr Opin Neurobiol 2007;17(6):622–628

Ting LH, van Antwerp KW, Scrivens JE, et al. Neuromechanical tuning of nonlinear postural control dynamics. Chaos 2009;19(2):026111

Tombari D, Loubinoux I, Pariente J, et al. A longitudinal fMRI study: in recovering and then in clinically stable sub-cortical stroke patients. Neuroimage 2004;23(3):827–839

Torres-Oviedo G, Macpherson JM, Ting LH. Muscle synergy organization is robust across a variety of postural perturbations. J Neurophysiol 2006;96(3):1530–1546

Trousselard M, Barraud PA, Nougier V, Raphel C, Cian C. Contribution of tactile and interoceptive cues to the perception of the direction of gravity. Brain Res Cogn Brain Res 2004;20(3):355–362

Tyson SF, Hanley M, Chillala J, Selley A, Tallis RC. Balance disability after stroke. Phys Ther 2006;86(1):30–38

Umphred D. Merging neurophysiologic approaches with contemporary theories. In: Lister MJ, ed. Contemporary Management of Motor Control Problems: Proceedings of the II STEP Conference. Alexandria, VA; Foundation for Physical Therapy; 1991:127–130

Vaitl D, Mittelstaedt H, Saborowski R, Stark R, Baisch F. Shifts in blood volume alter the perception of posture: further evidence for somatic graviception. Int J Psychophysiol 2002;44(1):1–11

van Kordelaar J, van Wegen EEH, Kwakkel G. Unraveling the interaction between pathological upper limb synergies and compensatory trunk movements during reach-to-grasp after stroke: a cross-sectional study. Exp Brain Res 2012;221(3):251–262

van Nes IJW, Nienhuis B, Latour H, Geurts AC. Posturographic assessment of sitting balance recovery in the subacute phase of stroke. Gait Posture 2008;28(3):507–512

van Vliet PM, Wulf G. Extrinsic feedback for motor learning after stroke: what is the evidence? Disabil Rehabil 2006;28(13-14):831–840

Vaugoyeau M, Viallet F, Aurenty R, Assaiante C, Mesure S, Massion J. Axial rotation in Parkinson's disease. J Neurol Neurosurg Psychiatry 2006;77(7):815–821

Verheyden G, van Duijnhoven HJ, Burnett M, Littlewood J, Kunkel D, Ashburn AM; Stroke Association Rehabilitation Research Centre. Kinematic analysis of head, trunk, and pelvis movement when people early after stroke reach sideways. Neurorehabil Neural Repair 2011;25(7):656–663

Virji-Babul N. Effects of post-operative environment on recovery of function following brain damage: a brief literature review. Physiotherapy 1991;77(9):587–590

Visser JE, Bloem BR. Role of the basal ganglia in balance control. Neural Plast 2005;12(2-3):161–174, discussion 263–272

Wade MG, Jones G. The role of vision and spatial orientation in the maintenance of posture. Phys Ther 1997;77(6):619–628

Wang TY, Lin SI. Sensitivity of plantar cutaneous sensation and postural stability. Clin Biomech (Bristol, Avon) 2008;23(4):493–499

Wassinger CA, Rockett A, Pitman L, Murphy MM, Peters C. Acute effects of rearfoot manipulation on dynamic standing balance in healthy individuals. Man Ther 2014;19(3):242–245

Whiting HTA, Vereijken B. The acquisition of coordination in skill learning. Int J Sport Psychol 1993;24(4):343–357

Winter DA. Human balance and posture standing and walking. Gait Posture 1995;3:193–214

Winzeler-Merçay U, Mudie H. The nature of the effects of stroke on trunk flexor and extensor muscles during work and at rest. Disabil Rehabil 2002;24(17):875–886

Wong JD, Kistemaker DA, Chin A, Gribble PL. Can proprioceptive training improve motor learning? J Neurophysiol 2012;108(12):3313–3321

Woodbury ML, Howland DR, McGuirk TE, et al. Effects of trunk restraint combined with intensive task practice on poststroke upper extremity reach and function: a pilot study. Neurorehabil Neural Repair 2009;23(1):78–91

Woollacott MH, Crenna P. Postural control in standing and walking in children with cerebral palsy. In: Hadders-Algra M, Brogren Carlberg E, eds. Postural Control: A Key Issue in Developmental Disorders. London, UK: MacKeith Press; 2008:97–130

World Health Organization. 2006. International classification of functioning, disability and health (ICF). http://www:who.int/classifications/icf/en

Wright WG, Horak FB. Interaction of posture and conscious perception of gravitational vertical and surface horizontal. Exp Brain Res 2007;182(3):321–332

Wright WG, Gurfinkel VS, Nutt J, Horak FB, Cordo PJ. Axial hypertonicity in Parkinson's disease: direct measurements of trunk and hip torque. Exp Neurol 2007;208(1):38–46

Wright WG, Ivanenko YP, Gurfinkel VS. Foot anatomy specialization for postural sensation and control. J Neurophysiol 2012;107(5):1513–1521

Yavuzer G, Ergin S. Effect of an arm sling on gait pattern in patients with hemiplegia. Arch Phys Med Rehabil 2002;83(7):960–963

Yekutiel M, Guttman E. A controlled trial of the retraining of the sensory function of the hand in stroke patients. J Neurol Neurosurg Psychiatry 1993;56(3):241–244

Yelnik AP, Kassouha A, Bonan IV, et al. Postural visual dependence after recent stroke: assessment by optokinetic stimulation. Gait Posture 2006;24(3):262–269

Yiou E, Caderby T, Hussein T. Adaptability of anticipatory postural adjustments associated with voluntary movement. World J Orthod 2012;3(6):75–86

Yiou E, Hamaoui A, Le Bozec S. Influence of base of support size on arm pointing performance and associated anticipatory postural adjustments. Neurosci Lett 2007;423(1):29–34

Yogev-Seligmann G, Hausdorff JM, Giladi N. Do we always prioritize balance when walking? Towards an integrated model of task prioritization. Mov Disord 2012;27(6):765–770

Zelik KE, La Scaleia V, Ivanenko YP, Lacquaniti F. Coordination of intrinsic and extrinsic foot muscles during walking. Eur J Appl Physiol 2015;115(4):691–701

Chapter 3
Assessment

American College of Sports Medicine (ARCM). Resource Manual for Guidelines for Exercise Testing and Prescription. Philadelphia, PA: Lea and Febiger; 1988

Baker SM, Marshak HH, Rice GT, Zimmerman GJ. Patient participation in physical therapy goal setting. Phys Ther 2001;81(5):1118–1126

Barry E, Galvin R, Keogh C, Horgan F, Fahey T. Is the Timed Up and Go test a useful predictor of risk of falls in community dwelling older adults: a systematic review and meta-analysis. BMC Geriatr 2014;14(1):14

Benaim C, Pérennou DA, Villy J, Rousseaux M, Pelissier JY. Validation of a standardized assessment of postural control in stroke patients: the Postural Assessment Scale for Stroke Patients (PASS). Stroke 1999;30(9):1862–1868

Berg K, Wood-Dauphine S, Williams JI, Gayton D. Measuring balance in the elderly: preliminary development of an instrument. Physiother Can 1989;41:304–311

Berg K, Wood-Dauphinee S, Williams JI. The Balance Scale: reliability assessment with elderly residents and patients with an acute stroke. Scand J Rehabil Med 1995;27(1):27–36

Berg KO, Wood-Dauphinee SL, Williams JI, Maki B. Measuring balance in the elderly: validation of an instrument. Can J Public Health 1992;83(Suppl 2):S7–11

Bilney B, Morris M, Webster K. Concurrent related validity of the GAITRite walkway system for quantification of the spatial and temporal parameters of gait. Gait Posture 2003;17(1):68–74

Blum L, Korner-Bitensky N. Usefulness of the Berg Balance Scale in stroke rehabilitation: a systematic review. Phys Ther 2008;88(5):559–566

Bogle Thorbahn LD, Newton RA. Use of the Berg Balance Test to predict falls in elderly persons. Phys Ther 1996;76(6):576–583, discussion 584–585

Borg G. Perceived exertion as an indicator of somatic stress. Scand J Rehabil Med 1970;2(2):92–98

Bovend'Eerdt TJH, Botell RE, Wade DT. Writing SMART rehabilitation goals and achieving goal attainment scaling: a practical guide. Clin Rehabil 2009;23(4):352–361

Braman JP, Engel SC, Laprade RF, Ludewig PM. In vivo assessment of scapulohumeral rhythm during unconstrained overhead reaching in asymptomatic subjects. J Shoulder Elbow Surg 2009;18(6):960–967

Brock K, Haase G, Rothacher G, Cotton S. Does physiotherapy based on the Bobath concept, in conjunction with a task practice, achieve greater improvement in walking ability in people with stroke compared to physiotherapy focused on structured task practice alone?: a pilot randomized controlled trial. Clin Rehabil 2011;25(10):903–912

Buckworth J, Dishman R. Perceived exertion. In: Buckworth J, Dishman RK, eds. Exercise Psychology. Champaign, IL: Human Kinetics; 2002:256–284

Cabanas-Valdés R, Cuchi GU, Bagur-Calafat C. Trunk training exercises approaches for improving trunk performance and functional sitting balance in patients with stroke: a systematic review. NeuroRehabilitation 2013;33(4):575–592

Carey LM, Matyas TA. Frequency of discriminative sensory loss in the hand after stroke in a rehabilitation setting. J Rehabil Med 2011;43(3):257–263

De Baets L, Van Deun S, Desloovere K, Jaspers E. Dynamic scapular movement analysis: is it feasible and reliable in stroke patients during arm elevation? PLoS ONE 2013;8(11):e79046

Duncan PW, Weiner DK, Chandler J, Studenski S. Functional reach: a new clinical measure of balance. J Gerontol 1990;45(6):M192–M197

Duncan PW, Wallace D, Lai SM, Johnson D, Embretson S, Laster LJ. The stroke impact scale version 2.0. Evaluation of reliability, validity, and sensitivity to change. Stroke 1999;30(10):2131–2140

Edwards I, Jones M, Carr J, Braunack-Mayer A, Jensen GM. Clinical reasoning strategies in physical therapy. Phys Ther 2004;84(4):312–330, discussion 331–335

Ertzgaard P, Ward AB, Wissel J, Borg J. Practical considerations for goal attainment scaling during rehabilitation following acquired brain injury. J Rehabil Med 2011;43(1):8–14

Finch E; Canadian Physiotherapy Association. Physical Rehabilitation Outcome Measures: A Guide to Enhanced Clinical Decision Making. 2nd ed. Philadelphia, PA: Lippincott Williams & Wilkins; 2002

Flatow EL, Soslowsky LJ, Ticker JB, et al. Excursion of the rotator cuff under the acromion. Patterns of subacromial contact. Am J Sports Med 1994;22(6):779–788

Geurts AC, Visschers BA, van Limbeek J, Ribbers GM. Systematic review of aetiology and treatment of post-stroke hand oedema and shoulder-hand syndrome. Scand J Rehabil Med 2000;32:4–10

Gjelsvik B, Breivik K, Verheyden G, Smedal T, Hofstad H, Strand LI. The Trunk Impairment Scale - modified to ordinal scales in the Norwegian version. Disabil Rehabil 2012;34(16):1385–1395

Guyatt GH, Townsend M, Pugsley SO, et al. Bronchodilators in chronic air-flow limitation. Effects on airway function, exercise capacity, and quality of life. Am Rev Respir Dis 1987;135(5):1069–1074

Hacmon RR, Krasovsky T, Lamontagne A, Levin MF. Deficits in intersegmental trunk coordination during walking are related to clinical balance and gait function in chronic stroke. J Neurol Phys Ther 2012;36(4):173–181

Hazard RG, Spratt KF, McDonough CM, et al. Patient-centered evaluation of outcomes from rehabilitation for chronic disabling spinal disorders: the impact of personal goal achievement on patient satisfaction. Spine J 2012;12(12):1132–1137

Hesse S, Jahnke M, Schaffrin A, Lucke D, Reiter F, Konrad M. immediate effects of therapeutic facilitation on the gait of hemiparetic patients as compared with walking with and without a cane. Electroencephalogr Clin Neurophysiol 1998;109(6):512–522

Hsieh C-L, Sheu CF, Hsueh IP, Wang CH. Trunk control as an early predictor of comprehensive activities of daily living function in stroke patients. Stroke 2002;33(11):2626–2630

International Bobath Instructors Training Association. Theoretical Assumptions and Clinical Practice. 2008. http://ibita.org/Accessed November 4, 2008

Jacobs JV, Horak FB, Tran VK, Nutt JG. Multiple balance tests improve the assessment of postural stability in subjects with Parkinson's disease. J Neurol Neurosurg Psychiatry 2006;77(3):322–326

Jandt SR, Caballero RM, Junior LA, Dias AS. Correlation between trunk control, respiratory muscle strength and spirometry in patients with stroke: an observational study. Physiother Res Int 2011;16(4):218–224

Jenkinson C, Fitzpatrick R, Crocker H, Peters M. The Stroke Impact Scale: validation in a UK setting and development of a SIS short form and SIS index. Stroke 2013;44(9):2532–2535

Karatas M, Cetin N, Bayramoglu M, Dilek A. Trunk muscle strength in relation to balance and functional disability in unihemispheric stroke patients. Am J Phys Med Rehabil 2004;83(2):81–87

Kavounoudias A, Roll R, Roll JP. The plantar sole is a 'dynamometric map' for human balance control. Neuroreport 1998;9(14):3247–3252

Kibler WB. The scapula in rotator cuff disease. Med Sport Sci 2012;57:27–40

Kim JS, Yi S-J. Comparison of Two-point Discrimination Perception in Stroke Patients with and without Diabetes Mellitus. J Phys Ther Sci 2013;25(8):1007–1009

Klit H, Finnerup NB, Jensen TS. Central post-stroke pain: clinical characteristics, pathophysiology, and management. Lancet Neurol 2009;8(9):857–868

Kumar S, Selim MH, Caplan LR. Medical complications after stroke. Lancet Neurol 2010;9(1):105–118

Lacasse Y, Wong E, Guyatt GH, King D, Cook DJ, Goldstein RS. Meta-analysis of respiratory rehabilitation in chronic obstructive pulmonary disease. Lancet 1996;348(9035):1115–1119

Lennon S. Gait re-education based on the Bobath concept in two patients with hemiplegia following stroke. Phys Ther 2001;81(3):924–935

Levin MF, Panturin E. Sensorimotor integration for functional recovery and the Bobath approach. Mot Contr 2011;15(2):285–301

Lindgren I, Jönsson AC, Norrving B, Lindgren A. Shoulder pain after stroke: a prospective population-based study. Stroke 2007;38(2):343–348

Lord SE, Halligan PW, Wade DT. Visual gait analysis: the development of a clinical assessment and scale. Clin Rehabil 1998;12(2):107–119

Lord SR, Menz HB. Physiologic, psychologic, and health predictors of 6-minute walk performance in older people. Arch Phys Med Rehabil 2002;83(7):907–911

Ludewig PM, Reynolds JF. The association of scapular kinematics and glenohumeral joint pathologies. J Orthop Sports Phys Ther 2009;39(2):90–104

Mao HF, Hsueh IP, Tang PF, Sheu CF, Hsieh CL. Analysis and comparison of the psychometric properties of three balance measures for stroke patients. Stroke 2002;33(4):1022–1027

Meyer PF, Oddsson LI, De Luca CJ. The role of plantar cutaneous sensation in unperturbed stance. Exp Brain Res 2004;156(4):505–512

Moe-Nilssen R. A new method for evaluating motor control in gait under real-life environmental conditions. Part 2: Gait analysis. Clin Biomech (Bristol, Avon) 1998;13(4-5):328–335

Monaghan J, Channell K, McDowell D, Sharma AK. Improving patient and carer communication, multidisciplinary team working and goal-setting in stroke rehabilitation. Clin Rehabil 2005;19(2):194–199

Morris M, Iansek R, Smithson F, Huxham F. Postural instability in Parkinson's disease: a comparison with and without a concurrent task. Gait Posture 2000;12(3):205–216

Neuls PD, Clark TL, Van Heuklon NC, et al. Usefulness of the Berg Balance Scale to predict falls in the elderly. J Geriatr Phys Ther 2011;34(1):3–10

Niessen M, Janssen T, Meskers C, Koppe P, Konijnenbelt M, Veeger D. Kinematics of the contralateral and ipsilateral shoulder: a possible relationship with post-stroke shoulder pain. J Rehabil Med 2008;40(6):482–486

Persson CU, Hansson PO, Danielsson A, Sunnerhagen KS. A validation study using a modified version of Postural Assessment Scale for Stroke Patients: Postural Stroke Study in Gothenburg (POSTGOT). J Neuroeng Rehabil 2011;8:57

Persson CU, Danielsson A, Sunnerhagen KS, Grimby-Ekman A, Hansson PO. Timed Up & Go as a measure for longitudinal change in mobility after stroke - Postural Stroke Study in Gothenburg (POSTGOT). J Neuroeng Rehabil 2014;11(1):83

Pertoldi S, Di Benedetto P. Shoulder-hand syndrome after stroke. A complex regional pain syndrome. Eura Medicophys 2005;41(4):283–292

Podsiadlo D, Richardson S. The timed "Up & Go": a test of basic functional mobility for frail elderly persons. J Am Geriatr Soc 1991;39(2):142–148

Proske U, Gandevia SC. The kinaesthetic senses. J Physiol 2009;587(Pt 17):4139–4146

Raine S, Meadows L, Lynch-Ellerington M. The current theoretical assumptions of the Bobath concept as determined by the members of BBTA. Physiother Theory Pract 2007;23(3):137–152

Raine S, Meadows L, Lynch-Ellerington M. Bobath Concept: Therory and Clinical Practice in Neurological Rehabilitation. Hoboken, NJ: Wiley-Blackwell; 2009

Reisman DS, Scholz JP. Workspace location influences joint coordination during reaching in post-stroke hemiparesis. Exp Brain Res 2006;170(2):265–276

Ringsberg KA, Gärdsell P, Johnell O, Jónsson B, Obrant KJ, Sernbo I. Balance and gait performance in an urban and a rural population. J Am Geriatr Soc 1998;46(1):65–70

Ryerson S, Byl NN, Brown DA, Wong RA, Hidler JM. Altered trunk position sense and its relation to balance functions in people post-stroke. J Neurol Phys Ther 2008;32(1):14–20

Schleichkorn J. The Bobaths: A Biography of Berta and Karel Bobath. Tucson, AZ: Communication Skill Builders; 1992

Shumway-Cook A, Woollacott MH. Motor Control: Translating Research into Clinical Practice. 3rd ed. Philadelphia, PA: Lippincott Williams & Wilkins; 2006

Solway S, Brooks D, Lacasse Y, Thomas S. A qualitative systematic overview of the measurement properties of functional walk tests used in the cardiorespiratory domain. Chest 2001;119(1):256–270

Stevens A, Beurskens A, Köke A, van der Weijden T. The use of patient-specific measurement instruments in the process of goal-setting: a systematic review of available instruments and their feasibility. Clin Rehabil 2013;27(11):1005–1019

Treede RD, Jensen TS, Campbell JN, et al. Neuropathic pain: redefinition and a grading system for clinical and research purposes. Neurology 2008;70(18):1630–1635

Turner-Stokes L. Goal attainment scaling and its relationship with standardized outcome measures: a commentary. J Rehabil Med 2011;43(1):70–72

Turner-Stokes L, Jackson D. Shoulder pain after stroke: a review of the evidence base to inform the devel-

opment of an integrated care pathway. Clin Rehabil 2002;16(3):276–298

Tyson S, Connell L. The psychometric properties and clinical utility of measures of walking and mobility in neurological conditions: a systematic review. Clin Rehabil 2009;23(11):1018–1033

Vasudevan JM, Browne BJ. Hemiplegic shoulder pain: an approach to diagnosis and management. Phys Med Rehabil Clin N Am 2014;25(2):411–437

Vellas BJ, Wayne SJ, Romero L, Baumgartner RN, Rubenstein LZ, Garry PJ. One-leg balance is an important predictor of injurious falls in older persons. J Am Geriatr Soc 1997;45(6):735–738

Verheyden G, Nieuwboer A, Feys H, Thijs V, Vaes K, De Weerdt W. Discriminant ability of the Trunk Impairment Scale: A comparison between stroke patients and healthy individuals. Disabil Rehabil 2005;27(17):1023–1028

Verheyden G, Nieuwboer A, Mertin J, Preger R, Kiekens C, De Weerdt W. The Trunk Impairment Scale: a new tool to measure motor impairment of the trunk after stroke. Clin Rehabil 2004;18(3):326–334

Verheyden G, Vereeck L, Truijen S, et al. Trunk performance after stroke and the relationship with balance, gait and functional ability. Clin Rehabil 2006;20(5):451–458

Verheyden G, Nieuwboer A, Van de Winckel A, De Weerdt W. Clinical tools to measure trunk performance after stroke: a systematic review of the literature. Clin Rehabil 2007;21(5):387–394

Wewers ME, Lowe NK. A critical review of visual analogue scales in the measurement of clinical phenomena. Res Nurs Health 1990;13(4):227–236

Winzeler-Merçay U, Mudie H. The nature of the effects of stroke on trunk flexor and extensor muscles during work and at rest. Disabil Rehabil 2002;24(17):875–886

Yi Y, Shim JS, Kim K, et al. Prevalence of the rotator cuff tear increases with weakness in hemiplegic shoulder. Ann Rehabil Med 2013;37(4):471–478

Chapter 4
Case Histories

Chapter 4.1
Chronic Stroke: Assessment, Treatment, and Evaluation

Allum JHJ, Carpenter MG, Honegger F, Adkin AL, Bloem BR. Age-dependent variations in the directional sensitivity of balance corrections and compensatory arm movements in man. J Physiol 2002;542(Pt 2):643–663

Anders C, Wagner H, Puta C, Grassme R, Petrovitch A, Scholle HC. Trunk muscle activation patterns during walking at different speeds. J Electromyogr Kinesiol 2007;17(2):245–252

Anson E, Rosenberg R, Agada P, Kiemel T, Jeka J. Does visual feedback during walking result in similar improvements in trunk control for young and older healthy adults? J Neuroeng Rehabil 2013;10(110):110

Arnold AS, Anderson FC, Pandy MG, Delp SL. Muscular contributions to hip and knee extension during the single limb stance phase of normal gait: a framework for investigating the causes of crouch gait. J Biomech 2005;38(11):2181–2189

Aruin AS. The effect of asymmetry of posture on anticipatory postural adjustments. Neurosci Lett 2006;401(1-2):150–153

Aruin AS, Hanke TA, Sharma A. Base of support feedback in gait rehabilitation. Int J Rehabil Res 2003;26(4):309–312

Aruin AS, Kanekar N, Lee YJ, Ganesan M. Enhancement of anticipatory postural adjustments in older adults as a result of a single session of ball throwing exercise. Exp Brain Res 2015;233(2):649–655

Baccini M, Rinaldi LA, Federighi G, Vannucchi L, Paci M, Masotti G. Effectiveness of fingertip light contact in reducing postural sway in older people. Age Ageing 2007;36(1):30–35

Beres-Jones JA, Harkema SJ. The human spinal cord interprets velocity-dependent afferent input during stepping. Brain 2004;127(Pt 10):2232–2246

Bolgla LA, Malone TR. Plantar fasciitis and the windlass mechanism: a biomechanical link to clinical practice. J Athl Train 2004;39(1):77–82

Bowden MG, Balasubramanian CK, Neptune RR, Kautz SA. Anterior-posterior ground reaction forces as a measure of paretic leg contribution in hemiparetic walking. Stroke 2006;37(3):872–876

Cheng P-T, Chen CL, Wang CM, Hong WH. Leg muscle activation patterns of sit-to-stand movement in stroke patients. Am J Phys Med Rehabil 2004;83(1):10–16

Chou S-W, Wong AM, Leong CP, Hong WS, Tang FT, Lin TH. Postural control during sit-to stand and gait in stroke patients. Am J Phys Med Rehabil 2003;82(1):42–47

Chung E-J, Kim J-H, Lee B-H. The effects of core stabilization exercise on dynamic balance and gait function in stroke patients. J Phys Ther Sci 2013;25(7):803–806

Clarkson H. Joint Motion and Function Assessment: A Research-Based Practical Guide. Philadelphia, PA: Lippincott Williams & Wilkins; 2005

Cooper A, Alghamdi GA, Alghamdi MA, Altowaijri A, Richardson S. The relationship of lower limb muscle strength and knee joint hyperextension during the stance phase of gait in hemiparetic stroke patients. Physiother Res Int 2012;17(3):150–156

Cote KP, Brunet ME, Gansneder BM, Shultz SJ. Effects of pronated and supinated foot postures on static and dynamic postural stability. J Athl Train 2005;40(1):41–46

Dyer J-O, Maupas E, Melo SdeA, Bourbonnais D, Forget R. Abnormal coactivation of knee and ankle extensors is related to changes in heteronymous spinal pathways after stroke. J Neuroeng Rehabil 2011;8(1):41

Fiolkowski P, Brunt D, Bishop M, Woo R, Horodyski M. Intrinsic pedal musculature support of the medial longitudinal arch: an electromyography study. J Foot Ankle Surg 2003;42(6):327–333

Francis CA, Lenz AL, Lenhart RL, Thelen DG. The modulation of forward propulsion, vertical support, and center of pressure by the plantarflexors during human walking. Gait Posture 2013;38(4):993–997

Franzén E, Gurfinkel VS, Wright WG, Cordo PJ, Horak FB. Haptic touch reduces sway by increasing axial tone. Neuroscience 2011;174(3):216–223

Frost R, Skidmore J, Santello M, Artemiadis P. Sensorimotor control of gait: a novel approach for the study of the interplay of visual and proprioceptive feedback. Front Hum Neurosci 2015;9:14

Gjelsvik B, Breivik K, Verheyden G, Smedal T, Hofstad H, Strand LI. The Trunk Impairment Scale - modified to ordinal scales in the Norwegian version. Disabil Rehabil 2012;34(16):1385–1395

Goldberg A, Schepens S, Wallace M. Concurrent validity and reliability of the maximum step length test in older adults. J Geriatr Phys Ther 2010;33(3):122–127

Goulart F, Valls-Solé J. Reciprocal changes of excitability between tibialis anterior and soleus during the sit-to-stand movement. Exp Brain Res 2001;139(4):391–397

Graham JV, Eustace C, Brock K, Swain E, Irwin-Carruthers S. The Bobath concept in contemporary clinical practice. Top Stroke Rehabil 2009;16(1):57–68

Hao WY, Chen Y. Backward walking training improves balance in school-aged boys. Sports Med Arthrosc Rehabil Ther Technol 2011;3(1):24

Headlee DL, Leonard JL, Hart JM, Ingersoll CD, Hertel J. Fatigue of the plantar intrinsic foot muscles increases navicular drop. J Electromyogr Kinesiol 2008;18(3):420–425

Hoogkamer W, Meyns P, Duysens J. Steps forward in understanding backward gait: from basic circuits to rehabilitation. Exerc Sport Sci Rev 2014;42(1):23–29

Hu H, Meijer OG, Hodges PW, et al. Control of the lateral abdominal muscles during walking. Hum Mov Sci 2012;31(4):880–896

Hyngstrom A, Onushko T, Chua M, Schmit BD. Abnormal volitional hip torque phasing and hip impairments in gait post stroke. J Neurophysiol 2010;103(3):1557–1568

IJmker T, Lamoth CJ, Houdijk H, van der Woude LH, Beek PJ. Postural threat during walking: effects on energy cost and accompanying gait changes. J Neuroeng Rehabil 2014;11(1):71

Karthikbabu S, Rao BK, Manikandan N, Solomon JM, Chakrapani M. Role of trunk rehabilitation on trunk control, balance and gait in patients with chronic stroke: a pre-post design. Neurosci Med 2011;2(2):61–67

Kaur N, Bhanot K, Brody LT, Bridges J, Berry DC, Ode JJ. Effects of lower extremity and trunk muscles recruitment on serratus anterior muscle activation in healthy male adults. Int J Sports Phys Ther 2014;9(7):924–937

Kavanagh JJ. Lower trunk motion and speed-dependence during walking. J Neuroeng Rehabil 2009;6(6):9

Liu MQ, Anderson FC, Pandy MG, Delp SL. Muscles that support the body also modulate forward progression during walking. J Biomech 2006;39(14):2623–2630

Lomaglio MJ, Eng JJ. Muscle strength and weight-bearing symmetry relate to sit-to-stand performance in individuals with stroke. Gait Posture 2005;22(2):126–131

McGowan CP, Neptune RR, Kram R. Independent effects of weight and mass on plantar flexor activity during walking: implications for their contributions to body support and forward propulsion. J Appl Physiol (1985) 2008;105(2):486–494

Menz HB, Lord SR, Fitzpatrick RC. Age-related differences in walking stability. Age Ageing 2003;32(2):137–142

Moon DC, Kim K, Lee SK. Immediate Effect of Short-foot Exercise on Dynamic Balance of Subjects with Excessively Pronated Feet. J Phys Ther Sci 2014;26(1):117–119

Moseley A, Wales A, Herbert R, Schurr K, Moore S. Observation and analysis of hemiplegic gait: stance phase. Aust J Physiother 1993;39(4):259–267

Mulligan EP, Cook PG. Effect of plantar intrinsic muscle training on medial longitudinal arch morphology and dynamic function. Man Ther 2013;18(5):425–430

Neptune RR, Zajac FE, Kautz SA. Muscle force redistributes segmental power for body progression during walking. Gait Posture 2004;19(2):194–205

Pandian S, Arya KN, Kumar D. Does motor training of the nonparetic side influences balance and function in chronic stroke? A pilot RCT. ScientificWorldJournal 2014;2014:769726

Perera S, Mody SH, Woodman RC, Studenski SA. Meaningful change and responsiveness in common physical performance measures in older adults. J Am Geriatr Soc 2006;54(5):743–749

Peterson CL, Cheng J, Kautz SA, Neptune RR. Leg extension is an important predictor of paretic leg

propulsion in hemiparetic walking. Gait Posture 2010;32(4):451–456

Platts MM, Rafferty D, Paul L. Metabolic cost of over ground gait in younger stroke patients and healthy controls. Med Sci Sports Exerc 2006;38(6):1041–1046

Porter R, Lemon RN. Corticospinal Function and Voluntary Movement. New York, NY: Oxford University Press; 1995

Purser JL, Weinberger M, Cohen HJ, et al. Walking speed predicts health status and hospital costs for frail elderly male veterans. J Rehabil Res Dev 2005;42(4):535–546

Qaquish J, McLean S. Foot type and tibialis anterior muscle activity during the stance phase of gait : A pilot study. Int J Physiother Rehabil 2010;1(1):19–29

Raine S, Meadows L, Lynch-Ellerington M. Bobath Concept: Theory and Clinical Practice in Neurological Rehabilitation. Hoboken, NJ: Wiley-Blackwell; 2009

Rossignol S, Dubuc R, Gossard JP. Dynamic sensorimotor interactions in locomotion. Physiol Rev 2006;86(1):89–154

Roy G, Nadeau S, Gravel D, Malouin F, McFadyen BJ, Piotte F. The effect of foot position and chair height on the asymmetry of vertical forces during sit-to-stand and stand-to-sit tasks in individuals with hemiparesis. Clin Biomech (Bristol, Avon) 2006;21(6):585–593

Sharrock C, Cropper J, Mostad J, Johnson M, Malone T. A pilot study of core stability and athletic performance: is there a relationship? Int J Sports Phys Ther 2011;6(2):63–74

Shepherd R, Gentile A. Initial trunk position and biomechanical consequences in standing up. Hum Mov Sci 1994;13:817–840

Shumway-Cook, Woollacott MH. Motor Control: Translating Research into Clinical Practice. 4th ed. Philadelphia, PA: Lippincott Williams & Wilkins; 2011

Silva A, Sousa AS, Pinheiro R, et al. Activation timing of soleus and tibialis anterior muscles during sit-to-stand and stand-to-sit in post-stroke vs. healthy subjects. Somatosens Mot Res 2013;30(1):48–55

Son SM, Park MK, Lee NK. Influence of Resistance Exercise Training to Strengthen Muscles across Multiple Joints of the Lower Limbs on Dynamic Balance Functions of Stroke Patients. J Phys Ther Sci 2014;26(8):1267–1269

Stewart SG, Jull GA, Ng JKF, et al. An initial analysis of thoracic spine movement during unilateral arm elevation. J Manual Manip Ther 1995;3(1):15–20

Stoquart G, Detrembleur C, Lejeune TM. The reasons why stroke patients expend so much energy to walk slowly. Gait Posture 2012;36(3):409–413

Teixeira-Salmela LF, Nadeau S, Mcbride I, Olney SJ. Effects of muscle strengthening and physical conditioning training on temporal, kinematic and kinetic variables during gait in chronic stroke survivors. J Rehabil Med 2001;33(2):53–60

Terrier P, Dériaz O. Kinematic variability, fractal dynamics and local dynamic stability of treadmill walking. J Neuroeng Rehabil 2011;8(1):12

Turns LJ, Neptune RR, Kautz SA. Relationships between muscle activity and anteroposterior ground reaction forces in hemiparetic walking. Arch Phys Med Rehabil 2007;88(9):1127–1135

Winter DA. Human balance and posture standing and walking. Gait and Posture 1995;3:193–214

Chapter 4.2
Cerebellar Ataxia: Assessment, Treatment, and Evaluation

Behm DG, Drinkwater EJ, Willardson JM, Cowley PM; Canadian Society for Exercise Physiology. Canadian Society for Exercise Physiology position stand: The use of instability to train the core in athletic and nonathletic conditioning. Appl Physiol Nutr Metab 2010;35(1):109–112

Clifford AM, Holder-Powell H. Postural control in healthy individuals. Clin Biomech (Bristol, Avon) 2010;25(6):546–551

Criscimagna-Hemminger SE, Bastian AJ, Shadmehr R. Size of error affects cerebellar contributions to motor learning. J Neurophysiol 2010;103(4):2275–2284

Danna-Dos-Santos A, Degani AM, Latash ML. Anticipatory control of head posture. Clin Neurophysiol 2007;118(8):1802–1814

Davis JR, Campbell AD, Adkin AL, Carpenter MG. The relationship between fear of falling and human postural control. Gait Posture 2009;29(2):275–279

Franzén E, Gurfinkel VS, Wright WG, Cordo PJ, Horak FB. Haptic touch reduces sway by increasing axial tone. Neuroscience 2011;174(3):216–223

Frost DM, Cronin JB. Stepping back to improve sprint performance: a kinetic analysis of the first step forwards. J Strength Cond Res 2011;25(10):2721–2728

Gill-Body KM, Popat RA, Parker SW, Krebs DE. Rehabilitation of balance in two patients with cerebellar dysfunction. Phys Ther 1997;77(5):534–552

Graham JV, Eustace C, Brock K, Swain E, Irwin-Carruthers S. The Bobath concept in contemporary clinical practice. Top Stroke Rehabil 2009;16(1):57–68

Grimaldi A. Assessing lateral stability of the hip and pelvis. Man Ther 2011;16(1):26–32

Gurfinkel VS, Levik YuS. The suppression of cervico-ocular response by the haptokinetic information about the contact with a rigid, immobile object. Exp Brain Res 1993;95(2):359–364

Gusi N, Carmelo Adsuar J, Corzo H, Del Pozo-Cruz B, Olivares PR, Parraca JA. Balance training reduces fear of falling and improves dynamic balance and isometric strength in institutionalised older people: a randomised trial. J Physiother 2012;58(2):97–104

Hibbs AE, Thompson KG, French D, Wrigley A, Spears I. Optimizing performance by improving core stability and core strength. Sports Med 2008;38(12):995–1008

Horak FB. Postural compensation for vestibular loss. Ann N Y Acad Sci 2009;1164(1):76–81

Horak FB. Postural orientation and equilibrium: what do we need to know about neural control of balance to prevent falls? Age Ageing 2006;35(Suppl 2):ii7–ii11

Horak FB, Diener HC. Cerebellar control of postural scaling and central set in stance. J Neurophysiol 1994;72(2):479–493

Horak FB, Wrisley DM, Frank J. The Balance Evaluation Systems Test (BESTest) to differentiate balance deficits. Phys Ther 2009;89(5):484–498

Ilg W, Golla H, Thier P, Giese MA. Specific influences of cerebellar dysfunctions on gait. Brain 2007;130(Pt 3):786–798

Ilg W, Synofzik M, Brötz D, Burkard S, Giese MA, Schöls L. Intensive coordinative training improves motor performance in degenerative cerebellar disease. Neurology 2009;73(22):1823–1830

Johnson MB, Van Emmerik R EA. Effect of head orientation on postural control during upright stance and forward lean. Mot Contr 2012;16(1):81–93

Kibler WB, Ludewig PM, McClure PW, Michener LA, Bak K, Sciascia AD. Clinical implications of scapular dyskinesis in shoulder injury: the 2013 consensus statement from the 'Scapular Summit'. Br J Sports Med 2013;47(14):877–885

Lackner JR, DiZio P, Jeka J, Horak F, Krebs D, Rabin E. Precision contact of the fingertip reduces postural sway of individuals with bilateral vestibular loss. Exp Brain Res 1999;126(4):459–466

Levin MF, Panturin E. Sensorimotor integration for functional recovery and the Bobath approach. Mot Contr 2011;15(2):285–301

Liu W, Santos MJ, McIntire K, Loudon J, Goist-Foley H, Horton G. Patterns of inter-joint coordination during a single-limb standing. Gait Posture 2012;36(3):614–618

Martin CL, Tan D, Bragge P, Bialocerkowski A. Effectiveness of physiotherapy for adults with cerebellar dysfunction: a systematic review. Clin Rehabil 2009;23(1):15–26

Mottram SL. Dynamic stability of the scapula. Man Ther 1997;2(3):123–131

Nitz JC, Choy NL. The efficacy of a specific balance-strategy training programme for preventing falls among older people: a pilot randomised controlled trial. Age Ageing 2004;33(1):52–58

Oshita K, Yano S. Low-frequency force steadiness practice in plantar flexor muscle reduces postural sway during quiet standing. J Physiol Anthropol 2011;30(6):233–239

Park E, Schöner G, Scholz JP. Functional synergies underlying control of upright posture during changes in head orientation. PLoS ONE 2012;7(8):e41583

Petrosini L, Graziano A, Mandolesi L, Neri P, Molinari M, Leggio MG. Watch how to do it! New advances in learning by observation. Brain Res Brain Res Rev 2003;42(3):252–264

Raine S, Meadows L, Lynch-Ellerington M. Bobath Concept: Theory and Clinical Practice in Neurological Rehabilitation. Hoboken, NJ: Wiley-Blackwell; 2009

Riemann BL, Schmitz R. The relationship between various modes of single leg postural control assessment. Int J Sports Phys Ther 2012;7(3):257–266

Saute JAM, Donis KC, Serrano-Munuera C, et al; Iberoamerican Multidisciplinary Network for the Study of Movement Disorders (RIBERMOV) Study Group. Ataxia rating scales—psychometric profiles, natural history and their application in clinical trials. Cerebellum 2012;11(2):488–504

Saywell N, Taylor D. The role of the cerebellum in procedural learning—are there implications for physiotherapists' clinical practice? Physiother Theory Pract 2008;24(5):321–328

Sharrock C, Cropper J, Mostad J, Johnson M, Malone T. A pilot study of core stability and athletic performance: is there a relationship? Int J Sports Phys Ther 2011;6(2):63–74

Storey E, Tuck K, Hester R, Hughes A, Churchyard A. Inter-rater reliability of the International Cooperative Ataxia Rating Scale (ICARS). Mov Disord 2004;19(2):190–192

Trouillas P, Takayanagi T, Hallett M, et al; The Ataxia Neuropharmacology Committee of the World Federation of Neurology. International Cooperative Ataxia Rating Scale for pharmacological assessment of the cerebellar syndrome. J Neurol Sci 1997;145(2):205–211

Uemura K, Yamada M, Nagai K, Tanaka B, Mori S, Ichihashi N. Fear of falling is associated with prolonged anticipatory postural adjustment during gait initiation under dual-task conditions in older adults. Gait Posture 2012;35(2):282–286

Vaz DV, Schettino RdeC, Rolla de Castro TR, Teixeira VR, Cavalcanti Furtado SR, de Mello Figueiredo E. Treadmill training for ataxic patients: a single-subject experimental design. Clin Rehabil 2008;22(3):234–241

Wei K, Dijkstra TM, Sternad D. Stability and variability: indicators for passive stability and active control in a rhythmic task. J Neurophysiol 2008;99(6):3027–3041

Wuehr M, Schniepp R, Ilmberger J, Brandt T, Jahn K. Speed-dependent temporospatial gait variability and long-range correlations in cerebellar ataxia. Gait Posture 2013;37(2):214–218

Yardley L, Beyer N, Hauer K, Kempen G, Piot-Ziegler C, Todd C. Development and initial validation of the Falls Efficacy Scale-International (FES-I). Age Ageing 2005;34(6):614–619

Yiou E, Caderby T, Hussein T. Adaptability of anticipatory postural adjustments associated with voluntary movement. World J Orthod 2012;3(6):75–86

Index

Page numbers in *italics* refer to illustrations; those in **bold** refer to tables.